Learning Disabilities Sourcebook, 3rd Edition
Leukemia Sourcebook
Liver Disorders Sourcebook
Lung Disorders Sourcebook
Medical Tests Sourcebook, 3rd Edition
Men's Health Concerns Sourcebook, 2nd Edition
Mental Health Disorders Sourcebook, 4th Edition
Mental Retardation Sourcebook
Movement Disorders Sourcebook, 2nd Edition
Multiple Sclerosis Sourcebook
Muscular Dystrophy Sourcebook
Obesity Sourcebook
Osteoporosis Sourcebook
Pain Sourcebook, 3rd Edition
Pediatric Cancer Sourcebook
Physical & Mental Issues in Aging Sourcebook
Podiatry Sourcebook, 2nd Edition
Pregnancy & Birth Sourcebook, 2nd Edition
Prostate Cancer Sourcebook
Prostate & Urological Disorders Sourcebook
Reconstructive & Cosmetic Surgery Sourcebook
Rehabilitation Sourcebook
Respiratory Disorders Sourcebook, 2nd Edition
Sexually Transmitted Diseases Sourcebook, 3rd Edition
Sleep Disorders Sourcebook, 2nd Edition
Smoking Concerns Sourcebook
Sports Injuries Sourcebook, 3rd Edition
Stress-Related Disorders Sourcebook, 2nd Edition
Stroke Sourcebook, 2nd Edition
Surgery Sourcebook, 2nd Edition
Thyroid Disorders Sourcebook
Transplantation Sourcebook
Traveler's Health Sourcebook
Urinary Tract & Kidney Diseases & Disorders Sourcebook, 2nd Edition

Vegetar
Wo
Wor
Worl

Teen Health Series

Abuse & Violence Information for Teens
Accident & Safety Information for Teens
Alcohol Information for Teens, 2nd Edition
Allergy Information for Teens
Asthma Information for Teens
Body Information for Teens
Cancer Information for Teens
Complementary & Alternative Medicine Information for Teens
Diabetes Information for Teens
Diet Information for Teens, 2nd Edition
Drug Information for Teens, 2nd Edition
Eating Disorders Information for Teens, 2nd Edition
Fitness Information for Teens, 2nd Edition
Learning Disabilities Information for Teens
Mental Health Information for Teens, 2nd Edition
Pregnancy Information for Teens
Sexual Health Information for Teens, 2nd Edition
Skin Health Information for Teens, 2nd Edition
Sleep Information for Teens
Sports Injuries Information for Teens, 2nd Edition
Stress Information for Teens
Suicide Information for Teens
Tobacco Information for Teens

Mental Health Disorders SOURCEBOOK

Fourth Edition

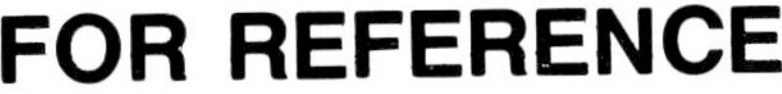

Health Reference Series

Fourth Edition

Mental Health Disorders SOURCEBOOK

Basic Consumer Health Information about the Causes and Symptoms of Mental Health Problems, Including Depression, Bipolar Disorder, Anxiety Disorders, Post-traumatic Stress Disorder, Obsessive-Compulsive Disorder, Eating Disorders, Addictions, and Personality and Schizophrenic Disorders

Along with Information about Medications and Treatments, Mental Health Concerns in Children and Adolescents, Tips on Living with Mental Health Disorders, a Glossary of Related Terms, and Directories of Resources for Additional Help and Information

Edited by
Amy L. Sutton

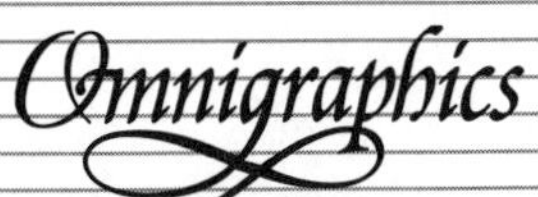

P.O. Box 31-1640, Detroit, MI 48231

Edited by Amy L. Sutton

Health Reference Series
Karen Bellenir, *Managing Editor*
David A. Cooke, M.D., *Medical Consultant*
Elizabeth Collins, *Research and Permissions Coordinator*
Cherry Edwards, *Permissions Assistant*
EdIndex, Services for Publishers, *Indexers*

* * *

Omnigraphics, Inc.
Matthew P. Barbour, *Senior Vice President*
Kevin M. Hayes, *Operations Manager*

* * *

Peter E. Ruffner, *Publisher*

ISBN 978-0-7808-1041-9

Library of Congress Cataloging-in-Publication Data

Mental health disorders sourcebook : basic consumer health information about the causes and symptoms of mental health problems, including depression, bipolar disorder, anxiety disorders, posttraumatic stress disorder, obsessive- compulsive disorder, eating disorders, addictions, and personality and schizophrenic disorders ... / edited by Amy L. Sutton. -- 4th ed.

p. cm.

Includes bibliographical references and index.

ISBN 978-0-7808-1041-9 (hardcover : alk. paper) 1. Mental illness. 2. Psychiatry. I. Sutton, Amy L.

RC454.4.M458 2009

616.89--dc22

2009012975

Printed in the United States

Table of Contents

Visit www.healthreferenceseries.com to view *A Contents Guide to the Health Reference Series*, a listing of more than 15,000 topics and the volumes in which they are covered.

Part II: Depression, Bipolar Disorder, and Other Mood Disorders

Part III: Anxiety Disorders

Part IV: Eating, Impulse Control, and Addiction Disorders

Part V: Personality and Schizophrenic Disorders

Part VI: Getting Help for Mental Health Disorders

Part VII: Living with Mental Health Disorders

Part VIII: Mental Health Concerns in Children and Adolescents

Part IX: Additional Help and Information

Preface

About This Book

Mental health disorders can cause serious distress and reduce a person's ability to function psychologically, socially, occupationally, and interpersonally. According to the U.S. Department of Health and Human Services, one person in four has been diagnosed with a mental health disorder within the last 12 months, and mental health disorders such as depression, bipolar disorder, obsessive-compulsive disorder, and schizophrenia rank among the leading causes of disability in the United States. Fortunately, however, developments in medications and behavioral therapies have improved health care professionals' ability to recognize, diagnose, and treat mental health conditions effectively.

Mental Health Disorders Sourcebook, Fourth Edition provides updated information about the prevalence of mental health disorders and their impact on children, adolescents, women, men, and older adults. It details the symptoms and treatments of mood disorders, such as depression and bipolar disorder; anxiety disorders, such as posttraumatic stress disorder and obsessive-compulsive disorder; eating, impulse control, and addiction disorders; and personality and schizophrenic disorders. Information on finding and paying for mental health treatment and tips on living with mental health disorders, locating housing and employment, and coping with stigma are also included. The book concludes with a glossary of related terms and directories of additional resources.

How to Use This Book

This book is divided into parts and chapters. Parts focus on broad areas of interest. Chapters are devoted to single topics within a part.

Part I: Understanding Mental Health Disorders provides general information about the prevalence and economic impact of mental health disorders on women, men, minorities, and the elderly in the United States. This part also debunks common myths about mental health disorders and discusses how stress, genetics, and exposure to violence influence mental health and the risk of suicide.

Part II: Depression, Bipolar Disorder, and Other Mood Disorders offers detailed facts on the types, causes, symptoms, and treatments of some of the most common mental health disorders, including depression, bipolar disorder, seasonal affective disorder, and premenstrual disorders.

Part III: Anxiety Disorders identifies the symptoms and treatments of anxiety disorders, including generalized anxiety disorder, panic disorder, phobias, posttraumatic stress disorder, and obsessive-compulsive disorder.

Part IV: Eating, Impulse Control, and Addiction Disorders defines and describes eating and body image disorders such as anorexia nervosa, bulimia nervosa, binge eating disorder, body dysmorphic disorder, and compulsive exercise. The part also examines disorders characterized by lack of impulse control, such as gambling, firesetting, hair pulling, and sexual compulsion, as well as addictions to drugs and alcohol.

Part V: Personality and Schizophrenic Disorders identifies and describes severe mental health problems, including antisocial, borderline, and paranoid personality disorder, dissociative disorders, and Munchausen by proxy syndrome. The symptoms, causes, and treatment of schizophrenia and related disorders are also discussed.

Part VI: Getting Help for Mental Health Disorders offers tips on finding and paying for mental health care and choosing a psychotherapy method. It discusses using medications for mental health disorders, and it describes cutting-edge treatments for mental illnesses, such as deep brain stimulation and transcranial magnetic stimulation. Information on dietary supplements, spiritual practices, physical activities, and alternative and complementary therapies that may alleviate the symptoms of mental illness is also included.

Part VII: Living with Mental Health Disorders identifies the everyday concerns of people with mental health disorders and their caregivers. Tips on dealing with grief, coping with stigma, managing anger, dealing with relationships, finding employment and housing, and planning for mental incapacity are discussed.

Part VIII: Mental Health Concerns in Children and Adolescents offers parents and caregivers information about the incidence and treatment of depression, bipolar disorder, anxiety disorders, obsessive-compulsive disorder, conduct disorder, oppositional defiant disorders, and substance abuse in youth.

Part IX: Additional Help and Information includes a glossary of important terms, a directory of organizations for patients with mental health disorders and their families, and a directory of prescription drug assistance programs.

Bibliographic Note

This volume contains documents and excerpts from publications issued by the following U.S. government agencies: Agency for Healthcare Research and Quality (AHRQ); Centers for Medicare and Medicaid Services; National Cancer Institute (NCI); National Center for Complementary and Alternative Medicine (NCCAM); National Center for Posttraumatic Stress Disorder (NCPTSD); National Institute of Mental Health (NIMH); National Institute of Neurological Disorders and Stroke (NINDS); National Institute on Drug Abuse (NIDA); National Institutes of Health (NIH); National Library of Medicine; National Youth Violence Prevention Resource Center; Office of Minority Health; Office on Women's Health; Social Security Administration (SSA); Substance Abuse and Mental Health Services Administration (SAMHSA); U.S. Department of Health and Human Services (HHS); and the U.S. Food and Drug Administration (FDA).

In addition, this volume contains copyrighted documents from the following organizations: A.D.A.M., Inc.; AIDS InfoNet; Alzheimer's Association; American Federation for Aging Research; American Geriatrics Society Foundation for Health in Aging; American Psychological Association; Anxiety Disorders Association of America; Judge David L. Bazelon Center for Mental Health Law; BSCS; International Society for the Study of Trauma and Dissociation; Matrix Medical Communications; Mental Health America; NAMI: The Nation's Voice on Mental Illness; National Alliance on Mental Illness—New Hampshire;

National Coalition for the Homeless; National Mental Health Consumers' Self-Help Clearinghouse; National Sleep Foundation; The Nemours Foundation; Parkinson's Disease Foundation; Quadrant HealthCom Inc.; Queensland Health; and the University of Florida Institute of Food and Agricultural Sciences.

Full citation information is provided on the first page of each chapter or section. Every effort has been made to secure all necessary rights to reprint the copyrighted material. If any omissions have been made, please contact Omnigraphics to make corrections for future editions.

Acknowledgements

Thanks go to the many organizations, agencies, and individuals who have contributed materials for this *Sourcebook* and to medical consultant Dr. David Cooke and document engineer Bruce Bellenir. Special thanks go to managing editor Karen Bellenir and research and permissions coordinator Liz Collins for their help and support.

About the Health Reference Series

The *Health Reference Series* is designed to provide basic medical information for patients, families, caregivers, and the general public. Each volume takes a particular topic and provides comprehensive coverage. This is especially important for people who may be dealing with a newly diagnosed disease or a chronic disorder in themselves or in a family member. People looking for preventive guidance, information about disease warning signs, medical statistics, and risk factors for health problems will also find answers to their questions in the *Health Reference Series*. The *Series*, however, is not intended to serve as a tool for diagnosing illness, in prescribing treatments, or as a substitute for the physician/patient relationship. All people concerned about medical symptoms or the possibility of disease are encouraged to seek professional care from an appropriate health care provider.

A Note about Spelling and Style

Health Reference Series editors use *Stedman's Medical Dictionary* as an authority for questions related to the spelling of medical terms and the *Chicago Manual of Style* for questions related to grammatical structures, punctuation, and other editorial concerns. Consistent adherence is not always possible, however, because the individual volumes within the *Series* include many documents from a wide variety of different producers and copyright holders, and the editor's primary goal is to present material from each source as accurately as is possible following the terms specified by each document's producer. This sometimes means that information in different chapters or sections may follow other guidelines and alternate spelling authorities. For example, occasionally a copyright holder may require that eponymous terms be shown in possessive forms (Crohn's disease *vs.* Crohn disease) or that British spelling norms be retained (leukaemia *vs.* leukemia).

Locating Information within the Health Reference Series

The *Health Reference Series* contains a wealth of information about a wide variety of medical topics. Ensuring easy access to all the fact sheets, research reports, in-depth discussions, and other material contained within the individual books of the *Series* remains one of our highest priorities. As the *Series* continues to grow in size and scope, however, locating the precise information needed by a reader may become more challenging.

A Contents Guide to the Health Reference Series was developed to direct readers to the specific volumes that address their concerns. It presents an extensive list of diseases, treatments, and other topics of general interest compiled from the Tables of Contents and major index headings. To access *A Contents Guide to the Health Reference Series*, visit www.healthreferenceseries.com.

Medical Consultant

Medical consultation services are provided to the *Health Reference Series* editors by David A. Cooke, M.D. Dr. Cooke is a graduate of Brandeis University, and he received his M.D. degree from the University of Michigan. He completed residency training at the University of Wisconsin Hospital and Clinics. He is board-certified in Internal Medicine. Dr. Cooke currently works as part of the University of Michigan Health System and practices in Ann Arbor, MI. In his free time, he enjoys writing, science fiction, and spending time with his family.

Our Advisory Board

We would like to thank the following board members for providing guidance to the development of this *Series*:

- Dr. Lynda Baker, Associate Professor of Library and Information Science, Wayne State University, Detroit, MI
- Nancy Bulgarelli, William Beaumont Hospital Library, Royal Oak, MI
- Karen Imarisio, Bloomfield Township Public Library, Bloomfield Township, MI
- Karen Morgan, Mardigian Library, University of Michigan-Dearborn, Dearborn, MI
- Rosemary Orlando, St. Clair Shores Public Library, St. Clair Shores, MI

Health Reference Series *Update Policy*

The inaugural book in the *Health Reference Series* was the first edition of *Cancer Sourcebook* published in 1989. Since then, the *Series* has been enthusiastically received by librarians and in the medical community. In order to maintain the standard of providing high-quality health information for the layperson the editorial staff at Omnigraphics felt it was necessary to implement a policy of updating volumes when warranted.

Medical researchers have been making tremendous strides, and it is the purpose of the *Health Reference Series* to stay current with the most recent advances. Each decision to update a volume is made on an individual basis. Some of the considerations include how much new information is available and the feedback we receive from people who use the books. If there is a topic you would like to see added to the update list, or an area of medical concern you feel has not been adequately addressed, please write to:

Editor
Health Reference Series
Omnigraphics, Inc.
P.O. Box 31-1640
Detroit, MI 48231
E-mail: editorial@omnigraphics.com

Part One

Understanding Mental Health Disorders

Chapter 1

Defining Mental Health Disorders

We can all be "sad" or "blue" at times in our lives. We have all seen movies about the madman and his crime spree, with the underlying cause of mental illness. We sometimes even make jokes about people being crazy or nuts, even though we know that we shouldn't. We have all had some exposure to mental illness, but do we really understand it or know what it is? Many of our preconceptions are incorrect. A mental illness can be defined as a health condition that changes a person's thinking, feelings, or behavior (or all three) and that causes the person distress and difficulty in functioning. As with many diseases, mental illness is severe in some cases and mild in others. Individuals who have a mental illness don't necessarily look like they are sick, especially if their illness is mild. Other individuals may show more explicit symptoms such as confusion, agitation, or withdrawal. There are many different mental illnesses, including depression, schizophrenia, attention deficit hyperactivity disorder (ADHD), autism, and obsessive-compulsive disorder. Each illness alters a person's thoughts, feelings, and/or behaviors in distinct ways. In this text, we will at times discuss mental illness in general terms and at other times, discuss specific mental illnesses.

Not all brain diseases are categorized as mental illnesses. Disorders such as epilepsy, Parkinson's disease, and multiple sclerosis are brain disorders, but they are considered neurological diseases rather

---

than mental illnesses. Interestingly, the lines between mental illnesses and these other brain or neurological disorders is blurring somewhat. As scientists continue to investigate the brains of people who have mental illnesses, they are learning that mental illness is associated with changes in the brain's structure, chemistry, and function and that mental illness does indeed have a biological basis. This ongoing research is, in some ways, causing scientists to minimize the distinctions between mental illnesses and these other brain disorders. In this text, we will restrict our discussion of mental illness to those illnesses that are traditionally classified as mental illnesses, as listed in the previous paragraph.

Mental Illness in the Population

Many people feel that mental illness is rare, something that only happens to people with life situations very different from their own, and that it will never affect them. Studies of the epidemiology of mental illness indicate that this belief is far from accurate. In fact, the surgeon general reports that mental illnesses are so common that few U.S. families are untouched by them.

Mental Illness in Adults

Even if you or a family member has not experienced mental illness directly, it is very likely that you have known someone who has. Estimates are that at least one in four people is affected by mental illness either directly or indirectly. Consider the following statistics to get an idea of just how widespread the effects of mental illness are in society:

- According to recent estimates, approximately 20 percent of Americans, or about one in five people over the age of 18, suffer from a diagnosable mental disorder in a given year.
- Four of the 10 leading causes of disability—major depression, bipolar disorder, schizophrenia, and obsessive-compulsive disorder—are mental illnesses.
- About 3 percent of the population have more than one mental illness at a time.
- About 5 percent of adults are affected so seriously by mental illness that it interferes with their ability to function in society. These severe and persistent mental illnesses include

schizophrenia, bipolar disorder, other severe forms of depression, panic disorder, and obsessive-compulsive disorder.

- Approximately 20 percent of doctor's appointments are related to anxiety disorders such as panic attacks.
- Eight million people have depression each year.
- Two million Americans have schizophrenia disorders, and 300,000 new cases are diagnosed each year.

Mental Illness in Children and Adolescents

Mental illness is not uncommon among children and adolescents. Approximately 12 million children under the age of 18 have mental disorders. The National Mental Health Association has compiled some statistics about mental illness in children and adolescents:

- Mental health problems affect one in every five young people at any given time.
- An estimated two-thirds of all young people with mental health problems are not receiving the help they need.
- Less than one-third of the children under age 18 who have a serious mental health problem receive any mental health services.
- As many as 1 in every 33 children may be depressed. Depression in adolescents may be as high as 1 in 8.
- Suicide is the third leading cause of death for 15- to 24-years-olds and the sixth leading cause of death for 5- to 15-year-olds.
- Schizophrenia is rare in children under age 12, but it occurs in about 3 of every 1,000 adolescents.
- Between 118,700 and 186,600 youths in the juvenile justice system have at least one mental illness.
- Of the 100,000 teenagers in juvenile detention, an estimated 60 percent have behavioral, cognitive, or emotional problems.

Warning Signs for Mental Illness

Each mental illness has its own characteristic symptoms. However, there are some general warning signs that might alert you that someone needs professional help. Some of these signs include:

- marked personality change,
- inability to cope with problems and daily activities,
- strange or grandiose ideas,
- excessive anxieties,
- prolonged depression and apathy,
- marked changes in eating or sleeping patterns,
- thinking or talking about suicide or harming oneself,
- extreme mood swings—high or low,
- abuse of alcohol or drugs, and
- excessive anger, hostility, or violent behavior.

A person who shows any of these signs should seek help from a qualified health professional.

Diagnosing Mental Illness

Mental Health Professionals

To be diagnosed with a mental illness, a person must be evaluated by a qualified professional who has expertise in mental health. Mental health professionals include psychiatrists, psychologists, psychiatric nurses, social workers, and mental health counselors. Family doctors, internists, and pediatricians are usually qualified to diagnose common mental disorders such as depression, anxiety disorders, and ADHD. In many cases, depending on the individual and his or her symptoms, a mental health professional who is not a psychiatrist will refer the patient to a psychiatrist. A psychiatrist is a medical doctor (M.D.) who has received additional training in the field of mental health and mental illnesses. Psychiatrists evaluate the person's mental condition in coordination with his or her physical condition and can prescribe medication. Only psychiatrists and other M.D.s can prescribe medications to treat mental illness.

Mental Illnesses Are Diagnosed by Symptoms

Unlike some disease diagnoses, doctors can't do a blood test or culture some microorganisms to determine whether a person has a mental illness. Maybe scientists will develop discrete physiological tests for mental illnesses in the future; until then, however, mental health professionals will have to diagnose mental illnesses based on the symptoms that a person has. Basing a diagnosis on symptoms and not on a quantitative medical test, such as a blood chemistry test, a throat swab, X-rays, or urinalysis, is not unusual. Physicians diagnose many diseases, including migraines, Alzheimer's disease, and Parkinson's disease based on their symptoms alone. For other diseases, such as asthma or mononucleosis, doctors rely on analyzing symptoms to get a good idea of what the problem is and then use a physiological test to provide additional information or to confirm their diagnosis.

When a mental health professional works with a person who might have a mental illness, he or she will, along with the individual, determine what symptoms the individual has, how long the symptoms have persisted, and how his or her life is being affected. Mental health professionals often gather information through an interview during which they ask the patient about his or her symptoms, the length of time that the symptoms have occurred, and the severity of the symptoms. In many cases, the professional will also get information about the patient from family members to obtain a more comprehensive picture. A physician likely will conduct a physical exam and consult the patient's history to rule out other health problems.

Mental health professionals evaluate symptoms to make a diagnosis of mental illness. They rely on the criteria specified in the *Diagnostic and Statistical Manual of Mental Disorders* (*DSM-IV*; currently, the fourth edition), published by the American Psychiatric Association, to diagnose a specific mental illness. For each mental illness, the *DSM-IV* gives a general description of the disorder and a list of typical symptoms. Mental health professionals refer to the *DSM-IV* to confirm that the symptoms a patient exhibits match those of a specific mental illness. Although the *DSM-IV* provides valuable information that helps mental health professionals diagnose mental illness, these professionals realize that it is important to observe patients over a period of time to understand the individual's mental illness and its effects on his or her life.

Mental Illness and the Brain

The term mental illness clearly indicates that there is a problem with the mind. But is it just the mind in an abstract sense, or is there a physical basis to mental illness? As scientists continue to investigate mental illnesses and their causes, they learn more and more about how the biological processes that make the brain work are changed when a person has a mental illness.

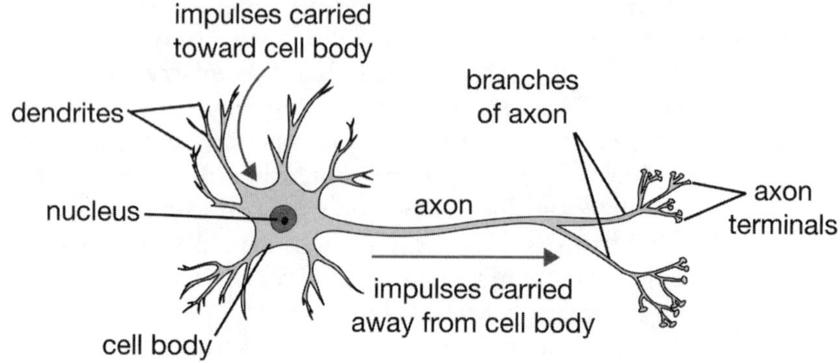

Figure 1.1. *The neuron, or nerve cell, is the functional unit of the nervous system. The neuron has processes called dendrites that receive signals and an axon that transmits signals to another neuron.*

The Basics of Brain Function

Before thinking about the problems that occur in the brain when someone has a mental illness, it is helpful to think about how the brain functions normally. The brain is an incredibly complex organ. It makes up only 2 percent of our body weight, but it consumes 20 percent of the oxygen we breathe and 20 percent of the energy we take in. It controls virtually everything we as humans experience, including movement, sensing our environment, regulating our involuntary body processes such as breathing, and controlling our emotions. Hundreds of thousands of chemical reactions occur every second in the brain; those reactions underlie the thoughts, actions, and behaviors with which we respond to environmental stimuli. In short, the brain dictates the internal processes and behaviors that allow us to survive.

How does the brain take in all this information, process it, and cause a response? The basic functional unit of the brain is the neuron. A neuron is a specialized cell that can produce different actions because of its precise connections with other neurons, sensory receptors, and muscle cells. A typical neuron has four structurally and functionally defined regions: the cell body, dendrites, axons, and the axon terminals.

The cell body is the metabolic center of the neuron. The nucleus is located in the cell body and most of the cell's protein synthesis occurs here.

A neuron usually has multiple fibers called dendrites that extend from the cell body. These processes usually branch out somewhat like tree branches and serve as the main apparatus for receiving input from other nerve cells.

The cell body also gives rise to the axon. The axon is usually much longer than the dendrites; in some cases, an axon can be up to 1 meter long. The axon is the part of the neuron that is specialized to carry messages away from the cell body and to relay messages to other cells. Some large axons are surrounded by a fatty insulating material called myelin, which enables the electrical signals to travel down the axon at higher speeds.

Near its end, the axon divides into many fine branches that have specialized swellings called axon terminals or presynaptic terminals. The axon terminals end near the dendrites of another neuron. The dendrites of one neuron receive the message sent from the axon terminals of another neuron.

The site where an axon terminal ends near a receiving dendrite is called the synapse. The cell that sends out information is called the presynaptic neuron, and the cell that receives the information is called the postsynaptic neuron. It is important to note that the synapse is not a physical connection between the two neurons; there is no cytoplasmic connection between the two neurons. The intercellular space between the presynaptic and postsynaptic neurons is called the synaptic space or synaptic cleft. An average neuron forms approximately 1,000 synapses with other neurons. It has been estimated that there are more synapses in the human brain than there are stars in our galaxy. Furthermore, synaptic connections are not static. Neurons form new synapses or strengthen synaptic connections in response to life experiences. This dynamic change in neuronal connections is the basis of learning.

Neurons communicate using both electrical signals and chemical messages. Information in the form of an electrical impulse is carried away from the neuron's cell body along the axon of the presynaptic neuron toward the axon terminals. When the electrical signal reaches the presynaptic axon terminal, it cannot cross the synaptic space, or synaptic cleft. Instead, the electrical signal triggers chemical changes that can cross the synapse to affect the postsynaptic cell. When the electrical impulse reaches the presynaptic axon terminal, membranous sacs called vesicles move toward the membrane of the axon terminal. When the vesicles reach the membrane, they fuse with the membrane and release their contents into the synaptic space. The molecules contained in the vesicles are chemical compounds called neurotransmitters. Each vesicle contains many molecules of a neurotransmitter. The released neurotransmitter molecules drift across the synaptic cleft and then bind to special proteins, called receptors, on the postsynaptic neuron. A neurotransmitter molecule will bind only to a specific kind of receptor.

The binding of neurotransmitters to their receptors causes that neuron to generate an electrical impulse. The electrical impulse then moves away from the dendrite ending toward the cell body. After the neurotransmitter stimulates an electrical impulse in the postsynaptic neuron, it releases from the receptor back into the synaptic space. Specific proteins called transporters or reuptake pumps carry the neurotransmitter back into the presynaptic neuron. When the neurotransmitter molecules are back in the presynaptic axon terminal, they can be repackaged into vesicles for release the next time an electrical impulse reaches the axon terminal. Enzymes present in the synaptic space degrade neurotransmitter molecules that are not taken back up into the presynaptic neuron.

The nervous system uses a variety of neurotransmitter molecules, but each neuron specializes in the synthesis and secretion of a single type of neurotransmitter. Some of the predominant neurotransmitters in the brain include glutamate, GABA [gamma aminobutyric acid], serotonin, dopamine, and norepinephrine. Each of these neurotransmitters has a specific distribution and function in the brain.

Investigating Brain Function

Mental health professionals base their diagnosis and treatment of mental illness on the symptoms that a person exhibits. The goal for these professionals in treating a patient is to relieve the symptoms that are interfering with the person's life so that the person can function well. Research scientists, on the other hand, have a different goal. They want to learn about the chemical or structural changes that occur in the brain when someone has a mental illness. If scientists can determine what happens in the brain, they can use that knowledge to develop better treatments or find a cure.

The techniques that scientists use to investigate the brain depend on the questions they are asking. For some questions, scientists use molecular or biochemical methods to investigate specific genes or proteins in the neurons. For other questions, scientists want to visualize changes in the brain so that they can learn more about how the activity or structure of the brain changes. Historically, scientists could examine brains only after death, but new imaging procedures enable scientists to study the brain in living animals, including humans. It is important to realize that these brain imaging techniques are not used for diagnosing mental illness. Mental illnesses are diagnosed by the set of symptoms that an individual exhibits. The imaging techniques described in the following paragraphs would not enable the mental health professional to diagnose or treat the patient more effectively. Some of the techniques are also invasive and expose patients to small amounts of radiation. Research studies using these tests are generally not conducted with children or adolescents.

One extensively used technique to study brain activity and how mental illness changes the brain is positron emission tomography (PET). PET measures the spatial distribution and movement of a radioactive chemical injected into the tissues of living subjects. Because the patient is awake, the technique can be used to investigate the relationship between behavioral and physiological effects and changes in brain activity. PET scans can detect very small (nanomolar) concentrations of tracer molecules and achieve spatial resolution of about 4 millimeters. In addition, computers can reconstruct images obtained from a PET scan in two or three dimensions.

PET requires the use of compounds that are labeled with positron-emitting isotopes. A positron has the same mass and spin as an electron but the opposite charge; an electron has a negative charge and a positron has a positive charge. A cyclotron accelerates protons into the nucleus of nitrogen, carbon, oxygen, or fluorine to generate these isotopes. The additional proton makes the isotope unstable. To become stable again, the proton must break down into a neutron and a positron. The unstable positron travels away from the site of generation and dissipates energy along the way. Eventually, the positron collides with an electron, leading to the emission of two gamma rays at 180 degrees from one another. The gamma rays reach a pair of detectors that record the event. Because the detectors respond only to simultaneous emissions, scientists can precisely map the location where the gamma rays were generated. The radioactive chemicals used for PET are very short lived. The half-life (the time for half of the radioactive label to disintegrate) of the commonly used radioisotopes ranges from approximately two minutes to less than two hours, depending on the specific compound. Because a PET scan requires only small amounts (a few micrograms) of short-lived radioisotopes, this technique can be used safely in humans.

PET scans can answer a variety of questions about brain function, including where the neurons are most active. Scientists use different radiolabeled compounds to investigate different biological questions. For example, radiolabeled glucose can identify parts of the brain that become more active in response to a specific stimulus. Active neurons metabolize more glucose than inactive neurons. Active neurons emit more positrons, and this shows as red or yellow on PET scans compared with blue or purple in areas where the neurons are not highly active. (Different computer enhancement techniques may use a different color scheme, but the use of a spectrum with red indicating high activity and blue indicating low activity is common.) Scientists can use PET to measure changes in the activity of specific brain areas in a person who has a mental illness. Scientists can also investigate how the mentally ill brain changes after a person receives treatment.

PET imaging is not the only technique that researchers use to investigate how mental illness changes the brain. Different techniques provide different information to scientists. Another important technique is magnetic resonance imaging (MRI). Unlike PET, which reveals changes in activity level, MRI is used to look at structural changes in the brain. For example, MRI studies reveal that the ventricles, or spaces within the brain, are larger in individuals who have schizophrenia compared with those of healthy individuals.

Other techniques that scientists use to investigate function in the living brain include single photon emission computed tomography (SPECT), functional magnetic resonance imaging (fMRI), and electroencephalography (EEG). Each technique has its own advantages, and each provides different information about brain structure and function. Scientists often use more than one technique when conducting their research.

The Causes of Mental Illnesses

At this time, scientists do not have a complete understanding of what causes mental illnesses. If you think about the structural and organizational complexity of the brain together with the complexity of effects that mental illnesses have on thoughts, feelings, and behaviors, it is hardly surprising that figuring out the causes of mental illnesses is a daunting task. The fields of neuroscience, psychiatry, and psychology address different aspects of the relationship between the biology of the brain and individuals' behaviors, thoughts, and feelings, and how their actions sometimes get out of control. Through this multidisciplinary research, scientists are trying to find the causes of mental illnesses. Once scientists can determine the causes of a mental illness, they can use that knowledge to develop new treatments or to find a cure.

The Biology of Mental Illnesses

Most scientists believe that mental illnesses result from problems with the communication between neurons in the brain (neurotransmission).

For example, the level of the neurotransmitter serotonin is lower in individuals who have depression. This finding led to the development of certain medications for the illness. Selective serotonin reuptake inhibitors (SSRIs) work by reducing the amount of serotonin that is taken back into the presynaptic neuron. This leads to an increase in the amount of serotonin available in the synaptic space for binding to the receptor on the postsynaptic neuron. Changes in other neurotransmitters (in addition to serotonin) may occur in depression, thus adding to the complexity of the cause underlying the disease.

Scientists believe that there may be disruptions in the neurotransmitters dopamine, glutamate, and norepinephrine in individuals who have schizophrenia. One indication that dopamine might be an important neurotransmitter in schizophrenia comes from the observation that cocaine addicts sometimes show symptoms similar to schizophrenia. Cocaine acts on dopamine-containing neurons in the brain to increase the amount of dopamine in the synapse.

Risk Factors for Mental Illnesses

Although scientists at this time do not know the causes of mental illnesses, they have identified factors that put individuals at risk. Some of these factors are environmental, some are genetic, and some are social. In fact, all these factors most likely combine to influence whether someone becomes mentally ill. Genetic, environmental, and social factors interact to influence whether someone becomes mentally ill.

Environmental factors such as head injury, poor nutrition, and exposure to toxins (including lead and tobacco smoke) can increase the likelihood of developing a mental illness. Genes also play a role in determining whether someone develops a mental illness. The illnesses that are most likely to have a genetic component include autism, bipolar disorder, schizophrenia, and ADHD. For example, the observation that children with ADHD are much more likely to have a sibling or parent with ADHD supports a role for genetics in determining whether someone is at risk for ADHD. In studies of twins, ADHD is significantly more likely to be present in an identical twin than a fraternal twin. The same can be said for schizophrenia and depression. Mental illnesses are not triggered by a change in a single gene; scientists believe that the interaction of several genes may trigger mental illness. Furthermore, the combination of genetic, environmental, and social factors might determine whether a case of mental illness is mild or severe.

Social factors also present risks and can harm an individual's, especially a child's, mental health. Social factors include:

- severe parental discord,
- death of a family member or close friend,
- parent's mental illness,
- parent's criminality,
- overcrowding,
- economic hardship,
- abuse,
- neglect, and
- exposure to violence.

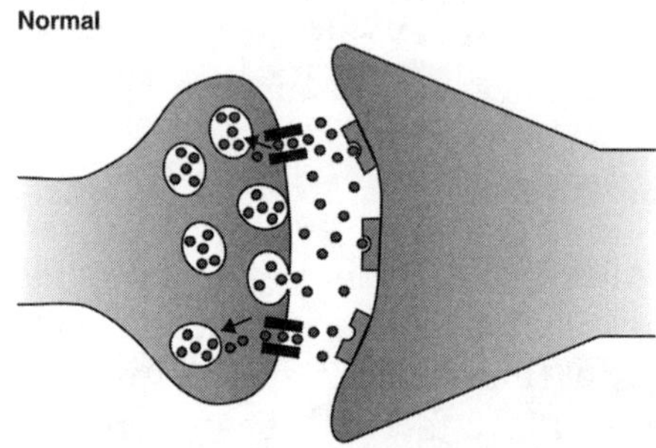

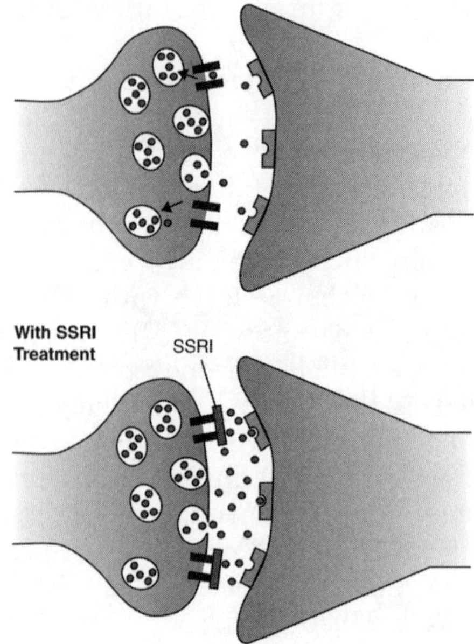

Figure 1.2. *Scientists understand that mental illnesses are associated with changes in neurochemicals. For example, in people who have depression, less of the transmitter serotonin (small circles) is released into the synaptic space than in people who do not have depression. Certain medications called selective serotonin reuptake inhibitors (SSRIs) relieve symptoms of depression by causing an increase in the amount of serotonin in the synaptic space.*

Treating Mental Illnesses

At this time, most mental illnesses cannot be cured, but they can usually be treated effectively to minimize the symptoms and allow the individual to function in work, school, or social environments. To begin treatment, an individual needs to see a qualified mental health professional. The first thing that the doctor or other mental health professional will do is speak with the individual to find out more about his or her symptoms, how long the symptoms have lasted, and how the person's life is being affected. The physician will also do a physical examination to determine whether there are other health problems. For example, some symptoms (such as emotional swings) can be caused by neurological or hormonal problems associated with chronic illnesses such as heart disease, or they can be a side effect of certain medications. After the individual's overall health is evaluated and the condition diagnosed, the doctor will develop a treatment plan. Treatment can involve both medications and psychotherapy, depending on the disease and its severity.

Medications

Medications are often used to treat mental illnesses. Through television commercials and magazine advertisements, we are becoming more aware of those medications. To become fully effective, medications for treating mental illness must be taken for a few days or a few weeks. When a patient begins taking medication, it is important for a doctor to monitor the patient's health. If the medication causes undesirable side effects, the doctor may change the dose or switch to a different medication that produces fewer side effects. If the medication does not relieve the symptoms, the doctor may prescribe a different medication. Sometimes, individuals who have a mental illness do not want to take their medications because of the side effects. It is important to remember that all medications have both positive and negative effects. For example, antibiotics have revolutionized treatment for some bacterial diseases. However, antibiotics often affect beneficial bacteria in the human body, leading to side effects such as nausea and diarrhea. Psychiatric drugs, like other medications, can alleviate symptoms of mental illness but can also produce unwanted side effects. People who take a medication to treat an illness, whether it is a mental illness or another disease, should work with their doctors to understand what medication they are taking, why they are taking it, how to take it, and what side effects to watch for.

Occasionally, the media reports stories in which the side effects of a psychiatric medication are tied to a potentially serious consequence, such as suicide. In these cases, it is usually very difficult to determine how much suicidal behavior was due to the mental disorder and what the role of the medication might have been. Medications for treating mental illness can, like other medications, have side effects. The psychiatrist or physician can usually adjust the dose or change the medication to alleviate side effects.

Psychotherapy

Psychotherapy is a treatment method in which a mental health professional (psychiatrist, psychologist, or other mental health professional) and the patient discuss problems and feelings. This discussion helps patients understand the basis of their problems and find solutions. Psychotherapy may take different forms. The therapy can help patients"

- change thought or behavior patterns,
- understand how past experiences influence current behaviors,
- solve other problems in specific ways, or
- learn illness self-management skills.

Psychotherapy may occur between a therapist and an individual; a therapist and an individual and his or her family members; or a therapist and a group. Often, treatment for mental illness is most successful when psychotherapy is used in combination with medications. For severe mental illnesses, medication relieves the symptoms and psychotherapy helps individuals cope with their illness.

Just as there are no medications that can instantly cure mental illnesses, psychotherapy is not a one-time event. The amount of time a person spends in psychotherapy can range from a few visits to a few years, depending on the nature of the illness or problem. In general, the more severe the problem, the more lengthy the psychotherapy should be.

The Stigma of Mental Illness

"Mentally ill people are nuts, crazy, wacko." "Mentally ill people are morally bad." "Mentally ill people are dangerous and should be locked in an asylum forever." "Mentally ill people need somebody to take care of them." How often have we heard comments like these or seen these types of portrayals in movies, television shows, or books? We may even be guilty of making comments like them ourselves. Is there any truth behind these portrayals, or is that negative view based on our ignorance and fear?

Stigmas are negative stereotypes about groups of people. Common stigmas about people who are mentally ill are:

- Individuals who have a mental illness are dangerous.
- Individuals who have a mental illness are irresponsible and can't make life decisions for themselves.
- People who have a mental illness are childlike and must be taken care of by parents or guardians.
- People who have a mental illness should just get over it.

Each of those preconceptions about people who have a mental illness is based on false information. Very few people who have a mental illness are dangerous to society. Most can hold jobs, attend school, and live independently. A person who has a mental illness cannot simply decide to get over it any more than someone who has a different chronic disease such as diabetes, asthma, or heart disease can. A mental illness, like those other diseases, is caused by a physical problem in the body.

Stigmas against individuals who have a mental illness lead to injustices, including discriminatory decisions regarding housing, employment, and education. Overcoming the stigmas commonly associated with mental illness is yet one more challenge that people who have a mental illness must face. Indeed, many people who successfully manage their mental illness report that the stigma they face is in many ways more disabling than the illness itself. The stigmatizing attitudes toward mental illness held by both the public and those who have a mental illness lead to feelings of shame and guilt, loss of self-esteem, social dependence, and a sense of isolation and hopelessness. One of the worst consequences of stigma is that people who are struggling with a mental illness may be reluctant to seek treatment that, in most cases, would significantly relieve their symptoms.

Providing accurate information is one way to reduce stigmas about mental illness. Advocacy groups protest stereotypes imposed upon those who are mentally ill. They demand that the media stop presenting inaccurate views of mental illness and that the public stops believing these negative views. A powerful way of countering stereotypes about mental illness occurs when members of the public meet people who are effectively managing a serious mental illness: holding jobs, providing for themselves, and living as good neighbors in a community. Interaction with people who have mental illnesses challenges a person's assumptions and changes a person's attitudes about mental illness.

Attitudes about mental illness are changing, although there is a long way to go before people accept that mental illness is a disease with a biological basis. A survey by the National Mental Health Association found that 55 percent of people who have never been diagnosed with depression recognize that depression is a disease and not something people should "snap out of." This is a substantial increase over the 38 percent of survey respondents in 1991 who recognized depression as a disease.

The Consequences of Not Treating Mental Illness

Most people don't think twice before going to a doctor if they have an illness such as bronchitis, asthma, diabetes, or heart disease. However, many people who have a mental illness don't get the treatment that would alleviate their suffering. Studies estimate that two-thirds of all young people with mental health problems are not receiving the help they need and that less than one-third of the children under age 18 who have a serious mental health problem receive any mental health services. Mental illness in adults often goes untreated, too. What are the consequences of letting mental illness go untreated?

In September 2000, the U.S. surgeon general held a conference on children's mental health. The former surgeon general, Dr. David Satcher, emphasized the importance of mental health in children by stating, " Children and families are suffering because of missed opportunities for prevention and early identification, fragmented services, and low priorities for resources. Overriding all of this is the issue of stigma, which continues to surround mental illness."

The consequences of mental illness in children and adolescents can be substantial. Many mental health professionals speak of accrued deficits that occur when mental illness in children is not treated. To begin with, mental illness can impair a student's ability to learn. Adolescents whose mental illness is not treated rapidly and aggressively tend to fall further and further behind in school. They are more likely to drop out of school and are less likely to be fully functional members of society when they reach adulthood. We also now know that depressive disorders in young people confer a higher risk for illness and interpersonal and psychosocial difficulties that persist after the depressive episode is over. Furthermore, many adults who suffer from mental disorders have problems that originated in childhood. Depression in youth may predict more severe illness in adult life. Attention deficit hyperactivity disorder, once thought to affect children and adolescents only, may persist into adulthood and may be associated with social, legal, and occupational problems. Mental illness impairs a student's ability to learn. Adolescents whose mental illness is not treated rapidly and aggressively tend to fall further and further behind in school.

The high incidence of mental illness has a great impact on society. Depression alone causes employers to lose over $23 billion each year due to decreased productivity and absenteeism of employees. The Global Burden of Disease Study, conducted by the World Health Organization, assessed the burden of all diseases in units that measure lost years of healthy life due to premature death or disability (disability-adjusted life years, or DALYs). Over 15 percent of the total DALYs were due to mental illness. In 1996, the United States spent more than $69 billion for the direct treatment of mental illnesses. Indirect costs of mental illness due to lost productivity in the workplace, schools, or homes represented a $79 billion loss for the U.S. economy in 1990.

Treatment, including psychotherapy and medication management, is cost-effective for patients, their families, and society. The benefits include fewer visits to other doctors' offices, diagnostic laboratories, and hospitals for physical ailments that are based in psychological distress; reduced need for psychiatric hospitalization; fewer sick days and disability claims; and increased job stability. Conversely, the costs of not treating mental disorders can be seen in ruined relationships, job loss or poor job performance, personal anguish, substance abuse, unnecessary medical procedures, psychiatric hospitalization, and suicide.

Chapter 2

Common Myths about Mental Health Disorders

What is mental illness?

- Mental illnesses and severe emotional disturbances are biologically based disorders, just as are diabetes, cancer, and heart disease. Mental and emotional disorders disrupt a person's ability to think, feel, and relate to others.
- Mental illness is the nation's second leading cause of disability after heart disease.[1]

Who does mental illness affect?

- Twenty percent (20%) of adults, or about 40 million (40,000,000) Americans, experience some type of mental disorder every year.[2]
- Five percent (5%) of adults, or about 10 million (10,000,000) Americans, have a serious mental illness, such as schizophrenia, major depression, or bipolar disorder.[1]
- Ten percent (10%) of children and adolescents suffer from mental illness severe enough to cause some level of impairment.[2]
- Young people between 15 and 24 years old are the age group most likely to experience a major depressive episode.[2]

"Take Action: Mental Illness Facts & Myths," © 2004 National Alliance on Mental Illness—New Hampshire (www.naminh.org). Reprinted with permission. The copyright holder considers this information to be current.

- Depression in elders accounts for a majority of suicidal ideation, inpatient admissions, medical outpatient visits, emergency room use, and medical co-morbidity.[3]
- Fifty to sixty percent (50–60%) of individuals with severe mental disorders are also affected by substance abuse. This compares with ten percent (10%) in the general population.[4]
- People with mental illness have a higher incidence of medical disorders, including obesity, heart disease, and diabetes.[5]

How well are mental illness treatment needs met?

- Less than one third of adults and half of children with a diagnosable mental disorder receive any level of treatment in any one year.[2]
- It is estimated that only 1 in 5 children (20%) suffering from a mental illness receives mental health services, the same level it was 20 years ago.[2]
- Health care insurers place arbitrary and more restrictive caps on benefits for some mental illness than medical disorders.[2]

What is the impact of mental illness?

- Suicide is the third leading cause of death among teens, exceeded only by accidents and homicides.[2]
- Untreated mental illnesses contribute to employee absenteeism and turnover, increased disability claims, lower productivity, and lower work quality.
- Employers firmly believe that early, appropriate treatment of mental illness is essential to productivity in the workplace, and is vital to employees and their families.[6]
- It is estimated that 80–90% of people with serious brain disorders are unemployed.[7]
- It is estimated that 60% of all persons with mental illness are willing to work but unable to overcome the barriers.
- Individuals receiving treatment for schizophrenia are no more prone to violence than the general public.
- De-institutionalization has moved many people with serious mental illness from hospitals to homeless shelters, the streets, jails, and prisons.[2]

- Jails, prisons, and juvenile facilities are too often the treatment facilities for adults, children, and adolescents with mental illness.[2]
- Sixteen percent (16%) of people in jails and prisons suffer from a serious mental illness.[2]
- Between 50 and 75% of youth in juvenile justice facilities suffer from a diagnosable mental health disorder and frequently do not receive counseling, treatment, or support.[2]
- It is estimated that at least 25% of homeless people suffer from serious mental illness.[2]
- It is estimated that 21% of persons in all hospital beds, at any one time, are there because of mental illness.
- Twenty-three percent (23%) of parents and caregivers of children with mental illness were forced by state regulations to consider relinquishing custody of their child in order to access mental health services and 20% actually did so.[2]

What are the costs of mental illness?

- Direct costs, including hospitalizations and medications, to the nation for mental illness are estimated to be $70 billion annually.
- Indirect costs to the Nation for mental illness, including lost wages, family care-giving and lost productivity due to suicide, are estimated to be an additional $80 billion annually.
- Approximately 53% of all mental health and substance abuse treatment costs are publicly funded, compared to 47% of total health care spending.[2]
- Medicaid accounts for more than 50% of state and local mental health spending and is expected to reach 60% by 2007. Medicaid is nearly 15% of many state budgets, second only to education.[2]

How effective is mental health treatment?

- Diagnoses of mental disorders made using specific criteria are as reliable as those for general medical disorders.[1]
- Mental disorders are as treatable today as general medical conditions.[2]
- Treatment success for schizophrenia, bipolar illness, major depression, panic disorder and obsessive-compulsive disorder compare

favorably with general medical or surgical treatments, such as angioplasty or atherectomy for heart disease, which have success rates at or below 50%.[2]

- Some cases of mental illness are long-term, severe, and persistent, similar to diabetes and other medical conditions. The quality of life for such individuals can be improved by their focusing on their recovery and well-being and by access to services.[2]
- For individuals with mental illness and addictive disorders, integrated treatment delivered simultaneously at the same treatment facility by staff trained in both is more effective than sequential or parallel treatment of each disorder.[2]
- A growing body of evidence shows that most mentally ill persons in need of treatment can be served more effectively and at less cost in community settings than in traditional psychiatric hospitals.[2]
- The most effective treatment for mental disorders addresses all relevant issues, which may include securing affordable housing, income support, health care services, employment training, social services, social and recreational opportunities, and appropriate medications.[2]

Is treatment for mental illness accessible?

- Stigma discourages many individuals and their families from even seeking treatment for mental illness and severe emotional disturbances.[2]
- Only one fifth of children and adolescents who need mental health treatment receive it.
- Forty million (40,000,000) Americans do not have health coverage. Mental health services for the indigent population in NH [New Hampshire] are limited, if available at all. Only limited emergency services are available, and that is often provided in hospital emergency rooms that are costly and ill-prepared for such emergencies.

Common Myths about Mental Illness

Myth: If I have a mental health problem I should be able to take care of it myself.

Reality: Some mental health problems, such as mild depression or anxiety, can be relieved with support, self-help, and proper care.

However, if problems or symptoms persist, a person should consult with their primary doctor or a qualified mental health professional.

Myth: If I have a mental illness, it is a sign of weakness—it's my fault.

Reality: Mental illness is not anyone's fault, anymore than heart disease or diabetes is a person's fault. According to the Surgeon General's report: "Mental disorders are health conditions that are characterized by alterations in thinking, mood, or behavior (or some combination thereof), associated with distress and/ or impaired functioning."

Mental illnesses are not a condition that people choose to have or not have. Mental illnesses are not results of willful, petulant behavior. No one should have to feel ashamed of this condition any more than any other medical condition.

Myth: If I seek help for my mental health problem, others will think I am crazy.

Reality: No one should delay getting treatment for a mental health problem that is not getting better, just as one would not wait to take care of a medical condition that needed treatment. Some people worry that others will avoid them if they seek treatment for their mental illness. Early treatment can produce better results. Seeking appropriate help is a sign of strength not weakness.

Myth: People diagnosed with a mental illness are always ill and out of touch with reality.

Reality: Most people suffering from even the most severe of mental illnesses are in touch with reality more often than they are not. Many people quietly bear the symptoms of mental illness without ever showing signs of their illness to others, and most people with mental illness live productive, active lives.

Myth: Stress causes mental illness.

Reality: This is only partially true. Stress may occasionally trigger an episode or cause symptoms such as anxiety or depression, but persistent symptoms appear to be biological in nature. There are probably many things that can contribute to mental illness—the cause is not yet fully understood.

Myth: A person can recover from a mental illness by turning his or her thoughts positively and with prayer.

Reality: Recovery is possible when the person receives the necessary treatment and support. Spirituality can also be an important source of strength for some individuals.

Myth: People who have mental illness are dangerous.

Reality: People who have mental illness are not more violent than is someone suffering from cancer or any other serious disease.

Myth: Most people with mental illness live on the streets or are in mental hospitals.

Reality: Over two-thirds of Americans who have a mental illness live in the community and lead productive lives. Most people who need hospitalization are only there for brief periods to get treatment and are then able to return home, just like people hospitalized for other conditions. Some people with mental illness do become homeless and could benefit from treatment and services.

Note: The facts presented in this publication have been compiled from recognized sources and nationwide surveys that, evidence suggests, equally reflect conditions in New Hampshire.

References

1. Mental Health: A Report of the Surgeon General, 12/1999.
2. NAMI Policymaker's Fact Sheet on Mental Illness. No. 01-02, 9/26/2002.
3. "Integrated Mental health and the Primary Care for Older Persons," Stephen J. Bartels, M.D., Presentation to NASMHPD Older Persons Division, 8/26/2002.
4. "Epidemiology of Substance Abuse Among Persons with Chronic Mental Illness," Mueser, K.T., Bennett, M, Kushner, MG, (1995). In Integrated Dual Disorders Treatment, Evidenced Based Practices Project, Resource Kit, 2002.
5. Ken Duckworth, M.D., "A Mind and a Body: Another Dimension of Recovery," *NAMI Advocate*, Fall 2002.

6. Anthony WA, Blanch A., "Supported Employment for Persons who are Psychiatrically Disabled: An Historical and Conceptual Perspective"; *Psychosocial Rehabilitation Journal* 11(2): 5–23, 1987.

7. Report on the Surgeon General's Conference on Children's Mental Health: A National Action Agenda; 9/2000.

Chapter 3

Mental Health Disorders in the United States

Mental disorders are common in the United States and internationally. An estimated 26.2 percent of Americans ages 18 and older—about one in four adults—suffer from a diagnosable mental disorder in a given year.[1] When applied to the 2004 U.S. Census residential population estimate for ages 18 and older, this figure translates to 57.7 million people.[2] Even though mental disorders are widespread in the population, the main burden of illness is concentrated in a much smaller proportion—about 6 percent, or 1 in 17—who suffer from a serious mental illness.[1] In addition, mental disorders are the leading cause of disability in the U.S. and Canada for ages 15–44.[3] Many people suffer from more than one mental disorder at a given time. Nearly half (45 percent) of those with any mental disorder meet criteria for two or more disorders, with severity strongly related to comorbidity.[1]

In the United States, mental disorders are diagnosed based on the *Diagnostic and Statistical Manual of Mental Disorders, Fourth Edition (DSM-IV)*.[4]

Mood Disorders

Mood disorders include major depressive disorder, dysthymic disorder, and bipolar disorder.

"The Numbers Count: Mental Disorders in America," from the National Institute of Mental Health (NIMH, www.nimh.nih.gov), part of the National Institutes of Health, June 26, 2008.

- Approximately 20.9 million American adults, or about 9.5 percent of the U.S. population age 18 and older in a given year, have a mood disorder.[1]
- The median age of onset for mood disorders is 30 years.[5]
- Depressive disorders often co-occur with anxiety disorders and substance abuse.[5]

Major Depressive Disorder

- Major depressive disorder is the leading cause of disability in the United States for ages 15–44.[3]
- Major depressive disorder affects approximately 14.8 million American adults, or about 6.7 percent of the U.S. population age 18 and older in a given year.[1]
- While major depressive disorder can develop at any age, the median age at onset is 32.[5]
- Major depressive disorder is more prevalent in women than in men.[6]

Dysthymic Disorder

- Symptoms of dysthymic disorder (chronic, mild depression) must persist for at least 2 years in adults (one year in children) to meet criteria for the diagnosis. Dysthymic disorder affects approximately 1.5 percent of the U.S. population age 18 and older in a given year.[1] This figure translates to about 3.3 million American adults.[2]
- The median age of onset of dysthymic disorder is 31.[1]

Bipolar Disorder

- Bipolar disorder affects approximately 5.7 million American adults, or about 2.6 percent of the U.S. population age 18 and older in a given year.[1]
- The median age of onset for bipolar disorders is 25 years.[5]

Suicide

- In 2004, 32,439 (approximately 11 per 100,000) people died by suicide in the United States.[7]

- More than 90 percent of people who kill themselves have a diagnosable mental disorder, most commonly a depressive disorder or a substance abuse disorder.[8]
- The highest suicide rates in the United States are found in white men over age 85.[9]
- Four times as many men as women die by suicide[9]; however, women attempt suicide two to three times as often as men.[10]

Schizophrenia

- Approximately 2.4 million American adults, or about 1.1 percent of the population age 18 and older in a given year,[11] have schizophrenia.
- Schizophrenia affects men and women with equal frequency.[12]
- Schizophrenia often first appears in men in their late teens or early twenties. In contrast, women are generally affected in their twenties or early thirties.[12]

Anxiety Disorders

Anxiety disorders include panic disorder, obsessive-compulsive disorder, post-traumatic stress disorder, generalized anxiety disorder, and phobias (social phobia, agoraphobia, and specific phobia).

- Approximately 40 million American adults ages 18 and older, or about 18.1 percent of people in this age group in a given year, have an anxiety disorder.[1]
- Anxiety disorders frequently co-occur with depressive disorders or substance abuse.[1]
- Most people with one anxiety disorder also have another anxiety disorder. Nearly three quarters of those with an anxiety disorder will have their first episode by age 21.[5]

Panic Disorder

- Approximately 6 million American adults ages 18 and older, or about 2.7 percent of people in this age group in a given year, have panic disorder.[1]
- Panic disorder typically develops in early adulthood (median age of onset is 24), but the age of onset extends throughout adulthood.[5]

- About one in three people with panic disorder develops agoraphobia, a condition in which the individual becomes afraid of being in any place or situation where escape might be difficult or help unavailable in the event of a panic attack.[12]

Obsessive-Compulsive Disorder (OCD)

- Approximately 2.2 million American adults age 18 and older, or about 1.0 percent of people in this age group in a given year, have OCD.[1]
- The first symptoms of OCD often begin during childhood or adolescence, however, the median age of onset is 19.[5]

Posttraumatic Stress Disorder (PTSD)

- Approximately 7.7 million American adults age 18 and older, or about 3.5 percent of people in this age group in a given year, have PTSD.[1]
- PTSD can develop at any age, including childhood, but research shows that the median age of onset is 23 years.[5]
- About 19 percent of Vietnam veterans experienced PTSD at some point after the war.[13] The disorder also frequently occurs after violent personal assaults such as rape, mugging, or domestic violence; terrorism; natural or human-caused disasters; and accidents.

Generalized Anxiety Disorder (GAD)

- Approximately 6.8 million American adults, or about 3.1 percent of people age 18 and over, have GAD in a given year.[1]
- GAD can begin across the life cycle, though the median age of onset is 31 years old.[5]

Social Phobia

- Approximately 15 million American adults age 18 and over, or about 6.8 percent of people in this age group in a given year, have social phobia.[1]
- Social phobia begins in childhood or adolescence, typically around 13 years of age.[5]

Agoraphobia

Agoraphobia involves intense fear and anxiety of any place or situation where escape might be difficult, leading to avoidance of situations such as being alone outside of the home; traveling in a car, bus, or airplane; or being in a crowded area.[5]

- Approximately 1.8 million American adults age 18 and over, or about 0.8 percent of people in this age group in a given year, have agoraphobia without a history of panic disorder.[1]
- The median age of onset of agoraphobia is 20 years of age.[5]

Specific Phobia

Specific phobia involves marked and persistent fear and avoidance of a specific object or situation.

- Approximately 19.2 million American adults age 18 and over, or about 8.7 percent of people in this age group in a given year, have some type of specific phobia.[1]
- Specific phobia typically begins in childhood; the median age of onset is 7 years.[5]

Eating Disorders

The three main types of eating disorders are anorexia nervosa, bulimia nervosa, and binge-eating disorder.

- Females are much more likely than males to develop an eating disorder. Only an estimated 5 to 15 percent of people with anorexia or bulimia[14] and an estimated 35 percent of those with binge-eating disorder[15] are male.
- In their lifetime, an estimated 0.5 percent to 3.7 percent of females suffer from anorexia, and an estimated 1.1 percent to 4.2 percent suffer from bulimia.[16]
- Community surveys have estimated that between 2 percent and 5 percent of Americans experience binge-eating disorder in a 6-month period.[15,17]
- The mortality rate among people with anorexia has been estimated at 0.56 percent per year, or approximately 5.6 percent per decade, which is about 12 times higher than the annual

death rate due to all causes of death among females ages 15–24 in the general population.[18]

Attention Deficit Hyperactivity Disorder (ADHD)

- ADHD, one of the most common mental disorders in children and adolescents, also affects an estimated 4.1 percent of adults, ages 18–44, in a given year.[1]
- ADHD usually becomes evident in preschool or early elementary years. The median age of onset of ADHD is 7 years, although the disorder can persist into adolescence and occasionally into adulthood.[5]

Autism

Autism is part of a group of disorders called autism spectrum disorders (ASDs), also known as pervasive developmental disorders. ASDs range in severity, with autism being the most debilitating form while other disorders, such as Asperger syndrome, produce milder symptoms.

- Estimating the prevalence of autism is difficult and controversial due to differences in the ways that cases are identified and defined, differences in study methods, and changes in diagnostic criteria. A recent study reported the prevalence of autism in 3–10 year-olds to be about 3.4 cases per 1000 children.[19]
- Autism and other ASDs develop in childhood and generally are diagnosed by age 3.[20]
- Autism is about four times more common in boys than girls. Girls with the disorder, however, tend to have more severe symptoms and greater cognitive impairment.[19,20]

Alzheimer Disease

- AD affects an estimated 4.5 million Americans. The number of Americans with AD has more than doubled since 1980.[21]
- AD is the most common cause of dementia among people age 65 and older.[22]
- Increasing age is the greatest risk factor for Alzheimer disease. In most people with AD, symptoms first appear after age 65. One in 10 individuals over 65 and nearly half of those over 85

are affected.[23] Rare, inherited forms of Alzheimer disease can strike individuals as early as their 30s and 40s.[24]

- From the time of diagnosis, people with AD survive about half as long as those of similar age without dementia.[25]

References

1. Kessler RC, Chiu WT, Demler O, Walters EE. Prevalence, severity, and comorbidity of twelve-month DSM-IV disorders in the National Comorbidity Survey Replication (NCS-R). *Archives of General Psychiatry,* 2005 Jun;62(6):617–27.
2. U.S. Census Bureau Population Estimates by Demographic Characteristics. Table 2: Annual Estimates of the Population by Selected Age Groups and Sex for the United States: April 1, 2000 to July 1, 2004 (NC-EST2004-02) Source: Population Division, U.S. Census Bureau Release Date: June 9, 2005. http://www.census.gov/popest/national/asrh
3. The World Health Organization. *The World Health Report 2004: Changing History*, Annex Table 3: Burden of disease in DALYs by cause, sex, and mortality stratum in WHO regions, estimates for 2002. Geneva: WHO, 2004.
4. *American Psychiatric Association. Diagnostic and Statistical Manual on Mental Disorders, fourth edition (DSM-IV).* Washington, DC: American Psychiatric Press, 1994.
5. Kessler RC, Berglund PA, Demler O, Jin R, Walters EE. Lifetime prevalence and age-of-onset distributions of *DSM-IV* disorders in the National Comorbidity Survey Replication (NCS-R). *Archives of General Psychiatry.* 2005 Jun;62(6):593–602.
6. Kessler RC, Berglund P, Demler O, Jin R, Koretz D, Merikangas KR, Rush AJ, Walters EE, Wang PS. The epidemiology of major depressive disorder: results from the National Comorbidity Survey Replication (NCS-R). *Journal of the American Medical Association,* 2003; Jun 18;289(23): 3095–105.
7. Centers for Disease Control and Prevention, National Center for Injury Prevention and Control (producer). Web-based Injury Statistics Query and Reporting System (WISQARS). Available online from: URL: http://www.cdc.gov/ncipc/wisqars/default.htm accessed December 2006.

8. Conwell Y, Brent D. Suicide and aging I: patterns of psychiatric diagnosis. *International Psychogeriatrics*, 1995; 7(2): 149–64.

9. Kochanek KD, Murphy SL, Anderson RN, Scott C. Deaths: final data for 2002. *National Vital Statistics Reports*. 2004 Oct 12;53 (5):1–115.

10. Weissman MM, Bland RC, Canino GJ, et al. Prevalence of suicide ideation and suicide attempts in nine countries. *Psychological Medicine,* 1999; 29(1): 9–17.

11. Regier DA, Narrow WE, Rae DS, Manderscheid RW, Locke BZ, Goodwin FK. The de facto mental and addictive disorders service system. Epidemiologic Catchment Area prospective 1-year prevalence rates of disorders and services. *Archives of General Psychiatry.* 1993 Feb;50(2):85–94.

12. Robins LN, Regier DA, eds. *Psychiatric Disorders in America: The Epidemiologic Catchment Area Study*. New York: The Free Press, 1991.

13. Dohrenwend BP, Turner JB, Turse NA, Adams BG, Koen KC, Marshall R. The psychological risk of Vietnam for U.S. veterans: A revisit with new data and methods. *Science.* 2006; 313(5789):979–982.

14. Andersen AE. Eating disorders in males. In: Brownell KD, Fairburn CG, eds. *Eating Disorders and Obesity: A Comprehensive Handbook*. New York: Guilford Press, 1995;177–87.

15. Spitzer RL, Yanovski S, Wadden T, Wing R, Marcus MD, Stunkard A, Devlin M, Mitchell J, Hasin D, Horne RL. Binge eating disorder: its further validation in a multisite study. *International Journal of Eating Disorders.* 1993 Mar;13(2):137–53.

16. American Psychiatric Association Work Group on Eating Disorders. Practice guideline for the treatment of patients with eating disorders (revision). *American Journal of Psychiatry.* 2000 Jan;157(1 Suppl):1–39.

17. Bruce B, Agras WS. Binge eating in females: a population-based investigation. *International Journal of Eating Disorders.* 1992;12:365–73.

18. Sullivan PF. Mortality in anorexia nervosa. *American Journal of Psychiatry.* 1995 Jul;152(7):1073-4.

19. Yeargin-Allsopp M, Rice C, Karapurkar T, Doernberg N, Boyle C, Murphy C. Prevalence of Autism in a US Metropolitan Area. *The Journal of the American Medical Association.* 2003 Jan 1;289(1):49–55.

20. Fombonne E. Epidemiology of autism and related conditions. In: Volkmar FR, ed. *Autism and pervasive developmental disorders.* Cambridge, England: Cambridge University Press, 1998; 32–63.

21. Hebert LE, Scherr PA, Bienias JL, Bennett DA, Evans DA. Alzheimer disease in the US population: prevalence estimates using the 2000 census. *Archives of Neurology.* 2003 Aug;60(8):1119–22.

22. National Institute on Aging, Progress Report on Alzheimer's Disease 2004-2005. NIH Publication No. 05-5724. Bethesda, MD: National Institute on Aging, 2005. Available from http://www.alzheimers.org/pr04-05/index.asp

23. Evans DA, Funkenstein HH, Albert MS, Scherr PA, Cook NR, Chown MJ, Hebert LE, Hennekens CH, Taylor JO. Prevalence of Alzheimer's disease in a community population of older persons: Higher than previously reported. *The Journal of the American Medical Association.* 1989 Nov 10;262(18):2551–6.

24. Bird TD, Sumi SM, Nemens EJ, Nochlin D, Schellenberg G, Lampe TH, Sadovnick A, Chui H, Miner GW, Tinklenberg J. Phenotypic heterogeneity in familial Alzheimer's disease: a study of 24 kindreds. *Annals of Neurology.* 1989 Jan;25(1):12–25.

25. Larson EB, Shadlen MF, Wang L, McCormick WC, Bowen JD, Teri L, Kukull WA. Survival after initial diagnosis of Alzheimer disease. *Annals of Internal Medicine.* 2004 Apr 6;140(7):501–9.

Chapter 4

The Economic Cost of Mental Health Disorders

Chapter Contents

Section 4.1

Mental Disorders Cost Society Billions in Unearned Income

"Mental Disorders Cost Society Billions in Unearned Income," from the National Institute of Mental Health (NIMH, www.nimh.nih.gov), part of the National Institutes of Health, May 7, 2008.

Major mental disorders cost the nation at least $193 billion annually in lost earnings alone, according to a new study funded by the National Institutes of Health's National Institute of Mental Health (NIMH). The study was published May 7, 2008, in the *American Journal of Psychiatry*.

"Lost earning potential, costs associated with treating coexisting conditions, Social Security payments, homelessness, and incarceration are just some of the indirect costs associated with mental illnesses that have been difficult to quantify," said NIMH Director Thomas R. Insel, M.D. "This study shows us that just one source of these indirect costs is staggeringly high."

Direct costs associated with mental disorders like medication, clinic visits, and hospitalization are relatively easy to quantify, but they reveal only a small portion of the economic burden these illnesses place on society. Indirect costs like lost earnings likely account for enormous expenses, but they are very difficult to define and estimate.

In the study, Ronald C. Kessler, Ph.D., of Harvard University, and colleagues analyzed data from the 2002 National Comorbidity Survey Replication (NCS-R), a nationally representative study of Americans age 18 to 64.

Using data from 4,982 respondents, the researchers calculated the amount of earnings lost in the year prior to the survey among people with serious mental illness (SMI). SMI is a broad category of illnesses that includes mood and anxiety disorders that have seriously impaired a person's ability to function for at least 30 days in the year prior to the survey. It also includes cases of any mental disorder associated with life-threatening suicidal behaviors or repeated acts of violence.

Eighty-six percent of respondents reported earning income in the previous year. But those with SMI reported earning significantly less—around $22,545—than respondents without SMI, who averaged $38,852. Although men with SMI took a greater hit in earnings than women with SMI, men still earned more overall than women with and without SMI.

By extrapolating these results to the general population, the researchers calculated that SMI costs society $193.2 billion annually in lost earnings. The researchers attributed about 75 percent of this total to the reduced income that people with SMI likely earn, while 25 percent is attributed to the increased likelihood that people with SMI would have no earnings.

"The results of this study confirm the belief that mental disorders contribute to enormous losses of human productivity," said Kessler. "Yet this estimate is probably conservative because the NCS-R did not assess people in hospitals or prisons, and included very few participants with autism, schizophrenia, or other chronic illnesses that are known to greatly affect a person's ability to work. The actual costs are probably higher than what we have estimated."

The researchers concluded by recommending that future studies on the effectiveness of treatments should consider measuring employment status and earnings over the long term to document the effects of mental disorders on a person's functioning and ability to remain productive.

Reference

Kessler, RC, Heeringa S, Lakoma MD, Petukhova M, Rupp AE, Schoenbaum M, Wang PS, Zaslavsky AM. The individual-level and societal-level effects of mental disorders on earnings in the United States: Results from the National Comorbidity Survey Replication. *American Journal of Psychiatry,* May 7, 2008.

Section 4.2

Mental Disorders Account for Large Percentage of Adult Disability

"Mental Disorders Account for Large Percentage of Adult Role Disability," from the National Institute of Mental Health (NIMH, www.nimh.nih.gov), part of the National Institutes of Health, October 1, 2007.

An NIMH-funded study finds that more than half of U.S. adults have a mental or physical condition that prevents them from working or conducting their usual duties (e.g., role disability) for several days each year, and a large portion of those days can be attributed to mental disorders. The study, published in the October 2007 issue of the *Archives of General Psychiatry,* is based on data from the National Comorbidity Survey Replication (NCS-R), a nationwide survey among 9,282 Americans ages 18 and older.

Role disability is increasingly recognized as a major source of the societal costs of illness, but these indirect costs—the result of impaired functioning and lost productivity—are not easily measured, making it difficult to estimate the total costs of illness. To help quantify these costs, NIMH researcher Kathleen Merikangas, Ph.D., Ronald Kessler, Ph.D., of Harvard University, and colleagues analyzed data from 5,962 respondents of the NCS-R to determine the rate and frequency of role disability. They asked respondents how many days they were completely unable to work or carry out their usual activities as a result of a mental or chronic physical condition, such as an anxiety or mood disorder, substance or alcohol dependence, cancer, cardiovascular illness, musculoskeletal conditions, or others.

They found that over a 1-year period, 53 percent of U.S. adults have one or more mental or physical conditions that result in role disability. Among those adults, each experienced an average of 32 days of disability per year. Nationwide, about 2.4 billion disability days resulted from physical conditions, and about 1.3 billion disability days resulted from mental conditions. "These figures suggest an enormous burden on the people who have one or more of these conditions, their families and their employers," said Dr. Merikangas.

Estimating the impact of specific diseases on disability is difficult because people tend to have more than one illness or disorder at a time, such as depression and heart disease. By accounting for the likelihood of coexisting disorders, the authors found that musculoskeletal disorders, especially back and neck pain, resulted in the greatest number of disability days (1.2 billion) while major depression resulted in the second greatest number of disability days (387 million).

This research documents that the level of disability associated with chronic mental conditions is as large as that associated with many chronic physical conditions. By documenting the impact and cost of chronic mental and physical disorders, this research may be useful to health care providers and policymakers.

Reference

Merikangas KR. Ames M, Cui L, Stang PE, Ustun TB, von Korff M, Kessler, RC. The impact of comorbidity of mental and physical conditions on role disability in the U.S. adult population. *Archives of General Psychiatry,* Oct 2007; vol. 64(10).

Chapter 5

Stress and Mental Health Disorders

Neuroscientists at Harvard Medical School and its affiliate McLean Hospital have shown that long-term exposure to stress hormone in mice directly results in the anxiety that often comes with depression. After years of circumstantial evidence linking stress and depression, this evidence may be the "smoking gun" of what, for some, causes some types of mood disorders. The research appears in the April 2006 issue of *Behavioral Neuroscience*, which is published by the American Psychological Association.

The findings are important for understanding the causes and improving the treatment of depression. Scientists already knew that many people with depression have high levels of cortisol, a human stress hormone, but it wasn't clear whether that was a cause or effect. Now it appears likely that long-term exposure to cortisol actually contributes to the symptoms of depression.

Paul Ardayfio, PhD candidate, and Kwang-Soo Kim, PhD, of the Molecular Neurobiology Laboratory at McLean Hospital, made their discovery by exposing mice to both short-term and long-term durations of stress hormone, which in rodents is corticosterone. In humans,

---

"Chronic Exposure to Stress Hormone Causes Anxious Behavior in Mice, Confirming the Mechanism by Which Long-Term Stress Can Lead to Mood Disorders," reprinted with permission from http://www.apa.org/releases/stressmood0406.html.

usually ongoing, chronic stress, such as caring for a spouse with dementia, rather than acute stress, has been associated with depression.

Using 58 mice, the researchers gave the hormone in drinking water so as not to confound the results with the stress of injection. Chronic doses were 17 to 18 days of exposure; acute doses were 24 hours of exposure.

Compared with mice given stress hormone for a day, mice given stress hormone for more than two weeks took significantly longer to emerge from a small dark compartment into a brightly lit open field, a common behavioral test of anxiety in animals. In other words, they seemed more fearful and were less willing to explore the new environment. Chronic but not acute treatment also dulled reactions to a startling stimulus, another sign their nervous systems were overwhelmed.

To the best of the authors' knowledge, this was the first experiment to compare the effects of chronic corticosterone with the effects of acute corticosterone on anxiety-like behavior.

Given four related lines of evidence, the findings were not a complete surprise. First, more than half the people with Cushing's disease, in which a disordered adrenal system releases too much cortisol, have depression and anxiety. Second, the "anxious-retarded" subtype of depression is commonly associated with disruption of that same hormonal system. Third, people getting corticosteroid therapy for inflammatory and other disorders have increased mood-related side effects, including anxiety and depression. Fourth, higher glucocorticoid levels for chronic periods have been linked to increased activity in anxiety-related brain regions such as the amygdala in both rodents and humans.

Now the pieces fit together around a central axiom: Stress hormone can cause anxiety, which appears with depression. Having found this causal link in a controlled laboratory setting, the authors say, "Our results suggest that chronically high levels of cortisol, which occurs in Cushing's disease and some subtypes of depression, can increase anxiety on the one hand and dull responses to external stimuli on the other." The difference between the responses to acute and chronic hormone exposure strengthen the view that very-short-term or acute exposure, they add, "may be adaptive, whereas chronic exposure has detrimental effects on brain and behavior."

Ardayfio and Kim say that outlining the relationship between physiological disruptions and subsequent behavior may help researchers to design new psychiatric drugs that treat the causes of disease rather than peripheral disease-related phenomena. The authors speculate that drugs that reverse or block the deleterious effects of chronically elevated stress hormones may help guard against some types of anxiety symptoms in depression, citing preclinical evidence in rats.

Article: "Anxiogenic-like Effect of Chronic Corticosterone in the Light-Dark Emergence Task in Mice," Paul Ardayfio, PhD candidate, and Kwang-Soo Kim, PhD, McLean Hospital and Harvard Medical School; *Behavioral Neuroscience*, Vol. 120, No. 2.

Chapter 6

What Genes Tell Us about the Risk of Mental Health Disorders

New tests that scan all of a person's genes—that person's "genome"—or large parts of his or her genome are now on the market. Anyone who can afford the new scans can buy one, without a prescription or a health professional's advice, by mailing a saliva sample to a company that sells the scans. Advertisements suggest that the company then can provide information about clients' risks of developing specific diseases, based on variations found in their genes.

It's too early for these new genome scans to give people a complete picture of their risk of mental illnesses or to diagnose them. Scientists don't yet know all of the gene variations that contribute to mental illnesses, and those that are known, so far, raise the risk by very small amounts.

Genetic research might make it possible—one day—to provide a more complete picture of a person's risk of getting a particular kind of mental illness or to diagnose it, based on his or her genes. That day isn't here yet, although studies are underway now.

In the meantime, it's important to know the difference between the new genome scans being advertised today and the kinds of traditional genetic tests doctors have been ordering for many years. Traditional genetic tests look for specific variations clearly shown by research to be the cause of certain rare diseases, such as cystic fibrosis, that generally are caused by variations in a single gene.

From "Looking at My Genes: What Can They Tell Me?" by the National Institute of Mental Health (NIMH, www.nimh.nih.gov), part of the National Institutes of Health, 2008.

Doctors order traditional genetic testing for people they think are at high risk of one of these rare diseases; for example, if the neurological disorder Huntington disease runs in a person's family. The results enable patients and their doctors to make health-care decisions together.

But people who buy the new genome scans may not have any reason, such as family history, to suspect they're at risk of one of these rare diseases. They may just want to randomly look at all of their genes with the hope of finding out if they're at risk of any diseases. As noted, when it comes to common diseases, like mental illness or adult-onset diabetes, not enough is known about which gene variations are involved to give a complete picture of a person's risk.

Also, the genetics of mental illnesses and other common diseases are much more complex than the genetics of many of the rare, single-gene diseases. Mental illnesses appear to involve variations in many genes combined with other factors, such as stress.

People who are thinking about buying one of the new genome scans, to look at all or most of their genes with the hope of finding out if they're at risk of a mental illness or another common disease, may want to get their health-care providers' advice before taking that step.

People who suspect they have a rare disease strongly tied to their genetic make-up—for example, if a rare disease runs in their family—may want to ask their health-care providers about genetic testing. Their providers can tell them whether or not the disease can be detected through genetic testing at this time and, if so, what kind of test and follow-up care are needed.

What are the new genome scans on the market?

In recent years, scientists identified almost all of the genes in humans and the most common variations in many of them. This has proven to be a valuable tool for research.

Some companies are using this new information to market genome scans directly to consumers, which anyone can buy without a doctor's advice. Clients send their saliva to the company, and the company examines the saliva for variations in the clients' genes.

The company tells the client what gene variations he or she has, and offers to analyze the results or to allow the client to analyze the results on an interactive website.

Can the new genome scans tell me what diseases I might get?

To date, no gene variants are known that can predict with certainty whether or not someone will get a number of common diseases, including mental illnesses. Scientists haven't yet discovered whether many of the gene variations that occur in humans are connected to specific diseases or how much they raise or lower the risk.

For example, a genome scan might show that a person has one or more gene variations related to a common disease, such as adult-onset diabetes. But it's likely that many other gene variations also contribute to this disease, and it's not yet known which ones. The variations associated with most common diseases, to date, raise the risk only very slightly and, by themselves, don't yet provide medically useful information.

An example using heart disease suggests how the results of the new genome scans might confuse consumers. Early research might have shown that certain gene variations are associated with a common kind of heart disease. People whose scans showed they didn't have these variations might think they weren't at risk.

They might think it would be safer for them than for other people to forego some of the healthiest, heart-protecting habits known to science: exercising, not smoking, and avoiding obesity. But it's likely that, as with mental illnesses, this kind of heart disease involves many variations in many genes, and scientists don't yet know what all of them are. Foregoing healthy lifestyle changes based on this incomplete genetic picture could contribute to illness that might have been prevented.

What is traditional genetic testing?

Like the new genome scans being marketed to consumers, traditional genetic testing looks for variations in a person's genes by examining body fluids or tissues. A major difference is that traditional genetic tests focus on specific variations in a single gene known with certainty to be the cause of a rare disease, and genetic testing usually is ordered by a doctor working closely with a patient.

Doctors are looking for evidence of a specific disease when they order traditional genetic testing; for example, if they know that a disease runs in a person's family.

Can traditional genetic testing tell me what diseases I might get?

Genetic tests for some rare diseases clearly tied to a specific, single gene, like cystic fibrosis, fragile X syndrome (a heritable cause of mental retardation), or sickle cell disease, give people definitive answers about their risk of getting these rare illnesses. Doctors have ordered genetic tests for these kinds of illnesses for many years.

The results have given people valuable health information that has helped them get the right treatments or, if no treatment is available, to plan their lives and care, in consultation with their health-care team.

Should I have traditional genetic testing?

Your health-care provider can help you decide whether to have traditional genetic testing; for example, if you know that a rare disease with a clearly identified genetic basis runs in your family, and you want to know if your parents passed on to you the gene variations that cause the disease—and whether you're at risk of passing the variations to your children.

Your provider can determine exactly which test is needed and can arrange genetic counseling—an important part of genetic testing.

Test results may put your mind at ease if they show you don't carry the genetic variation that causes the disease. If the results show that you do have the variation, that may help you make life plans, such as whether to have children or adopt. Your health-care team will play a key role, interpreting the test results for you and helping you decide how the results will affect important life decisions.

Some rare genetic diseases, or their symptoms, can be prevented or treated, and genetic testing can help you and your health-care provider take action. If there is no effective treatment, you and your provider can take measures to improve your health and your life.

What is genetic counseling?

Genetic counseling provides information and support to people who have, or may be at risk of, inherited disorders. A genetics professional (medical geneticist, genetics counselor, or genetics nurse) discusses your risk with you and may or may not suggest genetic testing.

Genetics professionals:

- assess your risk by looking at your family's health history and medical records;
- provide support and information to help you decide whether to be tested;
- explain what the results of genetic tests mean;
- provide counseling or refer you to support services;
- explain options for treatment or prevention; and/or
- explain how test results could affect decisions about having children.

If your test shows that you do have a genetic variation clearly associated with a specific disease, you may be referred to a doctor or researcher who specializes in that illness. Both your primary care provider and a genetics professional can help you with decisions about testing and can help you interpret your test results.

Some genetics professionals specialize in a disease category (such as cancer), age group (such as adolescents), or type of counseling (such as prenatal).

Are there risks associated with genetic testing?

Some people who know they're at risk of a serious disease, because the disease runs in the family, avoid having genetic testing. They're afraid their insurance companies or employers will drop them if tests show they have the gene variation that may lead to the disease. They fear they might have trouble getting insurance or a job.

As of March 2008, efforts are underway to enact federal legislation that would make it illegal to discriminate on the basis of genetic test results.

For the rare, single-gene diseases, genetic testing is important. It leads to early detection and therapy for these diseases.

What can research about gene variations tell us about disease risk?

As they continue to discover combinations of gene variations and external factors that contribute to specific diseases, scientists are building a more complete picture of how to detect which people are at risk of common diseases.

This research also is helping to reveal the biological pathways through which gene variations contribute to disease. Scientists can use this information to design better screening and prevention for specific diseases, and find more precise molecular targets at which to aim as they develop new medications.

Does family history give you good clues about your risk?

Your family history is one of your best clues about your risk of developing many common illnesses, including mental disorders.

For example, bipolar disorder and schizophrenia tend to run in families. At this time, no type of genetic testing can tell you whether or not you will develop mental illnesses. Not enough is known about which gene variations contribute to them, or the degree to which other factors contribute.

For now, your family history may be your best indicator. For example, studies show that if you have a close relative with bipolar disorder, you have about a 10 percent chance of getting a mood disorder, such as bipolar disorder or depression.

Now consider what the gene variations scientists have linked to mental disorders, so far, can tell you about your risk. Even the variations with the strongest ties raise the risk by only very small amounts. Knowing that you have one of these variations won't tell you nearly as much about your risk as your family history can.

Family history also provides a good clue about your risk of rare diseases that can be detected through genetic testing. If one of these rare diseases, such as cystic fibrosis, runs in your family, your risk is likely very high.

If a disease runs in your family, your health-care provider can tell you if it's the kind of illness that can be detected through genetic testing at this time.

Your provider can help you make decisions about whether to be tested and can help you understand test results and their implications.

What are genes?

Genes are pieces of DNA, in cells, that parents pass down to their children at conception. Genes turn on and off throughout life to transmit chemical instructions for making the body's proteins. Proteins are part of what gives us our characteristics; for example, our height, eye color, personality, and our chances of getting specific diseases.

Genes can have slight differences in their structure from person to person, and these variations can cause differences in people's characteristics. Gene variations help explain why members of the same family often look alike and have other characteristics in common, such as certain illnesses—because each child inherits a mixture of both parents' gene variations.

Some gene variations make people more vulnerable to different diseases, and some have protective effects against different diseases. Some rare diseases are caused by variations in a single gene. Most common diseases are caused by a mixture of many gene variations, some unknown, and external factors, such as stress or toxic substances.

Some gene variations appear to have no effect on risk of disease.

Chapter 7

Aging and Mental Health

Risk factors for late-life depression have been identified through a systematic review of the research literature and a longitudinal study. In a review of 20 studies, Cole and Dendukuri noted that bereavement, sleep disturbance, disability, prior depression, and female gender were all significant predictors of depression. Risk factors for depression have also been identified through a survey of older persons living in the community. In a second study of 1,947 older adults, Strawbridge and colleagues noted that older adults who were more likely to be depressed included those:

- with low and medium levels of physical activity;
- who possess a physical disability or mobility impairment;
- who have one or more chronic conditions;
- with fewer than three close friends or relatives; and
- those who were somewhat satisfied or not satisfied with friendships.

Several of these risk factors may be mitigated by preventive efforts, including programs for persons who are currently suffering from depression or have a history of recurrent depression. In addition,

---

Excerpted from "Depression and Anxiety Prevention for Older Adults," by the Older Americans Substance Abuse and Mental Health Technical Assistance Center (www.samhsa.gov), 2005.

undertreated conditions that commonly precipitate depression such as vascular disease, functional impairment, or nutritional deficiencies may be prevented through programs as well.

Did You Know?

- One in five older adults has a significant mental disorder. This includes more than 16% with a primary psychiatric illness and 3% with dementia complicated by psychiatric symptoms.
- Depression and anxiety disorders are among the most common mental health problems in older persons, affecting approximately 3–7% and 11% of the general older adult population, respectively. The prevalence of anxiety symptoms among older adults may be as high as 20%.
- Estimates suggest that sub-threshold or minor depression is present in 8–16% of older adults residing in the community, 15–20% of those receiving primary care services, 25–33% of older adults in an acute care hospital, and up to 50% of older adults in long-term care facilities.
- The prevalence of other mental health disorders among older adults such as schizophrenia and bipolar disorder is much lower (less than 1%), although these disorders impart significant functional impairments to older persons.

Preventing Depression in Older Adults

Exercise

Findings from at least two programs show that exercise can help prevent depression in older adults. Wallace and colleagues evaluated a multi-component intervention in which participants received a 30- to 60-minute visit at a senior center with a registered nurse to review risk factors for disability, develop a targeted health promotion plan, and introduce a supervised exercise program. This visit focused on current exercise habits, alcohol and tobacco use, dietary habits, and home safety issues. The nurse contacted subjects by telephone to review progress toward goals, motivate continued behavior change, and identify problems with compliance. The exercise program was conducted in groups of up to 10–15 older adults led by a trained exercise instructor. Positive outcomes included improved health functioning and a reduction in depressive symptoms.

A second study conducted by Penninx and colleagues evaluated the effectiveness of exercise in preventing depression in older adults with osteoarthritis. They compared a 3-month facility-based aerobic or resistance exercise program to a control group receiving education on arthritis management. The aerobic exercise program consisted of an indoor walking program that was conducted under the supervision of an exercise leader three times per week for 1 hour. The aerobic and resistance exercise programs were each followed by a 14-month home exercise program with support and supervision from an exercise leader. Evaluation of these programs found that aerobic exercise, but not resistance exercise, significantly reduced depressive symptoms. Not only do these findings support previous research showing that exercise is an effective treatment for late-life depression, but they illustrate the benefits of exercise in preventing depressive symptomatology in non-depressed older adults.

Educational Classes

Several educational programs were evaluated to determine their effectiveness in preventing depression, including two that were directly targeted at increasing knowledge regarding specific medical conditions. A 10-week arthritis education class was associated with significant reductions in depressive symptoms compared to a control group at 1 and 2-year followup evaluations. Similarly, a 6-week diabetes education class combined with a support group was associated with lower incidence of depression at 2-year followup compared to a control group. Finally, classroom and home-based multi-component mind-body wellness courses, including relaxation training, cognitive restructuring, problem solving, communication, behavioral treatment for insomnia, nutrition and exercise, and instruction on mind-body relationships, were associated with a reduction in depression and anxiety symptoms compared to a control group.

Life Review

Zauszniewski and colleagues examined the effectiveness of a focused reflection reminiscence program in reducing negative emotions in older adults living in retirement communities. The program, titled "Reflections for Seniors," included members of a retirement community who met for 2 hours per week over a 6-week period. A similar life review program evaluated by Haight and colleagues included nursing home residents who met for 1 hour per week over a 6-week period. Both studies found small effects on the reduction of depressive symptoms in older adults.

Evidence also suggests that screening alone may be associated with a lowering of depression levels. A study conducted in urban senior congregate housing settings also used gatekeepers to identify older adults at high risk of psychiatric problems. The Psychogeriatric Assessment and Treatment in City Housing (PATCH) model incorporates components of the Gatekeeper program and assertive community treatment. The PATCH psychiatric nurse met with the building administrator; an education program was provided to housing personnel to enhance recognition of high-risk residents; and to clarify procedures for making referrals of high-risk residents, and weekly nurse visits included in-home psychiatric evaluation and case management services for residents ages 60 and older. This study of the PATCH model found that outreach services were associated with a decrease in overall psychiatric symptom severity for individuals with a variety of psychiatric disorders.

Problem-Solving Therapy

Two studies have evaluated the effectiveness of problem-solving therapy (PST) for older adults with dysthymia or minor depression. The PEARLS program, evaluated by Ciechanowski and colleagues, was found to be associated with improved depressive symptoms and functional and emotional well-being. In addition, compared to a control group, those receiving PST were more likely to achieve remission of depressive symptoms (36% vs. 12%). In contrast, Williams and colleagues evaluated PST compared to an antidepressant medication (paroxetine) or a placebo.

They found that neither treatment was associated with a difference in rates of remission compared to placebo. However, for those patients with minor depression, both paroxetine and PST improved mental health functioning in patients with initial low functioning. Only paroxetine was associated with improvement for persons with dysthymia.

Interpersonal Therapy

One study found interpersonal therapy (IPT) to be effective at preventing an increase in depressive symptoms. Mossey and colleagues compared IPT to usual care. IPT was associated with improved self-rated health and after 6 months, three-fifths of the intervention group, compared to approximately one-third of the control group, had experienced a reduction in depressive symptoms.

Resistance Training

A study of older persons with pre-existing depressive symptoms (59% with minor depression or dysthymia) found that resistance training was more effective than health education alone in preventing the worsening of depression. Singh and colleagues noted that remission was achieved by six of seven (86%) participants in the resistance exercise group, compared to 4 of 10 (40%) participants in the health education control group.

Interventions for Care Providers

Two studies evaluate whether modifications to the provision of care can affect depressive symptoms. Cuijpers and colleagues evaluated a multifaceted education and support program administered in a residential care setting, compared to usual care. The intervention included training for caregivers and other employees of the residential home, informational meetings for residents and their relatives, support groups, and discussion and feedback sessions for care providers. The target population included older persons who were incapable of living independently due to physical, psychiatric, or psychosocial constraints, yet who did not require extensive nursing home care. Results indicate that providing education, support, and feedback to residential care providers can reduce depressive symptoms and maintain health-related quality of life for older persons. Waterreus and Blanchard evaluated the effectiveness of care delivered through a nurse case management system in which the care plan was developed through coordination of a multidisciplinary psychogeriatric team. Compared to a usual care control group, the intervention group exhibited greater reduction in depression severity, but the intervention was not associated with fewer cases of depression.

Interventions for Family Caregivers

Family caregivers, such as spouses or children caring for loved ones with dementia, are also at risk for developing depressive disorders. In the early 1990s, Mittelman and colleagues developed and tested an intervention consisting of scheduled individual and family counseling sessions, unlimited consultation on request, and continuous support group participation for family caregivers of persons with dementia. This intervention was found to delay nursing home placement by an average of 329 days, prompting researchers to develop, refine, and test similar interventions to support the capacity of natural caregivers to care for their loved one in the home environment. In addition to improving outcomes for the individual with Alzheimer's disease, this intervention also has been found to reduce stress and psychological symptoms for caregivers. The counseling and support provided to families is associated with greater satisfaction with assistance received from others, as well as decreased caregiver depression. In addition, PST has been successfully used to enhance the ability of caregivers to cope with stress and to decrease the incidence of depression and other adverse outcomes. For example, Teri and colleagues studied the effectiveness of PST as an intervention for reducing depression among individuals with dementia and their caregivers. Caregivers who participated in PST decreased their levels of depression and burden over a 6-month period.

Of note, a recent systematic review evaluated major outcomes in family caregiving interventions for dementia, as published in 43 studies since 1996. Findings indicate that the major impact on caregivers includes decreased incidence and severity of depression, moderate decreases in reported anger, moderate improvement in stress management, positive changes in clinical health indicators such as blood pressure and stress, and small improvements in caregiver burden.

Conclusions

This review highlights the scientific evidence for the prevention and early intervention of depression and anxiety in older adults. As shown, several programs have identified positive effects in preventing depression or reducing depression symptoms. The best evidence exists for the effectiveness of exercise and psychotherapeutic interventions, such as problem-solving therapy and interpersonal therapy. In addition, there is evidence to suggest that targeted outreach to older adults is effective in engaging isolated and vulnerable older persons in treatment for mental health and substance abuse problems. Other potentially effective strategies include life review, reminiscence therapy, educational classes, mind-body wellness, and provider education. Many of these approaches require further evaluation prior to establishing their effectiveness among older adults.

Our review also revealed that there is minimal evidence for programs that target the prevention of anxiety among older adults. As one in five older adults experiences symptoms of anxiety, programs are needed in this area.

It is important to acknowledge that several programs developed to prevent depression have not demonstrated effectiveness. For instance, among the brief interventions for older adults with minor depression reviewed by Cole and Dendukuri, several trials showed no effect in the prevention of depression. These studies were primarily focused on bereavement support groups or life review. The lack of effect on the prevention of depression was also noted in a social support network intervention for seniors. Finally, it is important to remember that late-life depression is often chronic or characterized by a relapse. Although this review focuses on the universal prevention of late-life depression and selective and indicated prevention of the exacerbation of minor depression into major depression, an important area of research addresses the prevention of further disability among older adults who have developed depression. Prevention strategies should focus attention on preventing relapse, recurrence, and residual symptoms among older adults with current or remittent major depression.

Chapter 8

Minorities and Mental Health

Almost 60 years ago, the World Health Organization (WHO) defined health as "a state of complete physical, mental and social well-being and not merely the absence of disease or infirmity." This definition opened the window to an increased recognition of the human as a holistic being of mind, body and spirit, and propelled the need to better understand the interrelationship between physical and mental health.

Mental health is how a person thinks, feels, and acts when faced with life's situations. It is how people look at themselves, their lives, and the other people in their lives, evaluate their challenges and problems, and explore choices. This includes handling stress, relating to other people, and making decisions.

The HHS Substance Abuse and Mental Health Administration's (SAMHSA) vision is "a life in the community for everyone." Their mission is to build resilience and facilitate recovery in the areas of substance abuse and mental illness.

Mental Health Problems

Mental health problems are real. They affect one's thoughts, body, feelings, and behavior. Mental health problems are not just a passing

---

From "Mental Health 101," by the Office of Minority Health (OMHRC, www.omhrc.gov), part of the U.S. Department of Health and Human Services, July 8, 2008.

phase. They can be severe, seriously interfere with a person's life, and even cause a person to become disabled.

Mental disorders constitute an immense burden on the U.S. population, with major depression now the leading cause of disability in the United States, and schizophrenia, bipolar disorder (manic depressive disorder), and obsessive-compulsive disorder ranked among the ten leading causes of disability. One person in four has been diagnosed with a mental disorder in the last 12 months and is consequently in need of services.

These disorders cause distress and result in a reduced ability to function psychologically, socially, occupationally, or interpersonally. People who have a mental illness might have trouble handling such things as daily activities, family responsibilities, relationships, or work and school responsibilities. You can have trouble with one area or all of them, to a greater or lesser degree. And you can have more than one type of mental illness at the same time.

What Are Risk and Protective Factors?

Risk factors increase the vulnerability of an individual, a group, or a community to substance abuse disorders or untreated mental health problems. Biology and heredity are among those risk factors for mental disorders; for example, children of parents with depression or schizophrenia are at greater risk for the disease, possibly due to a genetic predisposition. Similarly, the greater the number of drug abuse risk factors, the greater the risk for drug abuse. Additional risk factors might include a history of violence and or trauma, poverty, school problems, out of home placement, depression, and or suicide attempts. Although no one risk factor is disorder specific, multiple risk factors are often related to more negative outcomes such as mental disorders.

Protective factors build resiliency in the same individual, group, or community and increase the likelihood that substance abuse and its related effects can be resisted. These may include a positive self-esteem, an outgoing personality, supportive family relationships, and strong bonds to family, school, and community. Multiple protective factors improve one's chances for positive outcomes.

Resilience is a set of strengths internal to the individual and is highly influenced by protective factors. Resilient people are those who are better able to resist destructive behaviors, even in the presence of identified risk factors.

Minority populations are often over represented in our nation's most vulnerable populations, the poor, the uninsured, the homeless, and the incarcerated; they have little access and/or may under underutilize mental health services. For those who do receive mental health interventions, the appropriateness and quality of those treatments remain in question. These unmet needs and provision of poor quality mental health services to minority populations is impacting the well being of our nation.

Disparities in Mental Health

The United States population is composed of many diverse groups. Evidence indicates a persistent disparity in the health status of racial and ethnic minority populations, as compared with the overall health status of the U.S. population.

Over the next decade, the United States will continue to become more racially and ethnically diverse, increasing the demand for mental health services tailored to community needs. This will have significant consequences for the need and demand for providers of mental health services. Poverty, lack of adequate access to quality health services, few culturally and linguistically competent health providers and services, and lack of preventive health care are all factors that must be addressed.

A key finding of the *Surgeon General's Report on Mental Health: Culture, Race and Ethnicity* (2001) was that living in poverty has the most measurable effects on the rates of mental illness. Racial and ethnic minorities are overrepresented among the poor. People in the lowest socioeconomic positions are at least two to three times more likely than those in the highest positions to experience a mental disorder, and the overall rate of poverty among most racial and ethnic minority groups in the United States is much higher, than that of non-Hispanic Whites. Racism and discrimination are highly stressful and can adversely affect health and mental health.

With advances in research, the causes and treatments for mental illness are better known today than ever before. According to recent reports, the great majority of mental illnesses are treatable. Some have found that 80 percent of patients with depression can now recover (National Institute of Mental Health, 2004). With treatment and recovery more reachable, everyone regardless of age, sex, religion, race, ethnicity, primary language, or national origin should have the right and access to evidenced-based mental health services.

Addressing Stigma

Although mental illnesses are surprisingly common, affecting up to 28 percent of our nation, recovery is possible. Studies show that many people with mental illnesses recover completely (SAMHSA, 2003). With treatments and supports available now more than ever, people with mental illnesses can lead active, productive lives and contribute to their communities.

Yet stigma continues to be a major barrier to seeking out care. Many people are still confused between facts and myths. They don't understand what mental illnesses are and continue to believe that there is something shameful about them. In addition to shame, minorities often feel the legacy of racism and discrimination, leading to the distrust of health and mental health professionals. Feelings of stigma, discrimination, and mistrust of authorities preclude individuals in need from seeking out and receiving the help and treatments that can lead them to recovery.

Because the small numbers of minorities that do seek behavioral health care prefer seeking and receiving that care in primary care settings, it is in our best interest to nurture and further develop this entry point into treatment, and we must assure the presence of a sensitive workforce that is culturally and linguistically competent. As such, providers themselves will help to break down some of the barriers created by stigma, while providing needed care.

Mental Health Treatment

Treatment for mental health depends on the specific condition or combination of conditions, and should rely on evidence-based practices. These treatments have been studied and proven effective in reducing symptoms and promoting wellness.

Research has contributed to our ability to recognize, diagnose, and treat mental health conditions effectively in terms of symptom control and behavior management. Medication and other therapies can be independent, combined, or sequenced depending on the individual's diagnosis and personal preference. A new recovery perspective is supported by evidence on rehabilitation and treatment as well as by the personal experiences of consumers.

Substance abuse is a major co-occurring problem for adults with mental disorders. Evidence supports combined treatment, although there are substantial gaps between what research recommends and what typically is available in communities.

Although sensitivity to culture, race, gender, disability, poverty, and the need for consumer involvement are important considerations for care and treatment, barriers of access exist in the organization and financing of mental health services for adults.

Because of the lack of access to preventive care, early identification of mental illness and lack of quality interventions, the service needs of minorities may exceed those of Whites. Poverty and lack of (or insufficient) medical insurance hampers access to care, often leading to more chronic mental health conditions. High concentrations of poverty in inner cities and the combination of isolation and poverty in rural and frontier areas pose additional challenges for residents of these areas.

In a recent report titled: "Health Centers' Role in Answering the Behavioral Health Needs of the Medically Underserved" (2004), the Health Resources and Services Administration (HRSA) reported that community health centers (CHC) are the primary care providers to 15 million medically underserved individuals. They have become critical sources of behavioral health services to those most vulnerable, particularly minority populations, the poor, and the uninsured. According to the 2003 CHC Uniform Data System, health centers reported 2.1 million encounters for mental health conditions and 720,000 contacts for drug or alcohol dependence.

The Indian Health Service (IHS) is an integrated health care system that provides valuable mental health services to American Indians and Alaska Natives (AI/AN) through its Mental Health and Social Services program.

This program is community oriented, clinical, and preventive—providing care to more than 1.6 million consumers, both urban and reservation-based. Nevertheless, the accessibility of mental health and substance abuse treatments continue to be a problem. Proven and Carle (2000) found the greatest unmet needs for adult AI/ANs to include substance abuse and mental health outpatient counseling services.

Chapter 9

Mental Health Issues in Returning Veterans

Mental Health Concerns in Veterans and Their Families

When Sergeant (Sgt.) Dean Nist returned home to rural Somerset, PA, after Marine Reserve combat service in Iraq that included the battle of Fallujah, he found dealing with civilians difficult. "I ordered my wife and kids around like they were my Marines," he recalls.

Across the country, in Tucson, AZ, former Army Sgt. Abel Moreno returned home after combat service in both Iraq and Afghanistan. Initially, he found himself unable to land a job that paid enough to support his family.

The challenges facing Sgt. Nist and Mr. Moreno, along with troubling wartime memories and feelings of isolation from the civilians around them, added up to major stress. Before long, both veterans were using alcohol heavily to deal with the pressures of readjustment to civilian life.

With some 700,000 of their comrades now back in the United States, similar issues confront active duty military personnel, returning veterans, and their families and communities across the nation.

This chapter contains text from "Veterans & Their Families: A SAMHSA Priority," by Beryl Lieff Benderly, is from the Substance Abuse and Mental Health Services Administration (SAMHSA, www.samhsa.gov), part of the U.S. Department of Health and Human Services, January 2008 and "Male Veterans Have Double the Suicide Rate of Civilians," from the National Institute of Mental Health (NIMH, www.nimh.nih.gov), part of the National Institutes of Health, June 12, 2007.

Combined data from the Substance Abuse and Mental Health Services Administration (SAMHSA)'s 2004 to 2006 National Survey on Drug Use and Health (NSDUH) have documented that more than 20 percent of veterans age 18 to 25 suffered serious psychological distress in the preceding year, with females more vulnerable than males.

According to a NSDUH report, one quarter of veterans age 25 and under had suffered from substance use disorders in the preceding year, with those from low-income families especially vulnerable. The two disorders co-occurred in more than 8 percent of the veterans age 25 and under, and those in families earning less than $20,000 per year again faced the highest risk.

Consequences of Trauma

"Anyone who has been in combat experiences trauma," says A. Kathryn Power, M.Ed., Director of SAMHSA's Center for Mental Health Services (CMHS). Because the current conflicts lack clear front lines and rear guards, they are especially problematic, she adds.

In addition to the horrors of war, longer and multiple deployments, uncertainty of the length of deployments, and the relentless tension of counterinsurgency warfare compound the stress.

"Many people can deal with trauma in a very normalizing way. They can respond and act with resilience," Ms. Power says.

However, posttraumatic stress disorder (PTSD) affects a substantial number of individuals and can seriously interfere with a person's ability to function on a day-to-day basis.

Sgt. Nist remembers a friend employed in a metal shop. "Every time they drop a sheet of metal, he just about goes through the roof," Sgt. Nist says. "He's severely into alcohol and misses 2 or 3 days of work a week."

Military Culture

With the help of family members and friends, Sgt. Nist and Mr. Moreno got their lives back in order. Now, they are committed to helping other returning veterans do the same.

Sgt. Nist, now a member of the Pennsylvania National Guard, serves as president of the Somerset County Military Family Support Group, a voluntary organization. He also was instrumental in organizing a local veterans' center.

Mr. Moreno is a staff member at Vets4Vets, a nonprofit organization providing peer-to-peer services to Iraq and Afghanistan veterans.

Each wave of veterans, whether from World War II or Iraq, forms a special "brotherhood" with its own language, set of experiences, and feeling of community, Mr. Moreno says.

Many issues are similar across the generations, but effective services for veterans require understanding the particulars of their generation's experience.

"Veterans need a place to talk about feelings, to decompress, and also to know that others out there are feeling the same things," Mr. Moreno says. "That keeps people from becoming isolated, self-medicating, and worse."

For care providers who lack a military background, familiarity with the former service members' culture, jargon, and concerns is an important element in building trust, adds Sgt. Nist.

"We're very fortunate in our town that our mental health people here asked us, 'Will you teach us how to understand you?' " Sgt. Nist says. "They told me, 'We are not veterans. We are not going to pretend to know what you're going through. We want to learn from you so we can help others.' The first thing they need to do is let the veterans know they're willing to help them. Then, they need to learn the language [and] how to deal with them."

Arne Owens, M.S.S.M., Senior Advisor to the SAMHSA Administrator, agrees that providers "need to have some understanding of what the military is about and how it is organized, to be able to tell the difference between a sergeant and a sergeant major. Most people who haven't been in the military don't understand those things.

Challenges

Community providers and their local communities face significant challenges. "Today, only about 30 to 40 percent of veterans who are eligible for care actually seek care from Veterans Administration (VA)," Ms. Power says.

Mr. Moreno, for example, resisted getting help because, as a paratrooper trained to be tough and strong, he "didn't want to look weak," he says. Sgt. Nist notes that a roundtrip from Somerset for an appointment at the nearest VA facility "takes the whole day."

In addition, troubling issues related to trauma can arise years, even a decade or more, after the event. Service-related health care benefits for National Guard and Reserve members, however, currently last only 2 years.

Family members affected either by deployments or by issues related to returning veterans also may require mental health or substance abuse care in their communities.

Male Veterans Have Double the Suicide Rate of Civilians

Male veterans in the general U.S. population are twice as likely as their civilian peers to die by suicide, a large study shows. Results of the research by Mark S. Kaplan, DrPH, and colleagues from Portland State University and Oregon Health & Science University were published online June 11 in the *Journal of Epidemiology and Community Health* and will appear in the July issue.

To date, most studies on suicide among veterans have relied on data from those getting health care from the Department of Veterans Affairs (VA) system. However, 75 percent of veterans do not get their health care through the VA. This study included 320,890 men age 18 and older in the general population, 104,026 of them veterans, whom researchers followed for 12 years.

Veterans who were white, had at least 12 years of education, or whose daily-life activities were limited by health problems were at highest risk. Those who were overweight had a lower risk. By the end of the study, 197 of the veterans had died by suicide. During the same period, the risk of death from other causes was the same in the veterans as in civilian men.

Compared to civilian men who died by suicide, veterans were 58 percent more likely to use a firearm to end their lives.

"Veterans in the general U.S. population, whether or not they are affiliated with the VA, are at an elevated risk of suicide," the researchers reported.

The researchers also note that the number of veterans with daily-life activity limitations—one of the higher risk factors for suicide listed above—is likely to rise. They suggest that clinical and community interventions will be needed, and call for clinicians to be alert for signs that veterans might be contemplating suicide and to assess their access to firearms.

Kaplan MS, Huguet N, McFarland H, Newsom JT. Suicide Among Male Veterans: A Prospective Population-Based Study. *Journal of Epidemiology and Community Health,* online ahead of print, June 11, 2007.

Chapter 10

Violence and Mental Health

The discrimination and stigma associated with mental illnesses largely stem from the link between mental illness and violence in the minds of the general public, according to *Mental Health: A Report of the Surgeon General* (1999). "For instance, 61 percent of Americans think that people with schizophrenia are likely to be dangerous to others," notes the report of the *President's New Freedom Commission on Mental Health, Achieving the Promise: Transforming Mental Health Care in America* (2003).

This link is promoted by the news and entertainment media. For example, the National Mental Health Association reported that, according to a survey for the Screen Actors' Guild, characters in prime time television portrayed as having a mental illness are depicted as the most dangerous of all demographic groups: 60 percent were shown to be involved in crime or violence (three times the average rate). In addition, studies showed that as many as 75 percent of stories dealing with mental illness focus on violence. Although more recent research suggests the prevalence of these kinds of stories is diminishing, at least a third of stories continue to focus on dangerousness. Also, the vast majority of remaining stories on mental illness either focus on other negative characteristics related to people with the disorder (e.g., unpredictability and unsociability) or on medical treatments. Notably absent are positive stories that highlight recovery of many persons with even the most serious of mental illnesses.

Excerpted from "Understanding Mental Illness: Factsheet," from the Substance Abuse and Mental Health Services Administration (SAMHSA, www.samhsa.gov), part of the U.S. Department of Health and Human Services, April 20, 2007.

The average citizen finds these images persuasive. According to Americans' Views of Mental Health and Illness at Century's End: Continuity and Change, between 1950 and 1996, "the proportion of Americans who describe mental illness in terms consistent with violent or dangerous behavior nearly doubled."

As a result, Americans are hesitant to interact with people who have mental illnesses: 38 percent are unwilling to be friends with someone having mental health difficulties, 64 percent do not want someone who has schizophrenia as a close coworker, and more than 68 percent are unwilling to have someone with depression marry into their family.

But, in truth, people have little reason for such fears. A consensus statement signed by more than three dozen lawyers, advocates, consumers/survivors, and mental health professionals reads in part: "The results of several recent large-scale research projects conclude that only a weak association between mental disorders and violence exists in the community. Serious violence by people with major mental disorders appears concentrated in a small fraction of the total number, and especially in those who use alcohol and other drugs."

In addition:

- Research has shown that the vast majority of people who are violent do not suffer from mental illnesses.
- Clearly, mental health status makes at best a trivial contribution to the overall level of violence in society.
- The absolute risk of violence among the mentally ill as a group is still very small and—only a small proportion of the violence in our society can be attributed to persons who are mentally ill.
- Most people who suffer from a mental disorder are not violent—there is no need to fear them. Embrace them for who they are—normal human beings experiencing a difficult time, who need your open mind, caring attitude, and helpful support.
- Compared with the risk associated with the combination of male gender, young age, and lower socioeconomic status, the risk of violence presented by mental disorder is modest.
- People with psychiatric disabilities are far more likely to be victims than perpetrators of violent crime. A new study by researchers at North Carolina State University and Duke University has found that people with severe mental illness—schizophrenia, bipolar disorder, or psychosis—are 2½ times more likely to be attacked, raped, or mugged than the general population.

Chapter 11

Mental Health and the Risk of Suicide

Suicide is a major, preventable public health problem. In 2004, it was the eleventh leading cause of death in the United States, accounting for 32,439 deaths.[1] The overall rate was 10.9 suicide deaths per 100,000 people.[1] An estimated eight to 25 attempted suicides occur per every suicide death.[2]

Suicidal behavior is complex. Some risk factors vary with age, gender, or ethnic group and may occur in combination or change over time.

If you are in a crisis and need help right away, call this toll-free number, available 24 hours a day, every day: 800-273-TALK (8255). You will reach the National Suicide Prevention Lifeline, a service available to anyone. You may call for yourself or for someone you care about. All calls are confidential.

What are the risk factors for suicide?

Research shows that risk factors for suicide include:

- depression and other mental disorders, or a substance-abuse disorder (often in combination with other mental disorders). More than 90 percent of people who die by suicide have these risk factors.[2]
- stressful life events, in combination with other risk factors, such as depression. However, suicide and suicidal behavior are not

From "Suicide in the U.S.: Statistics and Prevention," by the National Institute of Mental Health (NIMH, www.nimh.nih.gov), part of the National Institutes of Health, June 26, 2008.

normal responses to stress; many people have these risk factors, but are not suicidal.

- prior suicide attempt
- family history of mental disorder or substance abuse
- family history of suicide
- family violence, including physical or sexual abuse
- firearms in the home,[3] the method used in more than half of suicides incarceration exposure to the suicidal behavior of others, such as family members, peers, or media figures.[2]

Research also shows that the risk for suicide is associated with changes in brain chemicals called neurotransmitters, including serotonin. Decreased levels of serotonin have been found in people with depression, impulsive disorders, and a history of suicide attempts, and in the brains of suicide victims.[4]

Are women or men at higher risk?

- Suicide was the eighth leading cause of death for males and the sixteenth leading cause of death for females in 2004.[1]
- Almost four times as many males as females die by suicide.[1]
- Firearms, suffocation, and poison are by far the most common methods of suicide, overall. However, men and women differ in the method used, as shown in Table 11.1.[1]

Table 11.1. Methods of Suicide

Suicide by:	Males (%)	Females (%)
Firearms	57	32
Suffocation	23	20
Poisoning	13	38

Is suicide common among children and young people?

In 2004, suicide was the third leading cause of death in each of the following age groups.[1] Of every 100,000 young people in each age group, the following number died by suicide:[1]

- Children ages 10 to 14—1.3 per 100,000
- Adolescents ages 15 to 19—8.2 per 100,000
- Young adults ages 20 to 24—12.5 per 100,000

As in the general population, young people were much more likely to use firearms, suffocation, and poisoning than other methods of suicide, overall. However, while adolescents and young adults were more likely to use firearms than suffocation, children were dramatically more likely to use suffocation.[1]

There were also gender differences in suicide among young people, as follows:

- Almost four times as many males as females ages 15 to 19 died by suicide.[1]
- More than six times as many males as females ages 20 to 24 died by suicide.[1]

Are older adults at risk?

Older Americans are disproportionately likely to die by suicide.

- Of every 100,000 people ages 65 and older, 14.3 died by suicide in 2004. This figure is higher than the national average of 10.9 suicides per 100,000 people in the general population.[1]
- Non-Hispanic white men age 85 or older had an even higher rate, with 17.8 suicide deaths per 100,000.[1]

Are some ethnic groups or races at higher risk?

Of every 100,000 people in each of the following ethnic/racial groups below, the following number died by suicide in 2004.[1]

- Highest rates:
    - Non-Hispanic Whites—12.9 per 100,000
    - American Indian and Alaska Natives—12.4 per 100,000
- Lowest rates:
    - Non-Hispanic Blacks—5.3 per 100,000
    - Asian and Pacific Islanders—5.8 per 100,000
    - Hispanics—5.9 per 100,000

What are some risk factors for nonfatal suicide attempts?

- As noted, an estimated eight to 25 nonfatal suicide attempts occur per every suicide death. Men and the elderly are more likely to have fatal attempts than are women and youth.[2]
- Risk factors for nonfatal suicide attempts by adults include depression and other mental disorders, alcohol abuse, cocaine use, and separation or divorce.[5,6]
- Risk factors for attempted suicide by youth include depression, alcohol or other drug-use disorder, physical or sexual abuse, and disruptive behavior.[6,7]
- Most suicide attempts are expressions of extreme distress, not harmless bids for attention. A person who appears suicidal should not be left alone and needs immediate mental-health treatment.

What can be done to prevent suicide?

Research helps determine which factors can be modified to help prevent suicide and which interventions are appropriate for specific groups of people. Before being put into practice, prevention programs should be tested through research to determine their safety and effectiveness.[8] For example, because research has shown that mental and substance-abuse disorders are major risk factors for suicide, many programs also focus on treating these disorders.

Studies showed that a type of psychotherapy called cognitive therapy reduced the rate of repeated suicide attempts by 50 percent during a year of follow-up. A previous suicide attempt is among the strongest predictors of subsequent suicide, and cognitive therapy helps suicide attempters consider alternative actions when thoughts of self-harm arise.[9]

Specific kinds of psychotherapy may be helpful for specific groups of people. For example, a recent study showed that a treatment called dialectical behavior therapy reduced suicide attempts by half, compared with other kinds of therapy, in people with borderline personality disorder (a serious disorder of emotion regulation).[10]

The medication clozapine is approved by the Food and Drug Administration for suicide prevention in people with schizophrenia.[11] Other promising medications and psychosocial treatments for suicidal people are being tested.

Since research shows that older adults and women who die by suicide are likely to have seen a primary care provider in the year before death, improving primary-care providers' ability to recognize and treat risk factors may help prevent suicide among these groups.[12] Improving outreach to men at risk is a major challenge in need of investigation.

What should I do if I think someone is suicidal?

If you think someone is suicidal, do not leave him or her alone. Try to get the person to seek immediate help from his or her doctor or the nearest hospital emergency room, or call 911. Eliminate access to firearms or other potential tools for suicide, including unsupervised access to medications.

References

1. Centers for Disease Control and Prevention, National Center for Injury Prevention and Control. Web-based Injury Statistics Query and Reporting System (WISQARS): www.cdc.gov/ncipc/wisqars
2. Moscicki EK. Epidemiology of completed and attempted suicide: toward a framework for prevention. *Clinical Neuroscience Research*, 2001; 1: 310-23.
3. Miller M, Azrael D, Hepburn L, Hemenway D, Lippmann SJ. The association between changes in household firearm ownership and rates of suicide in the United States, 1981-2002. *Injury Prevention* 2006;12:178-182; doi:10.1136/ip.2005.010850
4. Arango V, Huang YY, Underwood MD, Mann JJ. Genetics of the serotonergic system in suicidal behavior. *Journal of Psychiatric Research.* Vol. 37: 375-386. 2003.
5. Kessler RC, Borges G, Walters EE. Prevalence of and risk factors for lifetime suicide attempts in the National Comorbidity Survey. *Archives of General Psychiatry*, 1999; 56(7): 617-26.
6. Petronis KR, Samuels JF, Moscicki EK, Anthony JC. An epidemiologic investigation of potential risk factors for suicide attempts. *Social Psychiatry and Psychiatric Epidemiology*, 1990; 25(4): 193-9.
7. U.S. Public Health Service. National strategy for suicide prevention: goals and objectives for action. Rockville, MD: USDHHS, 2001.

8. Gould MS, Greenberg T, Velting DM, Shaffer D. Youth suicide risk and preventive interventions: a review of the past 10 years. *Journal of the American Academy of Child and Adolescent Psychiatry*, 2003; 42(4): 386-405.

9. Brown GK, Ten Have T, Henriques GR, Xie SX, Hollander JE, Beck AT. Cognitive therapy for the prevention of suicide attempts: a randomized controlled trial. *Journal of the American Medical Association*. 2005 Aug 3;294(5):563-70.

10. Linehan MM, Comtois KA, Murray AM, Brown MZ, Gallop RJ, Heard HL, Korslund KE, Tutek DA, Reynolds SK, Lindenboim N. Two-Year Randomized Controlled Trial and Follow-up of Dialectical Behavior Therapy vs Therapy by Experts for Suicidal Behaviors and Borderline Personality Disorder. *Archives of General Psychiatry*, 2006 Jul;63(7):757-766.

11. Meltzer HY, Alphs L, Green AI, Altamura AC, Anand R, Bertoldi A, Bourgeois M, Chouinard G, Islam MZ, Kane J, Krishnan R, Lindenmayer JP, Potkin S; International Suicide Prevention Trial Study Group. Clozapine treatment for suicidality in schizophrenia: International Suicide Prevention Trial (InterSePT). *Archives of General Psychiatry*, 2003; 60(1): 82-91.

12. Luoma JB, Pearson JL, Martin CE. Contact with mental health and primary care prior to suicide: a review of the evidence. *American Journal of Psychiatry*, 2002; 159: 909-16.

Chapter 12

Recognizing the Warning Signs of Mental Health Disorders

Most people believe that mental disorders are rare and "happen to someone else." In fact, mental disorders are common and widespread. An estimated 54 million Americans suffer from some form of mental disorder in a given year.

Most families are not prepared to cope with learning their loved one has a mental illness. It can be physically and emotionally trying, and can make us feel vulnerable to the opinions and judgments of others.

If you think you or someone you know may have a mental or emotional problem, it is important to remember there is hope and help.

What Is Mental Illness?

A mental illness is a disease that causes mild to severe disturbances in thought and/or behavior, resulting in an inability to cope with life's ordinary demands and routines.

There are more than 200 classified forms of mental illness. Some of the more common disorders are depression, bipolar disorder, dementia, schizophrenia, and anxiety disorders. Symptoms may include changes in mood, personality, personal habits, and/or social withdrawal.

Mental health problems may be related to excessive stress due to a particular situation or series of events. As with cancer, diabetes, and heart disease, mental illnesses are often physical as well as emotional and psychological. Mental illnesses may be caused by a reaction to environmental stresses, genetic factors, biochemical imbalances, or a combination of these. With proper care and treatment many individuals learn to cope or recover from a mental illness or emotional disorder.

How to Cope Day-to-Day

Accept Your Feelings

Despite the different symptoms and types of mental illnesses, many families who have a loved one with mental illness, share similar experiences. You may find yourself denying the warning signs, worrying what other people will think because of the stigma, or wondering what caused your loved one to become ill.

Accept that these feelings are normal and common among families going through similar situations. Find out all you can about your loved one's illness by reading and talking with mental health professionals. Share what you have learned with others.

Handling Unusual Behavior

The outward signs of a mental illness are often behavioral. Individuals may be extremely quiet or withdrawn. Conversely, he or she may burst into tears or have outbursts of anger. Even after treatment has started, individuals with a mental illness can exhibit antisocial behaviors. When in public, these behaviors can be disruptive and difficult to accept. The next time you and your family member visit your doctor or mental health professional, discuss these behaviors and develop a strategy for coping.

Establishing a Support Network

Whenever possible, seek support from friends and family members. If you feel you cannot discuss your situation with friends or other family members, find a self-help or support group. These groups provide an opportunity for you to talk to other people who are experiencing the same type of problems. They can listen and offer valuable advice.

Seeking Counseling

Therapy can be beneficial for both the individual with mental illness and other family members. A mental health professional can suggest ways to cope and better understand your loved one's illness.

When looking for a therapist, be patient and talk to a few professionals so you can choose the person that is right for you and your family. It may take time until you are comfortable, but in the long run you will be glad you sought help.

Taking Time Out

It is common for the person with the mental illness to become the focus of family life. When this happens, other members of the family may feel ignored or resentful. Some may find it difficult to pursue their own interests.

If you are the caregiver, you need some time for yourself. Schedule time away to prevent becoming frustrated or angry. If you schedule time for yourself it will help you to keep things in perspective and you may have more patience and compassion for coping or helping your loved one. Only when you are physically and emotionally healthy can you help others.

"Many families who have a loved one with mental illness share similar experiences": It is important to remember that there is hope for recovery and that with treatment many people with mental illness return to a productive and fulfilling life.

Warning Signs and Symptoms

To learn more about symptoms that are specific to a particular mental illness, refer to Mental Health America (www.nmha.org). The following are signs that your loved one may want to speak to a medical or mental health professional.

In adults:

- Confused thinking
- Prolonged depression (sadness or irritability)
- Feelings of extreme highs and lows
- Excessive fears, worries, and anxieties
- Social withdrawal
- Dramatic changes in eating or sleeping habits

- Strong feelings of anger
- Delusions or hallucinations
- Growing inability to cope with daily problems and activities
- Suicidal thoughts
- Denial of obvious problems
- Numerous unexplained physical ailments
- Substance abuse

In older children and pre-adolescents:

- Substance abuse
- Inability to cope with problems and daily activities
- Changes in sleeping and/or eating habits
- Excessive complaints of physical ailments
- Defiance of authority, truancy, theft, and/or vandalism
- Intense fear of weight gain
- Prolonged negative mood, often accompanied by poor appetite or thoughts of death
- Frequent outbursts of anger

In younger children:

- Changes in school performance
- Poor grades despite strong efforts
- Excessive worry or anxiety (i.e., refusing to go to bed or school)
- Hyperactivity
- Persistent nightmares
- Persistent disobedience or aggression
- Frequent temper tantrums

Part Two

Depression, Bipolar Disorder, and Other Mood Disorders

Chapter 13

Types of Depression and Their Treatment

What Is Depression?

Everyone occasionally feels blue or sad, but these feelings are usually fleeting and pass within a couple of days. When a person has a depressive disorder, it interferes with daily life, normal functioning, and causes pain for both the person with the disorder and those who care about him or her. Depression is a common but serious illness, and most who experience it need treatment to get better.

Many people with a depressive illness never seek treatment. But the vast majority, even those with the most severe depression, can get better with treatment. Intensive research into the illness has resulted in the development of medications, psychotherapies, and other methods to treat people with this disabling disorder.

What Are the Different Forms of Depression?

There are several forms of depressive disorders. The most common are major depressive disorder and dysthymic disorder.

Major depressive disorder, also called major depression, is characterized by a combination of symptoms that interfere with a person's ability to work, sleep, study, eat, and enjoy once-pleasurable activities. Major depression is disabling and prevents a person from functioning

---

Excerpted from "Depression," a booklet by the National Institute of Mental Health (NIMH, www.nimh.nih.gov), part of the National Institutes of Health, 2007.

normally. An episode of major depression may occur only once in a person's lifetime, but more often, it recurs throughout a person's life.

Dysthymic disorder, also called dysthymia, is characterized by long-term (2 years or longer) but less severe symptoms that may not disable a person but can prevent one from functioning normally or feeling well. People with dysthymia may also experience one or more episodes of major depression during their lifetimes.

Some forms of depressive disorder exhibit slightly different characteristics than those described above, or they may develop under unique circumstances. However, not all scientists agree on how to characterize and define these forms of depression. They include:

- **Psychotic depression**, which occurs when a severe depressive illness is accompanied by some form of psychosis, such as a break with reality, hallucinations, and delusions.
- **Postpartum depression**, which is diagnosed if a new mother develops a major depressive episode within one month after delivery. It is estimated that 10 to 15 percent of women experience postpartum depression after giving birth.
- **Seasonal affective disorder (SAD)**, which is characterized by the onset of a depressive illness during the winter months, when there is less natural sunlight. The depression generally lifts during spring and summer. SAD may be effectively treated with light therapy, but nearly half of those with SAD do not respond to light therapy alone. Antidepressant medication and psychotherapy can reduce SAD symptoms, either alone or in combination with light therapy.

What Are the Symptoms of Depression?

People with depressive illnesses do not all experience the same symptoms. The severity, frequency, and duration of symptoms will vary depending on the individual and his or her particular illness.

- Persistent sad, anxious, or "empty" feelings
- Feelings of hopelessness and/or pessimism
- Feelings of guilt, worthlessness, and/or helplessness
- Irritability, restlessness
- Loss of interest in activities or hobbies once pleasurable, including sex

- Fatigue and decreased energy
- Difficulty concentrating, remembering details and making decisions
- Insomnia, early-morning wakefulness, or excessive sleeping
- Overeating, or appetite loss
- Thoughts of suicide, suicide attempts
- Persistent aches or pains, headaches, cramps, or digestive problems that do not ease even with treatment

What Illnesses Often Coexist with Depression?

Depression often coexists with other illnesses. Such illnesses may precede the depression, cause it, and/or be a consequence of it. It is likely that the mechanics behind the intersection of depression and other illnesses differ for every person and situation. Regardless, these other co-occurring illnesses need to be diagnosed and treated.

Anxiety disorders, such as posttraumatic stress disorder (PTSD), obsessive-compulsive disorder, panic disorder, social phobia, and generalized anxiety disorder, often accompany depression. People experiencing PTSD are especially prone to having co-occurring depression. PTSD is a debilitating condition that can result after a person experiences a terrifying event or ordeal, such as a violent assault, a natural disaster, an accident, terrorism, or military combat.

People with PTSD often relive the traumatic event in flashbacks, memories, or nightmares. Other symptoms include irritability, anger outbursts, intense guilt, and avoidance of thinking or talking about the traumatic ordeal. In a National Institute of Mental Health (NIMH)-funded study, researchers found that more than 40 percent of people with PTSD also had depression at 1-month and 4-month intervals after the traumatic event.

Alcohol and other substance abuse or dependence may also co-occur with depression. In fact, research has indicated that the coexistence of mood disorders and substance abuse is pervasive among the U.S. population.

Depression also often coexists with other serious medical illnesses such as heart disease, stroke, cancer, HIV/AIDS [human immunodeficiency virus/acquired immunodeficiency syndrome], diabetes, and Parkinson disease. Studies have shown that people who have depression in addition to another serious medical illness tend to have more severe symptoms of both depression and the medical illness, more difficulty adapting to their medical condition, and more medical costs than those who do not have coexisting depression. Research has yielded increasing evidence that treating the depression can also help improve the outcome of treating the co-occurring illness.

What Causes Depression?

There is no single known cause of depression. Rather, it likely results from a combination of genetic, biochemical, environmental, and psychological factors.

Research indicates that depressive illnesses are disorders of the brain. Brain-imaging technologies, such as magnetic resonance imaging (MRI), have shown that the brains of people who have depression look different than those of people without depression. The parts of the brain responsible for regulating mood, thinking, sleep, appetite, and behavior appear to function abnormally. In addition, important neurotransmitters—chemicals that brain cells use to communicate—appear to be out of balance. But these images do not reveal why the depression has occurred.

Some types of depression tend to run in families, suggesting a genetic link. However, depression can occur in people without family histories of depression as well. Genetics research indicates that risk for depression results from the influence of multiple genes acting together with environmental or other factors.

In addition, trauma, loss of a loved one, a difficult relationship, or any stressful situation may trigger a depressive episode. Subsequent depressive episodes may occur with or without an obvious trigger.

How Do Women Experience Depression?

Depression is more common among women than among men. Biological, life cycle, hormonal and psychosocial factors unique to women may be linked to women's higher depression rate. Researchers have shown that hormones directly affect brain chemistry that controls emotions and mood. For example, women are particularly vulnerable to depression after giving birth, when hormonal and physical changes, along with the new responsibility of caring for a newborn, can be overwhelming. Many new mothers experience a brief episode of the "baby blues," but some will develop postpartum depression, a much more serious condition that requires active treatment and emotional support for the new mother. Some studies suggest that women who experience postpartum depression often have had prior depressive episodes.

Some women may also be susceptible to a severe form of premenstrual syndrome (PMS), sometimes called premenstrual dysphoric disorder (PMDD), a condition resulting from the hormonal changes that typically occur around ovulation and before menstruation begins. During the transition into menopause, some women experience an increased risk for depression. Scientists are exploring how the cyclical rise and fall of estrogen and other hormones may affect the brain chemistry that is associated with depressive illness.

Finally, many women face the additional stresses of work and home responsibilities, caring for children and aging parents, abuse, poverty, and relationship strains. It remains unclear why some women faced with enormous challenges develop depression, while others with similar challenges do not.

How Do Men Experience Depression?

Men often experience depression differently than women and may have different ways of coping with the symptoms. Men are more likely to acknowledge having fatigue, irritability, loss of interest in once-pleasurable activities, and sleep disturbances, whereas women are more likely to admit to feelings of sadness, worthlessness, and/or excessive guilt.

Men are more likely than women to turn to alcohol or drugs when they are depressed, or become frustrated, discouraged, irritable, angry, and sometimes abusive. Some men throw themselves into their work to avoid talking about their depression with family or friends, or engage in reckless, risky behavior. And even though more women attempt suicide, many more men die by suicide in the United States.

How Do Older Adults Experience Depression?

Depression is not a normal part of aging, and studies show that most seniors feel satisfied with their lives, despite increased physical ailments. However, when older adults do have depression, it may be overlooked because seniors may show different, less obvious symptoms, and may be less inclined to experience or acknowledge feelings of sadness or grief.

In addition, older adults may have more medical conditions such as heart disease, stroke, or cancer, which may cause depressive symptoms, or they may be taking medications with side effects that contribute to depression. Some older adults may experience what some doctors call vascular depression, also called arteriosclerotic depression or subcortical ischemic depression. Vascular depression may result when blood vessels become less flexible and harden over time, becoming constricted. Such hardening of vessels prevents normal blood flow to the body's organs, including the brain. Those with vascular depression may have, or be at risk for, a coexisting cardiovascular illness or stroke.

Although many people assume that the highest rates of suicide are among the young, older white males age 85 and older actually have the highest suicide rate. Many have a depressive illness that their doctors may not detect, despite the fact that these suicide victims often visit their doctors within 1 month of their deaths.

The majority of older adults with depression improve when they receive treatment with an antidepressant, psychotherapy, or a combination of both. Research has shown that medication alone and combination treatment are both effective in reducing the rate of depressive recurrences in older adults. Psychotherapy alone also can be effective in prolonging periods free of depression, especially for older adults with minor depression, and it is particularly useful for those who are unable or unwilling to take antidepressant medication.

How Do Children and Adolescents Experience Depression?

Scientists and doctors have begun to take seriously the risk of depression in children. Research has shown that childhood depression often persists, recurs, and continues into adulthood, especially if it goes untreated. The presence of childhood depression also tends to be a predictor of more severe illnesses in adulthood.

A child with depression may pretend to be sick, refuse to go to school, cling to a parent, or worry that a parent may die. Older children may sulk, get into trouble at school, be negative and irritable, and feel misunderstood. Because these signs may be viewed as normal mood swings typical of children as they move through developmental stages, it may be difficult to accurately diagnose a young person with depression.

Before puberty, boys and girls are equally likely to develop depressive disorders. By age 15, however, girls are twice as likely as boys to have experienced a major depressive episode.

Depression in adolescence comes at a time of great personal change—when boys and girls are forming an identity distinct from their parents, grappling with gender issues and emerging sexuality, and making decisions for the first time in their lives. Depression in adolescence frequently co-occurs with other disorders such as anxiety, disruptive behavior, eating disorders, or substance abuse. It can also lead to increased risk for suicide.

An NIMH-funded clinical trial of 439 adolescents with major depression found that a combination of medication and psychotherapy was the most effective treatment option. Other NIMH-funded researchers are developing and testing ways to prevent suicide in children and adolescents, including early diagnosis and treatment, and a better understanding of suicidal thinking.

How Is Depression Detected and Treated?

Depression, even the most severe cases, is a highly treatable disorder. As with many illnesses, the earlier that treatment can begin, the more effective it is and the greater the likelihood that recurrence can be prevented.

The first step to getting appropriate treatment is to visit a doctor. Certain medications, and some medical conditions such as viruses or a thyroid disorder, can cause the same symptoms as depression. A doctor can rule out these possibilities by conducting a physical examination, interview, and lab tests. If the doctor can eliminate a medical condition as a cause, he or she should conduct a psychological evaluation or refer the patient to a mental health professional.

The doctor or mental health professional will conduct a complete diagnostic evaluation. He or she should discuss any family history of depression, and get a complete history of symptoms, e.g., when they started, how long they have lasted, their severity, and whether they have occurred before and if so, how they were treated. He or she should also ask if the patient is using alcohol or drugs, and whether the patient is thinking about death or suicide.

Once diagnosed, a person with depression can be treated with a number of methods. The most common treatments are medication and psychotherapy.

Medication

Antidepressants work to normalize naturally occurring brain chemicals called neurotransmitters, notably serotonin and norepinephrine. Other antidepressants work on the neurotransmitter dopamine. Scientists studying depression have found that these particular chemicals are involved in regulating mood, but they are unsure of the exact ways in which they work.

The newest and most popular types of antidepressant medications are called selective serotonin reuptake inhibitors (SSRIs). SSRIs include fluoxetine (Prozac), citalopram (Celexa), sertraline (Zoloft), and several others. Serotonin and norepinephrine reuptake inhibitors (SNRIs) are similar to SSRIs and include venlafaxine (Effexor) and duloxetine (Cymbalta). SSRIs and SNRIs are more popular than the older classes of antidepressants, such as tricyclics—named for their chemical structure—and monoamine oxidase inhibitors (MAOIs) because they tend to have fewer side effects. However, medications affect everyone differently—no one-size-fits-all approach to medication exists. Therefore, for some people, tricyclics or MAOIs may be the best choice.

People taking MAOIs must adhere to significant food and medicinal restrictions to avoid potentially serious interactions. They must avoid certain foods that contain high levels of the chemical tyramine, which is found in many cheeses, wines, and pickles, and some medications including decongestants. MAOIs interact with tyramine in such a way that may cause a sharp increase in blood pressure, which could lead to a stroke. A doctor should give a patient taking an MAOI a complete list of prohibited foods, medicines, and substances.

For all classes of antidepressants, patients must take regular doses for at least 3 to 4 weeks before they are likely to experience a full therapeutic effect. They should continue taking the medication for the time specified by their doctor, even if they are feeling better, in order to prevent a relapse of the depression. Medication should be stopped only under a doctor's supervision. Some medications need to be gradually stopped to give the body time to adjust. Although antidepressants are not habit-forming or addictive, abruptly ending an antidepressant can cause withdrawal symptoms or lead to a relapse. Some individuals, such as those with chronic or recurrent depression, may need to stay on the medication indefinitely.

In addition, if one medication does not work, patients should be open to trying another. NIMH-funded research has shown that patients who did not get well after taking a first medication increased their chances of becoming symptom-free after they switched to a different medication or added another medication to their existing one.

Sometimes stimulants, anti-anxiety medications, or other medications are used in conjunction with an antidepressant, especially if the patient has a coexisting mental or physical disorder. However, neither anti-anxiety medications nor stimulants are effective against depression when taken alone, and both should be taken only under a doctor's close supervision.

What Are the Side Effects of Antidepressants?

Antidepressants may cause mild and often temporary side effects in some people, but they are usually not long-term. However, any unusual reactions or side effects that interfere with normal functioning should be reported to a doctor immediately.

The most common side effects associated with SSRIs and SNRIs include:

- Headache—usually temporary and will subside.
- Nausea—temporary and usually short-lived.
- Insomnia and nervousness (trouble falling asleep or waking often during the night)—may occur during the first few weeks but often subside over time or if the dose is reduced.
- Agitation (feeling jittery).
- Sexual problems—both men and women can experience sexual problems including reduced sex drive, erectile dysfunction, delayed ejaculation, or inability to have an orgasm.

Tricyclic antidepressants also can cause side effects including:

- Dry mouth—it is helpful to drink plenty of water, chew gum, and clean teeth daily.
- Constipation—it is helpful to eat more bran cereals, prunes, fruits, and vegetables.
- Bladder problems—emptying the bladder may be difficult, and the urine stream may not be as strong as usual. Older men with enlarged prostate conditions may be more affected. The doctor should be notified if it is painful to urinate.
- Sexual problems—sexual functioning may change, and side effects are similar to those from SSRIs.
- Blurred vision—often passes soon and usually will not require a new corrective lenses prescription.
- Drowsiness during the day—usually passes soon, but driving or operating heavy machinery should be avoided while drowsiness occurs. The more sedating antidepressants are generally taken at bedtime to help sleep and minimize daytime drowsiness.

Despite the relative safety and popularity of SSRIs and other antidepressants, some studies have suggested that they may have unintentional effects on some people, especially adolescents and young adults. In 2004, the Food and Drug Administration (FDA) conducted a thorough review of published and unpublished controlled clinical trials of antidepressants that involved nearly 4,400 children and adolescents. The review revealed that 4% of those taking antidepressants thought about or attempted suicide (although no suicides occurred), compared to 2% of those receiving placebos.

This information prompted the FDA, in 2005, to adopt a "black box" warning label on all antidepressant medications to alert the public about the potential increased risk of suicidal thinking or attempts in children and adolescents taking antidepressants. In 2007, the FDA proposed that makers of all antidepressant medications extend the warning to include young adults up through age 24. A "black box" warning is the most serious type of warning on prescription drug labeling.

The warning emphasizes that patients of all ages taking antidepressants should be closely monitored, especially during the initial weeks of treatment. Possible side effects to look for are worsening depression, suicidal thinking or behavior, or any unusual changes in behavior such as sleeplessness, agitation, or withdrawal from normal social situations. The warning adds that families and caregivers should also be told of the need for close monitoring and report any changes to the physician.

Results of a comprehensive review of pediatric trials conducted between 1988 and 2006 suggested that the benefits of antidepressant medications likely outweigh their risks to children and adolescents with major depression and anxiety disorders. The study was funded in part by the National Institute of Mental Health.

Also, the FDA issued a warning that combining an SSRI or SNRI antidepressant with one of the commonly used "triptan" medications for migraine headache could cause a life-threatening "serotonin syndrome," marked by agitation, hallucinations, elevated body temperature, and rapid changes in blood pressure. Although most dramatic in the case of the MAOIs, newer antidepressants may also be associated with potentially dangerous interactions with other medications.

Psychotherapy

Several types of psychotherapy—or "talk therapy"—can help people with depression. Some regimens are short-term (10 to 20 weeks) and other regimens are longer-term, depending on the needs of the individual. Two main types of psychotherapies—cognitive-behavioral therapy

(CBT) and interpersonal therapy (IPT)—have been shown to be effective in treating depression. By teaching new ways of thinking and behaving, CBT helps people change negative styles of thinking and behaving that may contribute to their depression. IPT helps people understand and work through troubled personal relationships that may cause their depression or make it worse.

For mild to moderate depression, psychotherapy may be the best treatment option. However, for major depression or for certain people, psychotherapy may not be enough. Studies have indicated that for adolescents, a combination of medication and psychotherapy may be the most effective approach to treating major depression and reducing the likelihood for recurrence. Similarly, a study examining depression treatment among older adults found that patients who responded to initial treatment of medication and IPT were less likely to have recurring depression if they continued their combination treatment for at least 2 years.

Electroconvulsive Therapy

For cases in which medication and/or psychotherapy does not help alleviate a person's treatment-resistant depression, electroconvulsive therapy (ECT) may be useful. ECT, formerly known as "shock therapy," once had a bad reputation. But in recent years, it has greatly improved and can provide relief for people with severe depression who have not been able to feel better with other treatments.

Before ECT is administered, a patient takes a muscle relaxant and is put under brief anesthesia. He or she does not consciously feel the electrical impulse administered in ECT. A patient typically will undergo ECT several times a week, and often will need to take an antidepressant or mood stabilizing medication to supplement the ECT treatments and prevent relapse. Although some patients will need only a few courses of ECT, others may need maintenance ECT, usually once a week at first, then gradually decreasing to monthly treatments for up to 1 year.

ECT may cause some short-term side effects, including confusion, disorientation, and memory loss. But these side effects typically clear soon after treatment. Research has indicated that after 1 year of ECT treatments, patients showed no adverse cognitive effects.

What Efforts Are Underway to Improve Treatment?

Researchers are looking for ways to better understand, diagnose, and treat depression among all groups of people. New potential treatments are being tested that give hope to those who live with depression that is particularly difficult to treat, and researchers are studying the risk factors for depression and how it affects the brain. NIMH continues to fund cutting-edge research into this debilitating disorder.

How Can I Help a Friend or Relative Who Is Depressed?

If you know someone who is depressed, it affects you, too. The first and most important thing you can do to help a friend or relative who has depression is to help him or her get an appropriate diagnosis and treatment. You may need to make an appointment on behalf of your friend or relative and go with him or her to see the doctor. Encourage him or her to stay in treatment, or to seek different treatment if no improvement occurs after 6 to 8 weeks.

- Offer emotional support, understanding, patience, and encouragement.
- Engage your friend or relative in conversation, and listen carefully.
- Never disparage feelings your friend or relative expresses, but point out realities and offer hope.
- Never ignore comments about suicide, and report them to your friend's or relative's therapist or doctor.
- Invite your friend or relative out for walks, outings, and other activities. Keep trying if he or she declines, but don't push him or her to take on too much too soon. Although diversions and company are needed, too many demands may increase feelings of failure.
- Remind your friend or relative that with time and treatment, the depression will lift.

How Can I Help Myself If I Am Depressed?

If you have depression, you may feel exhausted, helpless, and hopeless. It may be extremely difficult to take any action to help yourself. But it is important to realize that these feelings are part of the depression and do not accurately reflect actual circumstances. As you begin to recognize your depression and begin treatment, negative thinking will fade.

- Engage in mild activity or exercise. Go to a movie, a ballgame, or another event or activity that you once enjoyed. Participate in religious, social, or other activities.
- Set realistic goals for yourself.
- Break up large tasks into small ones, set some priorities, and do what you can as you can.
- Try to spend time with other people and confide in a trusted friend or relative. Try not to isolate yourself, and let others help you.
- Expect your mood to improve gradually, not immediately. Do not expect to suddenly "snap out of" your depression. Often during treatment for depression, sleep and appetite will begin to improve before your depressed mood lifts.
- Postpone important decisions, such as getting married or divorced or changing jobs, until you feel better. Discuss decisions with others who know you well and have a more objective view of your situation.
- Remember that positive thinking will replace negative thoughts as your depression responds to treatment.

Where Can I Go for Help?

If you are unsure where to go for help, ask your family doctor. Others who can help are listed below.

- Mental health specialists, such as psychiatrists, psychologists, social workers, or mental health counselors
- Health maintenance organizations
- Community mental health centers
- Hospital psychiatry departments and outpatient clinics
- Mental health programs at universities or medical schools
- State hospital outpatient clinics
- Family services, social agencies, or clergy
- Peer support groups
- Private clinics and facilities

- Employee assistance programs
- Local medical and/or psychiatric societies

You can also check the phone book under "mental health," "health," "social services," "hotlines," or "physicians" for phone numbers and addresses. An emergency room doctor also can provide temporary help and can tell you where and how to get further help.

What If I or Someone I Know Is in Crisis?

- If you are thinking about harming yourself, or know someone who is, tell someone who can help immediately.
- Call your doctor.
- Call 911 or go to a hospital emergency room to get immediate help or ask a friend or family member to help you do these things.
- Call the toll-free, 24-hour hotline of the National Suicide Prevention Lifeline at 800-273-TALK (800-273-8255); TTY: 800 799 4TTY (4889) to talk to a trained counselor.
- Make sure you or the suicidal person is not left alone.

Chapter 14

Women and Depression

Chapter Contents

Section 14.1

What Causes Depression in Women?

Excerpted from "Women and Depression: Discovering Hope," a booklet by the National Institute of Mental Health (NIMH, www.nimh.nih.gov), part of the National Institutes of Health, 2008. NIH Publication No. 08-4779.

What is depression?

Everyone occasionally feels blue or sad, but these feelings are usually fleeting and pass within a couple of days. When a woman has a depressive disorder, it interferes with daily life and normal functioning, and causes pain for both the woman with the disorder and those who care about her. Depression is a common but serious illness, and most who have it need treatment to get better.

Depression affects both men and women, but more women than men are likely to be diagnosed with depression in any given year. Efforts to explain this difference are ongoing, as researchers explore certain factors (biological, social, etc.) that are unique to women.

Many women with a depressive illness never seek treatment. But the vast majority, even those with the most severe depression, can get better with treatment.

What are the different forms of depression?

There are several forms of depressive disorders that occur in both women and men. The most common are major depressive disorder and dysthymic disorder. Minor depression is also common.

Major depressive disorder, also called major depression, is characterized by a combination of symptoms that interfere with a person's ability to work, sleep, study, eat, and enjoy once-pleasurable activities. Major depression is disabling and prevents a person from functioning normally. An episode of major depression may occur only once in a person's lifetime, but more often, it recurs throughout a person's life.

Dysthymic disorder, also called dysthymia, is characterized by depressive symptoms that are long-term (e.g., 2 years or longer) but less severe than those of major depression. Dysthymia may not disable a person, but it prevents one from functioning normally or feeling well. People with dysthymia may also experience one or more episodes of major depression during their lifetimes.

Minor depression may also occur. Symptoms of minor depression are similar to major depression and dysthymia, but they are less severe and/or are usually shorter term.

Some forms of depressive disorder have slightly different characteristics than those described above, or they may develop under unique circumstances. However, not all scientists agree on how to characterize and define these forms of depression. They include the following:

- **Psychotic depression** occurs when a severe depressive illness is accompanied by some form of psychosis, such as a break with reality; seeing, hearing, smelling, or feeling things that others can't detect (hallucinations); and having strong beliefs that are false, such as believing you are the president (delusions).
- **Seasonal affective disorder (SAD)** is characterized by a depressive illness during the winter months, when there is less natural sunlight. The depression generally lifts during spring and summer. SAD may be effectively treated with light therapy, but nearly half of those with SAD do not respond to light therapy alone. Antidepressant medication and psychotherapy also can reduce SAD symptoms, either alone or in combination with light therapy.

What causes depression in women?

Scientists are examining many potential causes for and contributing factors to women's increased risk for depression. It is likely that genetic, biological, chemical, hormonal, environmental, psychological, and social factors all intersect to contribute to depression.

Genetics: If a woman has a family history of depression, she may be more at risk of developing the illness. However, this is not a hard and fast rule. Depression can occur in women without family histories of depression, and women from families with a history of depression may not develop depression themselves. Genetics research indicates that the risk for developing depression likely involves the combination of multiple genes with environmental or other factors.

Chemicals and hormones: Brain chemistry appears to be a significant factor in depressive disorders. Modern brain-imaging technologies, such as magnetic resonance imaging (MRI), have shown that the brains of people suffering from depression look different than those of people without depression. The parts of the brain responsible for regulating mood, thinking, sleep, appetite and behavior don't appear to be functioning normally. In addition, important neurotransmitters—chemicals that brain cells use to communicate—appear to be out of balance. But these images do not reveal why the depression has occurred.

Scientists are also studying the influence of female hormones, which change throughout life. Researchers have shown that hormones directly affect the brain chemistry that controls emotions and mood. Specific times during a woman's life are of particular interest, including puberty; the times before menstrual periods; before, during, and just after pregnancy (postpartum); and just prior to and during menopause (perimenopause).

Premenstrual dysphoric disorder: Some women may be susceptible to a severe form of premenstrual syndrome called premenstrual dysphoric disorder (PMDD). Women affected by PMDD typically experience depression, anxiety, irritability and mood swings the week before menstruation, in such a way that interferes with their normal functioning. Women with debilitating PMDD do not necessarily have unusual hormone changes, but they do have different responses to these changes. They may also have a history of other mood disorders and differences in brain chemistry that cause them to be more sensitive to menstruation-related hormone changes. Scientists are exploring how the cyclical rise and fall of estrogen and other hormones may affect the brain chemistry that is associated with depressive illness.

Postpartum depression: Women are particularly vulnerable to depression after giving birth, when hormonal and physical changes and the new responsibility of caring for a newborn can be overwhelming. Many new mothers experience a brief episode of mild mood changes known as the "baby blues," but some will suffer from postpartum depression, a much more serious condition that requires active treatment and emotional support for the new mother. One study found that postpartum women are at an increased risk for several mental disorders, including depression, for several months after childbirth.

Some studies suggest that women who experience postpartum depression often have had prior depressive episodes. Some experience it during their pregnancies, but it often goes undetected. Research suggests that visits to the doctor may be good opportunities for screening for depression both during pregnancy and in the postpartum period.

Menopause: Hormonal changes increase during the transition between premenopause to menopause. While some women may transition into menopause without any problems with mood, others experience an increased risk for depression. This seems to occur even among women without a history of depression. However, depression becomes less common for women during the postmenopause period.

Stress: Stressful life events such as trauma, loss of a loved one, a difficult relationship, or any stressful situation—whether welcome or unwelcome—often occur before a depressive episode. Additional work and home responsibilities, caring for children and aging parents, abuse, and poverty also may trigger a depressive episode. Evidence suggests that women respond differently than men to these events, making them more prone to depression. In fact, research indicates that women respond in such a way that prolongs their feelings of stress more so than men, increasing the risk for depression. However, it is unclear why some women faced with enormous challenges develop depression, and some with similar challenges do not.

What illnesses often coexist with depression in women?

Depression often coexists with other illnesses that may precede the depression, follow it, cause it, be a consequence of it, or a combination of these. It is likely that the interplay between depression and other illnesses differs for every person and situation. Regardless, these other coexisting illnesses need to be diagnosed and treated.

Depression often coexists with eating disorders such as anorexia nervosa, bulimia nervosa, and others, especially among women. Anxiety disorders, such as posttraumatic stress disorder (PTSD), obsessive-compulsive disorder, panic disorder, social phobia and generalized anxiety disorder, also sometimes accompany depression. Women are more prone than men to having a coexisting anxiety disorder. Women suffering from PTSD, which can result after a person endures a terrifying ordeal or event, are especially prone to having depression.

Although more common among men than women, alcohol and substance abuse or dependence may occur at the same time as depression. Research has indicated that among both sexes, the coexistence of mood disorders and substance abuse is common among the U.S. population.

Depression also often coexists with other serious medical illnesses such as heart disease, stroke, cancer, HIV/AIDS [human immunodeficiency virus/acquired immunodeficiency syndrome], diabetes, Parkinson disease, thyroid problems and multiple sclerosis, and may even make symptoms of the illness worse. Studies have shown that both women and men who have depression in addition to a serious medical illness tend to have more severe symptoms of both illnesses. They also have more difficulty adapting to their medical condition, and more medical costs than those who do not have coexisting depression. Research has shown that treating the depression along with the coexisting illness will help ease both conditions.

How does depression affect adolescent girls?

Before adolescence, girls and boys experience depression at about the same frequency. By adolescence, however, girls become more likely to experience depression than boys.

Research points to several possible reasons for this imbalance. The biological and hormonal changes that occur during puberty likely contribute to the sharp increase in rates of depression among adolescent girls. In addition, research has suggested that girls are more likely than boys to continue feeling bad after experiencing difficult situations or events, suggesting they are more prone to depression. Another study found that girls tended to doubt themselves, doubt their problem-solving abilities, and view their problems as unsolvable more so than boys. The girls with these views were more likely to have depressive symptoms as well. Girls also tended to need a higher degree of approval and success to feel secure than boys.

Finally, girls may undergo more hardships, such as poverty, poor education, childhood sexual abuse, and other traumas than boys. One study found that more than 70 percent of depressed girls experienced a difficult or stressful life event prior to a depressive episode, as compared with only 14 percent of boys.

How does depression affect older women?

As with other age groups, more older women than older men experience depression, but rates decrease among women after menopause. Evidence suggests that depression in postmenopausal women generally occurs in women with prior histories of depression. In any case, depression is not a normal part of aging.

The death of a spouse or loved one, moving from work into retirement, or dealing with a chronic illness can leave women and men alike feeling sad or distressed. After a period of adjustment, many older women can regain their emotional balance, but others do not and may develop depression. When older women do suffer from depression, it may be overlooked because older adults may be less willing to discuss feelings of sadness or grief, or they may have less obvious symptoms of depression. As a result, their doctors may be less likely to suspect or spot it.

For older adults who experience depression for the first time later in life, other factors, such as changes in the brain or body, may be at play. For example, older adults may suffer from restricted blood flow, a condition called ischemia. Over time, blood vessels become less flexible. They may harden and prevent blood from flowing normally to the body's organs, including the brain. If this occurs, an older adult with no family or personal history of depression may develop what some doctors call "vascular depression." Those with vascular depression also may be at risk for a coexisting cardiovascular illness, such as heart disease or a stroke.

What if I or someone I know is in crisis?

Women are more likely than men to attempt suicide. If you are thinking about harming yourself or attempting suicide, tell someone who can help immediately.

- Call your doctor.
- Call 911 for emergency services.
- Go to the nearest hospital emergency room.
- Call the toll-free, 24-hour hotline of the National Suicide Prevention Lifeline at 800-273-TALK (800-273-8255); TTY: 800-799-4TTY (4889) to be connected to a trained counselor at a suicide crisis center nearest you.

Section 14.2

Depression during and after Pregnancy

Excerpted from "Depression During and After Pregnancy," by the Office on Women's Health (www.womenshealth.gov), part of the U.S. Health and Human Services Administration, April 2005.

How common is depression during and after pregnancy?

Depression is a common problem during and after pregnancy. About 13 percent of pregnant women and new mothers have depression.

What causes depression? What about postpartum depression?

There is no single cause. Rather, depression likely results from a combination of factors:

- Depression is a mental illness that tends to run in families.
- Women with a family history of depression are more likely to have depression.
- Changes in brain chemistry or structure are believed to play a big role in depression.
- Stressful life events, such as death of a loved one, caring for an aging family member, abuse, and poverty, can trigger depression.
- Hormonal factors unique to women may contribute to depression in some women. We know that hormones directly affect the brain chemistry that controls emotions and mood. We also know that women are at greater risk of depression at certain times in their lives, such as puberty, during and after pregnancy, and during perimenopause. Some women also have depressive symptoms right before their period.

Depression after childbirth is called postpartum depression. Hormonal changes may trigger symptoms of postpartum depression.

When you are pregnant, levels of the female hormones estrogen and progesterone increases greatly. In the first 24 hours after childbirth, hormone levels quickly return to normal. Researchers think the big change in hormone levels may lead to depression. This is much like the way smaller hormone changes can affect a woman's moods before she gets her period.

Levels of thyroid hormones may also drop after giving birth. The thyroid is a small gland in the neck that helps regulate how your body uses and stores energy from food. Low levels of thyroid hormones can cause symptoms of depression. A simple blood test can tell if this condition is causing your symptoms. If so, your doctor can prescribe thyroid medicine.

Other factors may play a role in postpartum depression. You may feel:

- tired after delivery;
- tired from a lack of sleep or broken sleep;
- overwhelmed with a new baby;
- doubts about your ability to be a good mother;
- stress from changes in work and home routines;
- an unrealistic need to be perfect mom;
- loss of who you were before having the baby;
- less attractive; or
- a lack of free time.

Are some women more at risk for depression during and after pregnancy?

Certain factors may increase your risk of depression during and after pregnancy:

- a personal history of depression or another mental illness;
- a family history of depression or another mental illness;
- a lack of support from family and friends;
- anxiety or negative feelings about the pregnancy;
- problems with a previous pregnancy or birth;
- marriage or money problems;

- stressful life events;
- young age; and
- substance abuse.

Women who are depressed during pregnancy have a greater risk of depression after giving birth.

If you take medicine for depression, stopping your medicine when you become pregnant can cause your depression to come back. Do not stop any prescribed medicines without first talking to your doctor. Not using medicine that you need may be harmful to you or your baby.

What is the difference between "baby blues," postpartum depression, and postpartum psychosis?

Many women have the baby blues in the days after childbirth. If you have the baby blues, you may:

- have mood swings;
- feel sad, anxious, or overwhelmed;
- have crying spells;
- lose your appetite; or
- have trouble sleeping.

The baby blues most often go away within a few days or a week. The symptoms are not severe and do not need treatment.

The symptoms of postpartum depression last longer and are more severe. Postpartum depression can begin anytime within the first year after childbirth. If you have postpartum depression, you may have any of the symptoms of depression. Symptoms may also include:

- thoughts of hurting the baby;
- thoughts of hurting yourself; or
- not having any interest in the baby.

Postpartum depression needs to be treated by a doctor.

Postpartum psychosis is rare. It occurs in about 1 to 4 out of every 1,000 births. It usually begins in the first 2 weeks after childbirth. Women who have bipolar disorder or another mental health problem called schizoaffective disorder have a higher risk for postpartum psychosis. Symptoms may include:

- seeing things that aren't there;
- feeling confused;
- having rapid mood swings; or
- trying to hurt yourself or your baby.

What should I do if I have symptoms of depression during or after pregnancy?

Call your doctor if:

- your baby blues don't go away after 2 weeks;
- symptoms of depression get more and more intense;
- strong feelings of sadness or anger come on 1 or 2 months after delivery;
- it is hard for you to perform tasks at work or at home;
- you cannot care for yourself or your baby; or
- you have thoughts of harming yourself or your baby.

Your doctor can ask you questions to test for depression. Your doctor can also refer you to a mental health professional who specializes in treating depression.

Some women don't tell anyone about their symptoms. They feel embarrassed, ashamed, or guilty about feeling depressed when they are supposed to be happy. They worry they will be viewed as unfit parents.

Any woman may become depressed during pregnancy or after having a baby. It doesn't mean you are a bad or "not together" mom. You and your baby don't have to suffer. There is help.

Here are some other helpful tips:

- Rest as much as you can. Sleep when the baby is sleeping.
- Don't try to do too much or try to be perfect.
- Ask your partner, family, and friends for help.
- Make time to go out, visit friends, or spend time alone with your partner.

- Discuss your feelings with your partner, family, and friends.
- Talk with other mothers so you can learn from their experiences.
- Join a support group. Ask your doctor about groups in your area.
- Don't make any major life changes during pregnancy or right after giving birth. Major changes can cause unneeded stress. Sometimes big changes can't be avoided. When that happens, try to arrange support and help in your new situation ahead of time.

How is depression treated?

The two common types of treatment for depression are:

- **Talk therapy:** This involves talking to a therapist, psychologist, or social worker to learn to change how depression makes you think, feel, and act.
- **Medicine:** Your doctor can prescribe an antidepressant medicine. These medicines can help relieve symptoms of depression.

If you are depressed, your depression can affect your baby. Getting treatment is important for you and your baby. Talk with your doctor about the benefits and risks of taking medicine to treat depression when you are pregnant or breastfeeding.

What can happen if depression is not treated?

Untreated depression can hurt you and your baby. Some women with depression have a hard time caring for themselves during pregnancy. They may:

- eat poorly;
- not gain enough weight;
- have trouble sleeping;
- miss prenatal visits;
- not follow medical instructions; or
- use harmful substances, like tobacco, alcohol, or illegal drugs.

Depression during pregnancy can raise the risk of:

- problems during pregnancy or delivery;
- having a low-birth-weight baby; or
- premature birth.

Untreated postpartum depression can affect your ability to parent. You may:

- lack energy;
- have trouble focusing;
- feel moody; and
- not be able to meet your child's needs.

As a result, you may feel guilty and lose confidence in yourself as a mother. These feelings can make your depression worse.

Researchers believe postpartum depression in a mother can affect her baby. It can cause the baby to have:

- delays in language development;
- problems with mother-child bonding;
- behavior problems; or
- increased crying.

It helps if your partner or another caregiver can help meet the baby's needs while you are depressed.

All children deserve the chance to have a healthy mom. And all moms deserve the chance to enjoy their life and their children. If you are feeling depressed during pregnancy or after having a baby, don't suffer alone. Please tell a loved one and call your doctor right away.

Chapter 15

Men and Depression

Researchers estimate that at least six million men in the United States suffer from a depressive disorder every year. Research and clinical evidence reveal that while both women and men can develop the standard symptoms of depression, they often experience depression differently and may have different ways of coping with the symptoms. Men may be more willing to acknowledge fatigue, irritability, loss of interest in work or hobbies, and sleep disturbances rather than feelings of sadness, worthlessness, and excessive guilt. Some researchers question whether the standard definition of depression and the diagnostic tests based upon it adequately capture the condition as it occurs in men.

Men are more likely than women to report alcohol and drug abuse or dependence in their lifetime; however, there is debate among researchers as to whether substance use is a "symptom" of underlying depression in men or a co-occurring condition that more commonly develops in men. Nevertheless, substance use can mask depression, making it harder to recognize depression as a separate illness that needs treatment.

Instead of acknowledging their feelings, asking for help, or seeking appropriate treatment, men may turn to alcohol or drugs when they are depressed, or become frustrated, discouraged, angry, irritable,

---

Excerpted from "Men and Depression," by the National Institute of Mental Health (NIMH, www.nimh.nih.gov), part of the National Institutes of Health, 2005.

and, sometimes, violently abusive. Some men deal with depression by throwing themselves compulsively into their work, attempting to hide their depression from themselves, family, and friends. Other men may respond to depression by engaging in reckless behavior, taking risks, and putting themselves in harm's way.

More than four times as many men as women die by suicide in the United States, even though women make more suicide attempts during their lives. In addition to the fact that men attempt suicide using methods that are generally more lethal than those used by women, there may be other factors that protect women against suicide death. In light of research indicating that suicide is often associated with depression, the alarming suicide rate among men may reflect the fact that men are less likely to seek treatment for depression. Many men with depression do not obtain adequate diagnosis and treatment that may be life saving.

More research is needed to understand all aspects of depression in men, including how men respond to stress and feelings associated with depression, how to make men more comfortable acknowledging these feelings and getting the help they need, and how to train physicians to better recognize and treat depression in men. Family members, friends, and employee assistance professionals in the workplace also can play important roles in recognizing depressive symptoms in men and helping them get treatment.

Depression in Older Men

Men must cope with several kinds of stress as they age. If they have been the primary wage earners for their families and have identified heavily with their jobs, they may feel stress upon retirement—loss of an important role, loss of self-esteem—that can lead to depression. Similarly, the loss of friends and family and the onset of other health problems can trigger depression.

Depression is not a normal part of aging. Depression is an illness that can be effectively treated, thereby decreasing unnecessary suffering, improving the chances for recovery from other illnesses, and prolonging productive life. However, health care professionals may miss depressive symptoms in older patients. Older adults may be reluctant to discuss feelings of sadness or grief, or loss of interest in pleasurable activities. They may complain primarily of physical symptoms. It may be difficult to discern a co-occurring depressive disorder in patients who present with other illnesses, such as heart disease, stroke, or cancer, which may cause depressive symptoms or may be treated with medications that have side effects that cause depression. If a depressive illness is diagnosed, treatment with appropriate medication and/or brief psychotherapy can help older adults manage both diseases, thus enhancing survival and quality of life.

Identifying and treating depression in older adults is critical. There is a common misperception that suicide rates are highest among the young, but it is older white males who suffer the highest rate. Over 70 percent of older suicide victims visit their primary care physician within the month of their death; many have a depressive illness that goes undetected during these visits. This fact has led to research efforts to determine how to best improve physicians' abilities to detect and treat depression in older adults.

Approximately 80 percent of older adults with depression improve when they receive treatment with antidepressant medication, psychotherapy, or a combination of both. In addition, research has shown that a combination of psychotherapy and antidepressant medication is highly effective for reducing recurrences of depression among older adults. Psychotherapy alone has been shown to prolong periods of good health free from depression, and is particularly useful for older patients who cannot or will not take medication. Improved recognition and treatment of depression in later life will make those years more enjoyable and fulfilling for the depressed elderly person, and his family and caregivers.

Depression in Boys and Adolescent Males

Only in the past two decades has depression in children been taken very seriously. Research has revealed that depression is occurring earlier in life today than in past decades. In addition, research has shown that early-onset depression often persists, recurs, and continues into adulthood, and that depression in youth may also predict more severe illness in adult life. An NIMH-sponsored study of 9- to 17-year-olds estimates that the prevalence of any depressive disorder is more than 6 percent in a six-month period, with 4.9 percent having major depression. Before puberty, boys and girls are equally likely to develop depressive disorders. After age 14, however, females are twice as likely as males to have major depression or dysthymia. The risk of developing bipolar disorder remains approximately equal for males and females throughout adolescence and adulthood.

The depressed younger child may say he is sick, refuse to go to school, cling to a parent, or worry that the parent may die. The depressed older child may sulk, get into trouble at school, be negative and grouchy, and feel misunderstood. Signs of depressive disorders in young people are often viewed as normal mood swings typical of a particular developmental stage. In addition, health care professionals may be reluctant to prematurely "label" a young person with a mental illness diagnosis. However, early diagnosis and treatment of depressive disorders are critical to healthy emotional, social, and behavioral development. Depression in young people frequently co-occurs with other mental disorders, most commonly anxiety, disruptive behavior, or substance abuse disorders, as well as with other serious illnesses such as diabetes.

Among both children and adolescents, depressive disorders confer an increased risk for illness and interpersonal and psychosocial difficulties that persist long after the depressive episode is resolved; in adolescents, there is also an increased risk for substance abuse and suicidal behavior. Unfortunately, these disorders often go unrecognized by families and physicians alike.

Although the scientific literature on treatment of children and adolescents with depression is far less extensive than that for adults, a number of recent studies have confirmed the short-term efficacy and safety of treatments for depression in youth. An NIMH-funded clinical trial of 439 adolescents with major depression found that a combination of medication and psychotherapy is the most effective treatment. Additional research is needed on how best to incorporate these treatments into primary care practice.

Bipolar disorder, although rare in young children, can appear in both children and adolescents. The unusual shifts in mood, energy, and functioning that are characteristic of bipolar disorder may begin with manic, depressive, or mixed manic and depressive symptoms. It is more likely to affect the children of parents who have the illness. Twenty to 40 percent of adolescents with major depression go on to reveal bipolar disorder within 5 years after the onset of depression.

Depression in children and adolescents is associated with an increased risk of suicidal behaviors. This risk may rise, particularly among adolescent males, if the depression is accompanied by conduct disorder and alcohol or other substance abuse. In 2002, suicide was the third leading cause of death among young males, age 15 to 24. NIMH-supported researchers found that among adolescents who develop major depressive disorder, as many as 7 percent may die by suicide in the young adult years. Therefore, it is important for doctors and parents to take seriously any remarks about suicide.

NIMH researchers are developing and testing various interventions to prevent suicide in children and adolescents. Early diagnosis and treatment, accurate evaluation of suicidal thinking, and limitations on young people's access to lethal agents—including firearms and medications—may hold the greatest suicide prevention value.

Suicide

Sometimes depression can cause people to feel like putting themselves in harm's way, or killing themselves. Although the majority of people with depression do not die by suicide, having depression does increase suicide risk compared to people without depression.

If you are thinking about suicide, get help immediately:

- Call your doctor's office.
- Call 911 for emergency services.
- Go to the emergency room of the nearest hospital.
- Ask a family member or friend to take you to the hospital or call your doctor.
- Call the toll-free, 24-hour hotline of the National Suicide Prevention Lifeline at 800-273-TALK (1-800-273-8255) to be connected to a trained counselor at the suicide crisis center nearest you.

Conclusion

A man can experience depression in many different ways. He may be grumpy or irritable, or have lost his sense of humor. He might drink too much or abuse drugs. It may be that he physically or verbally abuses his wife and his kids. He might work all the time, or compulsively seek thrills in high-risk behavior. Or, he may seem isolated, withdrawn, and no longer interested in the people or activities he used to enjoy.

Perhaps this man sounds like you. If so, it is important to understand that there is a brain disorder called depression that may be underlying these feelings and behaviors. It's real: scientists have developed sensitive imaging devices that enable us to see depression in the brain. And it's treatable: more than 80 percent of those suffering from depression respond to existing treatments, and new ones are continually becoming available and helping more people. Talk to a healthcare provider about how you are feeling, and ask for help.

Or perhaps this man sound like someone you care about. Try to talk to him, or to someone who has a chance of getting through to him.

Help him to understand that depression is a common illness among men and is nothing to be ashamed about. Encourage him to see a doctor and get an evaluation for depression.

For most men with depression, life doesn't have to be so dark and hopeless. Life is hard enough as it is; and treating depression can free up vital resources to cope with life's challenges effectively. When a man is depressed, he's not the only one who suffers. His depression also darkens the lives of his family, his friends, virtually everyone close to him. Getting him into treatment can send ripples of healing and hope into all of those lives.

Depression is a real illness; it is treatable; and men can have it. It takes courage to ask for help, but help can make all the difference.

Chapter 16

Older Adults and Depression

Chapter Contents

Section 16.1

Facts about Depression in Older Adults

Excerpted from "Older Adults: Depression and Suicide Facts," from the National Institute of Mental Health (NIMH, www.nimh.nih.gov), part of the National Institutes of Health, April 2007.

How Common Is Suicide among Older Adults?

Older Americans are disproportionately likely to die by suicide.

- Although they comprise only 12 percent of the U.S. population, people age 65 and older accounted for 16 percent of suicide deaths in 2004.
- 14.3 of every 100,000 people age 65 and older died by suicide in 2004, higher than the rate of about 11 per 100,000 in the general population.
- Non-Hispanic white men age 85 and older were most likely to die by suicide. They had a rate of 49.8 suicide deaths per 100,000 persons in that age group.

What Role Does Depression Play?

Depression, one of the conditions most commonly associated with suicide in older adults, is a widely under-recognized and undertreated medical illness. Studies show that many older adults who die by suicide—up to 75 percent—visited a physician within a month before death. These findings point to the urgency of improving detection and treatment of depression to reduce suicide risk among older adults.

- The risk of depression in the elderly increases with other illnesses and when ability to function becomes limited. Estimates of major depression in older people living in the community range from less than 1 percent to about 5 percent, but rises to 13.5 percent in those who require home healthcare and to 11.5 percent in elderly hospital patients.

- An estimated 5 million have subsyndromal depression, symptoms that fall short of meeting the full diagnostic criteria for a disorder.
- Subsyndromal depression is especially common among older persons and is associated with an increased risk of developing major depression.

Isn't Depression Just Part of Aging?

Depressive disorder is not a normal part of aging. Emotional experiences of sadness, grief, response to loss, and temporary "blue" moods are normal. Persistent depression that interferes significantly with ability to function is not.

Health professionals may mistakenly think that persistent depression is an acceptable response to other serious illnesses and the social and financial hardships that often accompany aging—an attitude often shared by older people themselves. This contributes to low rates of diagnosis and treatment in older adults.

Depression can and should be treated when it occurs at the same time as other medical illnesses. Untreated depression can delay recovery or worsen the outcome of these other illnesses.

What Are the Treatments for Depression in Older Adults?

Antidepressant medications or psychotherapy, or a combination of the two, can be effective treatments for late-life depression.

Medications

Antidepressant medications affect brain chemicals called neurotransmitters. For example, medications called SSRIs (selective serotonin reuptake inhibitors) affect the neurotransmitter serotonin. Different medications may affect different neurotransmitters.

Some older adults may find that newer antidepressant medications, including SSRIs, have fewer side effects than older medications, which include tricyclic antidepressants and monoamine oxidase inhibitors (MAOIs). However, others may find that these older medications work well for them.

It's important to be aware that there are several medications for depression, that different medications work for different people, and that it takes 4 to 8 weeks for the medications to work. If one medication doesn't help, research shows that a different antidepressant might.

Also, older adults experiencing depression for the first time should talk to their doctors about continuing medication even if their symptoms have disappeared with treatment. Studies showed that patients age 70 and older who became symptom-free and continued to take their medication for 2 more years were 60 percent less likely to relapse than those who discontinued their medications.

Psychotherapy

In psychotherapy, people interact with a specially trained health professional to deal with depression, thoughts of suicide, and other problems. Research shows that certain types of psychotherapy are effective treatments for late-life depression.

For many older adults, especially those who are in good physical health, combining psychotherapy with antidepressant medication appears to provide the most benefit. A study showed that about 80 percent of older adults with depression recovered with this kind of combined treatment and had lower recurrence rates than with psychotherapy or medication alone.

Another study of depressed older adults with physical illnesses and problems with memory and thinking showed that combined treatment was no more effective than medication alone.

Research can help further determine which older adults appear to be most likely to benefit from a combination of medication and psychotherapy or from either treatment alone.

Are Some Ethnic/Racial Groups at Higher Risk of Suicide?

For every 100,000 people age 65 and older in each of the ethnic/racial groups below, the following number died by suicide in 2004:

- Non-Hispanic Whites—15.8 per 100,000
- Asian and Pacific Islanders—10.6 per 100,000
- Hispanics—7.9 per 100,000
- Non-Hispanic Blacks—5.0 per 100,000

Section 16.2

Paying More for Prescriptions May Limit Seniors' Access to Antidepressants

From "Paying More for Prescriptions May Limit Seniors' Access to Antidepressants," by the National Institute of Mental Health (NIMH, www.nimh.nih.gov), part of the National Institutes of Health, April 2, 2008.

New cost-sharing policies may prevent some older adults diagnosed with depression from filling new antidepressant prescriptions, according to an analysis published in the April 2008 issue of *Psychiatric Services.*

The NIMH-funded study examined 8 years of data from a British Columbia, Canada, program that evolved from comprehensive prescription coverage to cost-sharing in which seniors were responsible for a part of the costs of their prescriptions.

Adults age 65 and older can suffer from major depression, but treating them with antidepressants can cause problems due to cost and potential interactions with other medications taken. As a result, many of those diagnosed with depression do not fill an antidepressant prescription.

Philip Wang, M.D., Dr. P.H., of NIMH's Division of Services and Intervention Research, and colleagues analyzed the province's prescription data from January 1997 to December 2005. After previously providing comprehensive prescription coverage, in January 2002 the province implemented a $10–25 Canadian co-pay with each prescription. Co-payments require the patient to pay a fixed amount for each prescription.

Then in May 2003, the co-pay policy was replaced with an income-based deductible and a 25 percent coinsurance payment after the deductible was met. Co-insurance requires the patient to pay a portion of the medication price, a potential hardship for people with many prescriptions. After meeting an out-of-pocket ceiling, full coverage kicked in. The transition is similar to what many U.S. retirees experience when they move from private insurance programs to Medicare, which also requires deductibles and coinsurance payments.

The researchers found that while neither policy change resulted in people discontinuing existing antidepressant prescriptions, each coverage policy change was associated with a decrease in the start of antidepressant therapy, suggesting that newly diagnosed seniors may not be filling new prescriptions.

The added costs likely prevented some from starting new prescriptions, said Wang and colleagues. Also, the researchers speculate that the stigma associated with antidepressants may have curtailed use, especially among those on lower fixed incomes. Wang and colleagues conclude that the consequences of decreases in antidepressant initiation are unclear and will require more research.

Reference

Wang PS, Patrick AR, Dormuth CR, Avorn M, Maclure M, Canning CF, Schneeweiss S. The impact of cost sharing on antidepressant use among older adults in British Columbia. *Psychiatric Services.* 2008 Apr: 59(4): pp. 377–383.

Chapter 17

Depression That Occurs with Other Illnesses

Chapter Contents

Section 17.1

Why Depression and Medical Illnesses Often Occur Together

Clinical depression is a common and serious medical illness that can be effectively treated. The risk of clinical depression is often higher in individuals with serious medical illnesses, such as heart disease, stroke, cancer, and diabetes. However, the warning signs are frequently discounted by patients and family members, who mistakenly assume feeling depressed is normal for people struggling with serious health conditions. In addition, the symptoms of depression are frequently masked by these other medical illnesses, resulting in treatment that addresses the symptoms but not the underlying depression. It is a myth that depression is a "normal" emotional response to another illness; it's extremely important to simultaneously treat both medical illnesses.

Impact of Depression in Primary Care Settings

- Nearly 74 percent of Americans who seek help for depression or symptoms of depression will go to a primary care physician rather than a mental health professional.[1]
- The rate of depression among those with medical illnesses in primary care settings is estimated at five to 10 percent. Among those hospitalized, the rate is estimated at 10 to 14 percent.[2]
- The more severe the medical condition, the more likely that the patient will experience clinical depression.[2]
- People with depression experience greater distress, an increase in impaired functioning and less ability to follow medical regimens, thus hindering the treatment of any other medical conditions.[2]

- Unfortunately, the diagnosis of depression is missed 50 percent of the time in primary care settings.[1]

Why Depression and Medical Illnesses Often Occur Together

- Medical disorders may contribute biologically to depression.[3]
- Medically ill people may become clinically depressed as a psychological reaction to the prognosis, the pain, and/or incapacity caused by the illness or its treatment.[3]
- Though occurring together, depression and a general medical disorder may be unrelated.[3]

Prevalence of Depression Co-Occurring with Other Medical Illnesses

Heart Disease and Depression

- Depression occurs in 40 to 65 percent of patients who have experienced a heart attack, and in 18 to 20 percent of people who have coronary heart disease, but who have not had a heart attack.[4]
- After a heart attack, patients with clinical depression have a three to four times greater chance of death within the next 6 months.[4]
- Men and women with depression are at increased risk for coronary artery disease but only men are at greater risk for dying.[5]

Stroke and Depression

- Depression occurs in 10 to 27 percent of stroke survivors and usually lasts about 1 year.[6]
- An additional 15-40 percent of stroke survivors experience some symptoms of depression within 2 months after the stroke.[6]
- Individuals reporting five or more depressive symptoms have more than a 50 percent risk of mortality due to stroke in the subsequent 29 years.[7]

Cancer and Depression

- One in four people with cancer also suffer from clinical depression.[8]

- Depression is sometimes mistaken as a side effect of corticosteroids or chemotherapy, both treatments for cancer.[8]
- Depressive symptoms can be mistakenly attributed to the cancer itself, which can also cause appetite and weight loss, insomnia, and loss of energy.[8]

Diabetes and Depression

- People with adult onset diabetes have a 25 percent chance of having depression.[9]
- Depression also affects as many as 70 percent of patients with diabetic complications.[9]

Eating Disorders and Depression

- Research shows a strong relationship between depression and eating disorders (anorexia and bulimia nervosa) in women.[10]

Alcohol/Drugs and Depression

- Research shows that one in three depressed people also suffer from some form of substance abuse or dependence.[1]

Common Symptoms of Depression and Other Medical Disorders

- Weight loss, sleep disturbances, and low energy may occur in people with diabetes, thyroid disorders, some neurological disorders, heart disease, cancer, and stroke—and also are common symptoms of depression.
- Apathy, poor concentration, and memory loss can occur in individuals with Parkinson's disease and Alzheimer's disease—and also are common symptoms of depression.
- Medications for high blood pressure, Parkinson's disease, and other medical problems can produce side effects similar to the symptoms of depression.

Importance of Treatment

- People who get treatment for co-occurring depression often experience an improvement in their overall medical condition, better compliance with general medical care, and a better quality of life.[9]

- More than 80 percent of people with depression can be treated successfully with medication, psychotherapy, or a combination of both.[2]
- Early diagnosis and treatment can reduce patient discomfort and morbidity, and can also reduce the costs associated with misdiagnosis, and the risks and costs associated with suicide.[1]

References

1. Montano B: "Recognition and Treatment of Depression in a Primary Care Setting," *Journal of Clinical Psychiatry* 1994; 55(12):18–33.
2. National Institute of Mental Health, "Co-occurrence of Depression with Medical, Psychiatric and Substance Abuse Disorders," Accessed July 1999. Netscape: http://www.nimh.nih.gov/depression/co_occur/abuse.htm.
3. National Institute of Mental Health, "Depression Co-occurring with General Medical Disorders," Accessed July 1999. Netscape: http://www.nimh.nih.gov/depression/co_occur/co_oc.htm.
4. National Institute of Mental Health, "Co-occurrence of Depression with Heart Disease," Accessed July 1999. Netscape: http://www.nimh.nih.gov/depression/co_occur/heart.htm.
5. Ferketich, A, Schwartzbaum, J, Frid, D, Moeschberger, M. Depression as an Antecedent to Heart Disease Among Women and Men in the NHANES I Study. *Archives of Internal Medicine* 2000; 160:1261–1268.
6. National Institute of Mental Health, "Co-occurrence of Depression with Stroke," Accessed July 1999. Netscape: http://www.nimh.nih.gov/depression/co_occur/stroke.htm.
7. Everson SA, Roberts RE, Goldberg DE, Kaplan GA: "Depressive Symptoms and Increased Risk of Stroke Mortality Over a 29-Year Period," *Archives of Internal Medicine* 1998; 158:1133–1138.
8. National Institute of Mental Health, "Co-occurrence of Depression with Cancer," Accessed July 1999. Netscape: http://www.nimh.nih.gov/depression/co_occur/cancer.htm.

9. Lamberg L: "Treating Depression in Medical Conditions May Improve Quality of Life." *JAMA* 1996; 276(Dec. 18):857–858.

10. Willcox M, Sattler DN: "The Relationship Between Eating Disorders and Depression," *Journal of Social Psychology* 1996; 136:269–271.

Section 17.2

Depression and Alzheimer Disease

"Depression and Alzheimer's," is reprinted with permission of the Alzheimer's Association. For additional information, call the Alzheimer's Association toll-free helpline, 800-272-2900, or visit their website at www.alz.org.

Introduction

Experts estimate that up to 40 percent of people with Alzheimer's disease suffer from significant depression. Fortunately, there are many effective non-drug and drug therapies available. Treatment of depression in Alzheimer's disease can improve a person's sense of well-being, quality of life, and individual function.

Symptoms of Depression

Men and women with Alzheimer's experience depression with about equal frequency. But identifying depression in someone with Alzheimer's can be difficult. There is no single test or questionnaire to detect the condition, and diagnosis requires careful evaluation of a variety of symptoms. Dementia itself can lead to certain symptoms commonly associated with depression, including:

- apathy
- loss of interest in activities and hobbies
- social withdrawal
- isolation

The cognitive impairment experienced by people with Alzheimer's often makes it difficult for them to articulate their sadness, hopelessness, guilt, and other feelings associated with depression.

Depression in Alzheimer's doesn't always look like depression in people without the disorder. For example, depression in Alzheimer's is sometimes less severe and may not last as long or recur as often.

Also, people with Alzheimer's and depression may be less likely to talk openly about wanting to kill themselves, and they are less likely to attempt suicide than depressed individuals without dementia. What's more, depressive symptoms in Alzheimer's may come and go, in contrast to memory and thinking problems that worsen steadily over time.

Diagnosing Depression in Alzheimer's Disease

The first step in diagnosis is a thorough professional evaluation. Side effects of medications or an unrecognized medical condition can sometimes produce symptoms of depression. Key elements of the evaluation will include:

- A review of the person's medical history
- A physical and mental examination
- Interviews with family members who know the person well

Because of the complexities involved in diagnosing depression in someone with Alzheimer's, it may be helpful to consult a geriatric psychiatrist who specializes in recognizing and treating depression in older adults.

To facilitate diagnosis and treatment of depression in people with Alzheimer's, the National Institute of Mental Health established a formal set of guidelines for diagnosing the condition. Although the criteria are similar to general diagnostic standards for major depression, they reduce emphasis on verbal expression and include irritability and social isolation.

For a person to be diagnosed with depression in Alzheimer's, he or she must have either depressed mood (sad, hopeless, discouraged, or tearful) or decreased pleasure in usual activities, along with two or more of the following symptoms over a two-week period:

- Social isolation or withdrawal
- Disruption in appetite that is not related to another medical condition

- Disruption in sleep
- Agitation or slowed behavior
- Irritability
- Fatigue or loss of energy
- Feelings of worthlessness or hopelessness, or inappropriate or excessive guilt
- Recurrent thoughts of death, suicide plans, or a suicide attempt

Treating Depression

The most common treatment for depression in Alzheimer's involves a combination of medicine, support, and gradual reconnection to activities and people the person finds pleasurable. Simply telling the person with Alzheimer's to "cheer up," "snap out of it," or "try harder" is seldom helpful. Depressed people with or without Alzheimer's are rarely able to make themselves better by sheer will, or without lots of support, reassurance, and professional help.

Non-Drug Approaches

- Schedule a predictable daily routine, taking advantage of the person's best time of day to undertake difficult tasks, such as bathing.
- Make a list of activities, people, or places that the person enjoys now and schedule these things more frequently.
- Help the person exercise regularly, particularly in the morning.
- Acknowledge the person's frustration or sadness, while continuing to express hope that he or she will feel better soon.
- Celebrate small successes and occasions.
- Find ways that the person can contribute to family life and be sure to recognize his or her contributions.
- Provide reassurance that the person is loved, respected, and appreciated as part of the family, and not just for what she or he can do now.
- Nurture the person with offers of favorite foods or soothing or inspirational activities.

- Reassure the person that he or she will not be abandoned.
- Consider supportive psychotherapy and/or a support group, especially an early-stage group for people with Alzheimer's who are aware of their diagnosis and prefer to take an active role in seeking help or helping others.

Medication to Treat Depression in Alzheimer's

Physicians may prescribe antidepressants for people with Alzheimer's who have depression. Examples include:

- bupropion (Wellbutrin®)
- citalopram (Celexa®)
- fluoxetine (Prozac®)
- mirtazapine (Remeron®)
- paroxetine (Paxil®)
- sertraline (Zoloft®)
- trazodone (Desyrel®)
- venlafaxine (Effexor®)

Antidepressants in a class called the tricyclics, which includes nortriptyline (Pamelor®) and desipramine (Norpramin®), are no longer used as first-choice treatments, but are sometimes used when individuals do not benefit from other medications.

Section 17.3

Depression and Cancer

Excerpted from PDQ® Cancer Information Summary. National Cancer Institute; Bethesda, MD. Depression (PDQ®): Supportive Care—Patient. Updated 12/2008. Available at: http://cancer.gov. Accessed January 2, 2009.

Overview

Depression is a disabling illness that affects about 15% to 25% of cancer patients. It affects men and women with cancer equally. People who face a diagnosis of cancer will experience different levels of stress and emotional upset. Important issues in the life of any person with cancer may include the following:

- fear of death;
- interruption of life plans;
- changes in body image and self-esteem;
- changes in social role and lifestyle; and
- money and legal concerns.

Everyone who is diagnosed with cancer will react to these issues in different ways and may not experience serious depression or anxiety.

Patients who are receiving palliative care for cancer may have frequent feelings of depression and anxiety, leading to a much lower quality of life. Patients in palliative care who suffer from depression report being more troubled about their physical symptoms, relationships, and beliefs about life. Depressed terminally ill patients have reported feelings of "being a burden" even when the actual amount of dependence on others is small.

Just as patients need to be evaluated for depression throughout their treatment, so do family caregivers. Caregivers have been found to experience a good deal more anxiety and depression than people who are not caring for patients with cancer. Children are also affected when a parent with cancer develops depression. A study of women with breast cancer showed that children of depressed patients were the most likely to have emotional and behavioral problems themselves.

There are many misconceptions about cancer and how people cope with it, such as the following:

- All people with cancer are depressed.
- Depression in a person with cancer is normal.
- Treatment does not help the depression.
- Everyone with cancer faces suffering and a painful death.

Sadness and grief are normal reactions to the crises faced during cancer, and will be experienced at times by all people. Because sadness is common, it is important to distinguish between normal levels of sadness and depression. An important part of cancer care is the recognition of depression that needs to be treated. Some people may have more trouble adjusting to the diagnosis of cancer than others may. Major depression is not simply sadness or a blue mood. Major depression affects about 25% of patients and has common symptoms that can be diagnosed and treated. Symptoms of depression that are noticed when a patient is diagnosed with cancer may be a sign that the patient had a depression problem before the diagnosis of cancer.

All people will experience reactions of sadness and grief periodically throughout diagnosis, treatment, and survival of cancer. When people find out they have cancer, they often have feelings of disbelief, denial, or despair. They may also experience difficulty sleeping, loss of appetite, anxiety, and a preoccupation with worries about the future. These symptoms and fears usually lessen as a person adjusts to the diagnosis. Signs that a person has adjusted to the diagnosis include an ability to maintain active involvement in daily life activities, and an ability to continue functioning as spouse, parent, employee, or other roles by incorporating treatment into his or her schedule. If the family of a patient diagnosed with cancer is able to express feelings openly and solve problems effectively, both the patient and family members have less depression. Good communication within the family reduces anxiety. A person who cannot adjust to the diagnosis after a long period of time, and who loses interest in usual activities, may be depressed. Mild symptoms of depression can be distressing and may be helped with counseling. Even patients without obvious symptoms of depression may benefit from counseling; however, when symptoms are intense and long-lasting, or when they keep coming back, more intensive treatment is important.

Diagnosis

The symptoms of major depression include the following:

- having a depressed mood for most of the day and on most days;
- loss of pleasure and interest in most activities;
- changes in eating and sleeping habits;
- nervousness or sluggishness;
- tiredness;
- feelings of worthlessness or inappropriate guilt;
- poor concentration; and
- constant thoughts of death or suicide.

To make a diagnosis of depression, these symptoms should be present on most days for at least 2 weeks. The diagnosis of depression can be difficult to make in people with cancer due to the difficulty of separating the symptoms of depression from the side effects of medications or the symptoms of cancer. This is especially true in patients undergoing active cancer treatment or those with advanced disease. Symptoms of guilt, worthlessness, hopelessness, thoughts of suicide, and loss of pleasure are the most useful in diagnosing depression in people who have cancer.

Some people with cancer may have a higher risk for developing depression. The cause of depression is not known, but the risk factors for developing depression are known. Risk factors may be cancer-related and noncancer-related.

Cancer-related risk factors:

- depression at the time of cancer diagnosis
- poorly controlled pain
- an advanced stage of cancer
- increased physical impairment or pain
- pancreatic cancer
- being unmarried and having head and neck cancer
- treatment with some anticancer drugs

Noncancer-related risk factors:

- history of depression

- lack of family support
- other life events that cause stress
- family history of depression or suicide
- previous suicide attempts
- history of alcoholism or drug abuse
- having many illnesses at the same time that produce symptoms of depression (such as stroke or heart attack)

The evaluation of depression in people with cancer should include a careful evaluation of the person's thoughts about the illness; medical history; personal or family history of depression or suicide; current mental status; physical status; side effects of treatment and the disease; other stresses in the person's life; and support available to the patient. Thinking of suicide, when it occurs, is frightening for the individual, for the health care worker, and for the family. Suicidal statements may range from an offhand comment resulting from frustration or disgust with a treatment course, such as "If I have to have one more bone marrow aspiration this year, I'll jump out the window," to a statement indicating deep despair and an emergency situation, such as, "I can't stand what this disease is doing to all of us, and I am going to kill myself." Exploring the seriousness of these thoughts is important. If the thoughts of suicide seem to be serious, then the patient should be referred to a psychiatrist or psychologist, and the safety of the patient should be secured.

The most common type of depression in people with cancer is called reactive depression. This shows up as feeling moody and being unable to perform usual activities. The symptoms last longer and are more pronounced than a normal and expected reaction but do not meet the criteria for major depression. When these symptoms greatly interfere with a person's daily activities, such as work, school, shopping, or caring for a household, they should be treated in the same way that major depression is treated (such as crisis intervention, counseling, and medication, especially with drugs that can quickly relieve distressing symptoms). Basing the diagnosis on just these symptoms can be a problem in a person with advanced cancer since the illness may be causing decreased functioning. It is important to identify the difference between fatigue and depression since they can be assessed and treated separately. In more advanced illness, focusing on despair, guilty thoughts, and a total lack of enjoyment of life is helpful in diagnosing depression.

Medical factors may also cause symptoms of depression in patients with cancer. Medication usually helps this type of depression more effectively than counseling, especially if the medical factors cannot be changed (for example, dosages of the medications that are causing the depression cannot be changed or stopped). Some medical causes of depression in patients with cancer include uncontrolled pain; abnormal levels of calcium, sodium, or potassium in the blood; anemia; vitamin B12 or folate deficiency; fever; and abnormal levels of thyroid hormone or steroids in the blood.

Treatment

Treatment with Drugs

Major depression may be treated with a combination of counseling and medications (drugs), such as antidepressants. A primary care doctor may prescribe medications for depression and refer the patient to a psychiatrist or psychologist for the following reasons:

- a physician or oncologist is not comfortable treating the depression (for example, the patient has suicidal thoughts);
- the symptoms of depression do not improve after 2 to 4 weeks of treatment;
- the symptoms are getting worse;
- the side effects of the medication keep the patient from taking the dosage needed to control the depression; and
- the symptoms are interfering with the patient's ability to continue medical treatment.

Antidepressants are usually effective in the treatment of depression and its symptoms. Unfortunately, antidepressants are not prescribed often for patients with cancer. About 25% of all patients are depressed, but only about 16% receive medication for the depression. The choice of antidepressant depends on the patient's symptoms, potential side effects of the antidepressant, and the person's individual medical problems and previous response to antidepressant drugs.

The Food and Drug Administration (FDA) has issued a warning that patients who are taking antidepressants, such as fluoxetine (Prozac), sertraline (Zoloft), paroxetine (Paxil), fluvoxamine (Luvox), citalopram (Celexa), escitalopram (Lexapro), bupropion (Wellbutrin), venlafaxine (Effexor), nefazodone (Serzone), and mirtazapine (Remeron), should be closely monitored for signs of worsening depression and suicidal thoughts. A Patient Medication Guide (MedGuide) should also be given to patients receiving antidepressants to warn them of the risk and suggest precautions that can be taken.

The FDA has also directed manufacturers of all antidepressant drugs to change the labeling for their products to include a boxed warning and more detailed warning statements about increased risk of suicidal thinking and behavior in children and adolescents being treated with antidepressants. Some studies show that the benefits of proper antidepressant use in children and adolescents, including careful monitoring for suicidal behavior, may outweigh the risks. However, for children younger than 12 years with major depression, only fluoxetine (Prozac) showed benefit compared to a placebo.

Patients with cancer may be treated with a number of drugs throughout their care. Some drugs do not mix safely with certain other drugs, foods, herbals, and nutritional supplements. Certain combinations may reduce or change how drugs work or cause life-threatening side effects. It is important that the patient's healthcare providers be told about all the drugs, herbals, and nutritional supplements the patient is taking, including drugs taken in patches on the skin. This can help prevent unwanted reactions.

St. John's wort (*Hypericum perforatum*) has been used as an over-the-counter supplement for mood enhancement. In the United States, dietary supplements are regulated as foods, not as drugs. The FDA does not require that supplements be approved before being put on the market. Because there are no standards for product manufacturing consistency, dose, or purity, the safety of St. John's wort is not known. The FDA has issued a warning that a significant drug interaction occurs between St. John's wort and indinavir (a drug used to treat HIV [human immunodeficiency virus] infection). When St. John's wort and indinavir are taken together, indinavir is less effective. Patients with symptoms of depression should be evaluated by a health professional and not self-treat with St. John's wort. St. John's wort is not recommended for major depression in patients who have cancer.

Most antidepressants take 3 to 6 weeks to begin working. The side effects must be considered when deciding which antidepressant to use. For example, a medication that causes sleepiness may be helpful in an anxious patient who is having problems sleeping, since the drug is both calming and sedating. Patients who cannot swallow pills may be able to take the medication as a liquid or as an injection. If the antidepressant helps the symptoms, treatment should continue for at least 6 months. Electroconvulsive therapy (ECT) is a useful and safe therapy when other treatments have been unsuccessful in relieving major depression.

Treatment with Psychotherapy

Several psychiatric therapies have been found to be helpful in the treatment of depression related to cancer. Most therapy programs for depression are given in 4 to 30 hours and are offered in both individual and group settings. They may include sessions about cancer education or relaxation skills. These therapies are often used in combination and include crisis intervention, psychotherapy, and thought/behavior techniques. Patients explore methods of lowering distress, improving coping and problem-solving skills; enlisting support; reshaping negative and self-defeating thoughts; and developing a close personal bond with an understanding health care provider. Talking with a clergy member may also be helpful for some people.

Specific goals of these therapies include the following:

- Assist people diagnosed with cancer and their families by answering questions about the illness and its treatment, explaining information, correcting misunderstandings, giving reassurance about the situation, and exploring with the patient how the diagnosis relates to previous experiences with cancer.
- Assist with problem solving, improve the patient's coping skills, and help the patient and family to develop additional coping skills. Explore other areas of stress, such as family role and lifestyle changes, and encourage family members to support and share concern with each other.
- Ensure that the patient and family understand that support will continue when the focus of treatment changes from trying to cure the cancer to relieving symptoms. The health care team will treat symptoms to help the patient control pain and remain comfortable, and will help the patient and his or her family members maintain dignity.

Cancer support groups may also be helpful in treating depression in patients with cancer, especially adolescents. Support groups have been shown to improve mood, encourage the development of coping skills, improve quality of life, and improve immune response. Support groups can be found through the wellness community, the American

Cancer Society, and many community resources, including the social work departments in medical centers and hospitals.

Recent studies of psychotherapy in patients with cancer, including training in problem solving, have shown that it helps decrease feelings of depression.

Section 17.4

Depression and Diabetes

This section includes text from "Patients who suffer from both diabetes and depression have a higher risk of dying," February 2006, and "Patients with diabetes and depression tend to skip self-care behaviors that would help keep their diabetes in check," March 2008. Both documents are from the Agency for Healthcare Research and Quality (AHRQ, www.ahrq.gov).

Patients Who Suffer from Both Diabetes and Depression Have a Higher Risk of Dying

An estimated 10 to 30 percent of people with diabetes also suffer from depression, and they have a higher risk of dying from all causes compared to patients with either condition alone, concludes a study supported by the Agency for Healthcare Research and Quality. More vigilance in recognizing and treating depression among patients with diabetes may improve their outcomes, suggest Leonard E. Egede, M.D., M.S., of the Medical University of South Carolina, and colleagues.

Researchers analyzed mortality rates for coronary heart disease (CHD) and all causes for 10,025 people who participated in the National Health and Nutrition Examination Survey I (1971-1975), then were interviewed in 1982 and followed until 1992. During 8 years of followup, nearly one-fifth of the group (1,925) died, with nearly one-fourth of deaths (522) due to CHD. Compared to patients without diabetes or depression, patients with depression only had a 29 percent and 20 percent higher risk of dying from CHD and all causes, respectively. Patients with diabetes had twice the risk of dying from CHD and all causes. Finally, patients who suffered from both depression and diabetes had more than twice the risk of dying from all causes and CHD.

Patients with Diabetes and Depression Tend to Skip Self-Care Behaviors That Would Help Keep Their Diabetes in Check

Many persons with diabetes also suffer from depression. In fact, a new study found that nearly one-fifth of patients with type 2 diabetes probably suffered from major depression and an additional two-thirds had at least some depressive symptoms. Both the very depressed patients and those with a few depressive symptoms (subclinical depression) were less likely than the 14 percent of patients who were not depressed to perform self-management tasks needed to control their blood-sugar levels.

For example, individuals with major depression (including those on antidepressants) spent fewer days than others following the recommended diet (such as eating lots of fruits and vegetables and spacing carbohydrates throughout the day), exercise, and glucose self-monitoring regimens. They were also 2.3 times more likely to miss medication doses in the prior week than patients who were not depressed.

Major depression was a better predictor of self-monitoring of blood-glucose levels. Yet the depression symptom severity score was a better predictor of not following diet, exercise, and medications. For example, a 1-point increase in the symptom severity score was associated with a 10 percent increase in the odds of missing one or more doses of prescribed medications over the prior week. Also, a symptom severity score of 6 was associated with a half-day less of exercise per week than a score of 1.

These findings challenge the current belief that only major depression is a risk factor for nonadherence to diabetes self-care. They suggest that there is a continuous relationship between symptoms of depression and nonadherence to self-care for diabetes that is evident even at subclinical levels. The findings were based on a survey of 879 patients with type 2 diabetes from two primary care clinics. The study was supported in part by the Agency for Healthcare Research and Quality.

Section 17.5

Depression and Epilepsy

Excerpted from "Seizures and Epilepsy: Hope Through Research," by the National Institute of Neurological Disorders and Stroke (NINDS, www.ninds.nih.gov), part of the National Institutes of Health, December 30, 2008.

What Is Epilepsy?

Epilepsy is a brain disorder in which clusters of nerve cells, or neurons, in the brain sometimes signal abnormally. Neurons normally generate electrochemical impulses that act on other neurons, glands, and muscles to produce human thoughts, feelings, and actions. In epilepsy, the normal pattern of neuronal activity becomes disturbed, causing strange sensations, emotions, and behavior, or sometimes convulsions, muscle spasms, and loss of consciousness. During a seizure, neurons may fire as many as 500 times a second, much faster than normal. In some people, this happens only occasionally; for others, it may happen up to hundreds of times a day.

More than 2 million people in the United States—about 1 in 100—have experienced an unprovoked seizure or been diagnosed with epilepsy. For about 80 percent of those diagnosed with epilepsy, seizures can be controlled with modern medicines and surgical techniques. However, about 25 to 30 percent of people with epilepsy will continue to experience seizures even with the best available treatment. Doctors call this situation intractable epilepsy. Having a seizure does not necessarily mean that a person has epilepsy. Only when a person has had two or more seizures is he or she considered to have epilepsy.

Epilepsy is not contagious and is not caused by mental illness or mental retardation. Some people with mental retardation may experience seizures, but seizures do not necessarily mean the person has or will develop mental impairment. Many people with epilepsy have normal or above-average intelligence.

Famous people who are known or rumored to have had epilepsy include the Russian writer Dostoyevsky, the philosopher Socrates, the military general Napoleon, and the inventor of dynamite, Alfred Nobel, who established the Nobel Prize. Several Olympic medalists and other athletes also have had epilepsy. Seizures sometimes do cause brain damage, particularly if they are severe. However, most seizures do not seem to have a detrimental effect on the brain. Any changes that do occur are usually subtle, and it is often unclear whether these changes are caused by the seizures themselves or by the underlying problem that caused the seizures.

While epilepsy cannot currently be cured, for some people it does eventually go away. One study found that children with idiopathic epilepsy, or epilepsy with an unknown cause, had a 68 to 92 percent chance of becoming seizure-free by 20 years after their diagnosis. The odds of becoming seizure-free are not as good for adults or for children with severe epilepsy syndromes, but it is nonetheless possible that seizures may decrease or even stop over time. This is more likely if the epilepsy has been well-controlled by medication or if the person has had epilepsy surgery.

What Causes Epilepsy?

Epilepsy is a disorder with many possible causes. Anything that disturbs the normal pattern of neuron activity—from illness to brain damage to abnormal brain development—can lead to seizures.

Epilepsy may develop because of an abnormality in brain wiring, an imbalance of nerve signaling chemicals called neurotransmitters, or some combination of these factors. Researchers believe that some people with epilepsy have an abnormally high level of excitatory neurotransmitters that increase neuronal activity, while others have an abnormally low level of inhibitory neurotransmitters that decrease neuronal activity in the brain. Either situation can result in too much neuronal activity and cause epilepsy. One of the most-studied neurotransmitters that plays a role in epilepsy is GABA, or gamma-aminobutyric acid, which is an inhibitory neurotransmitter. Research on GABA has led to drugs that alter the amount of this neurotransmitter in the brain or change how the brain responds to it. Researchers also are studying excitatory neurotransmitters such as glutamate.

In some cases, the brain's attempts to repair itself after a head injury, stroke, or other problem may inadvertently generate abnormal nerve connections that lead to epilepsy. Abnormalities in brain wiring that occur during brain development also may disturb neuronal activity and lead to epilepsy.

Research has shown that the cell membrane that surrounds each neuron plays an important role in epilepsy. Cell membranes are crucial for a neuron to generate electrical impulses. For this reason, researchers are studying details of the membrane structure, how molecules move in and out of membranes, and how the cell nourishes and repairs the membrane. A disruption in any of these processes may lead to epilepsy. Studies in animals have shown that, because the brain continually adapts to changes in stimuli, a small change in neuronal activity, if repeated, may eventually lead to full-blown epilepsy. Researchers are investigating whether this phenomenon, called kindling, may also occur in humans.

In some cases, epilepsy may result from changes in non-neuronal brain cells called glia. These cells regulate concentrations of chemicals in the brain that can affect neuronal signaling.

About half of all seizures have no known cause. However, in other cases, the seizures are clearly linked to infection, trauma, or other identifiable problems.

Mental Health Problems and Epilepsy

It is not uncommon for people with epilepsy, especially children, to develop behavioral and emotional problems. Sometimes these problems are caused by embarrassment or frustration associated with epilepsy. Other problems may result from bullying, teasing, or avoidance in school and other social settings. In children, these problems can be minimized if parents encourage a positive outlook and independence, do not reward negative behavior with unusual amounts of attention, and try to stay attuned to their child's needs and feelings.

Families must learn to accept and live with the seizures without blaming or resenting the affected person. Counseling services can help families cope with epilepsy in a positive manner. Epilepsy support groups also can help by providing a way for people with epilepsy and their family members to share their experiences, frustrations, and tips for coping with the disorder.

People with epilepsy have an increased risk of poor self-esteem, depression, and suicide. These problems may be a reaction to a lack of understanding or discomfort about epilepsy that may result in cruelty or avoidance by other people. Many people with epilepsy also live with an ever-present fear that they will have another seizure.

Section 17.6

Depression and Heart Disease

"Mind/Body Health: Heart Disease" reprinted with permission from http://apahelpcenter.org/articles/article.php?id=102. Copyright © 2004 by the American Psychological Association. Reproduced with permission. No further reproduction or distribution is permitted without written permission from the American Psychological Association.

You might think heart disease is linked only with physical activities—a lack of exercise, poor diet, smoking, and excessive drinking. While these habits do heighten the risk of high blood pressure, heart attacks, strokes, and other cardiovascular problems, your thoughts, attitudes, and emotions are just as important. They can not only accelerate the onset of heart disease, but also get in the way of taking positive steps to improve your health or that of a loved one.

Practicing Prevention

A healthy lifestyle can go a long way toward reducing the risk of heart disease or managing a diagnosed condition, even if you face a higher risk due to uncontrollable factors such as age, sex, or family history. But making changes in your daily life is not always easy. You may sense a loss of control over your life in having to give up favorite foods, make time for exercise in a busy schedule, or take regular medication.

It also takes personal discipline to ingrain these new habits into your lifestyle. Deviating from a prescribed diet or sneaking a cigarette when no one is looking may satisfy an immediate craving, but it won't achieve the long-term goal of improved health.

Coping with Life's Pressures

Heart disease has many other mind-body connections that you should consider. Prolonged stress due to the pressures at home, on the job, or from other sources can contribute to abnormally high blood pressure and circulation problems. As with many other diseases, the effects vary from person to person. Some people use stress as a motivator while others may "snap" at the slightest issue.

How you handle stress also influences how your cardiovascular system responds. Studies have shown that if stress makes you angry or irritable, you're more likely to have heart disease or a heart attack. In fact, the way you respond to stress may be a greater risk factor for heart problems than smoking, high blood pressure, and high cholesterol.

A Downward Spiral

Then there's depression, the persistent feeling of sadness and despair that can isolate you from the rest of the world. In its severest form, clinical depression, this condition can not only increase the risk of heart disease but also worsen an existing condition.

Research shows that while approximately 20 percent of us experience an episode of depression in our lifetimes, the figure climbs to 50 percent among people with heart disease. Long-term studies reveal that men and women diagnosed with clinical depression are more than twice as likely to develop coronary artery disease or suffer a heart attack. In addition, heart patients are three times as likely to be depressed at any given time than the population as a whole.

And happy people have healthier levels of fibrinogen and cortisol in their blood, making them less vulnerable to cardiovascular disease and other ailments.

Left untreated, depression can put you at substantially greater risk of suffering a heart attack or stroke. In fact, clinically depressed people are twice as likely to suffer a heart attack as long as 10 years after the initial depressive episode.

The Struggle to Rebound

Depression can also complicate the aftermath of a heart attack, stroke, or invasive procedure such as open-heart surgery. The immediate shock of coming so close to death is compounded by the prospect of a long recuperation, as well as the fear that another, potentially more serious event could occur without warning.

The result is often feelings of depression, anxiety, isolation, and diminished self-esteem. According to the National Institutes of Mental Health (NIMH), up to 65 percent of coronary heart disease patients with a history of heart attack experience various forms of depression. Though such emotions are not unusual, they should be addressed as quickly as possible. Major depression can complicate the recovery process and actually worsen your condition. Prolonged depression in patients with cardiovascular disease has been shown to contribute to subsequent heart attacks and strokes.

What You Can Do

Although heart disease is a serious condition that requires constant monitoring, there are many things you can do to reduce your risk for cardiovascular problems and live a full, active life, even if you should suffer a heart attack.

- **Talk to your doctor.** No two people are alike, and some treatment or risk reduction strategies may be inappropriate or even harmful if you attempt to do too much too quickly.
- **Avoid trying to fix every problem at once, if possible.** Focus instead on changing one existing habit (e.g., eating habits, inactive lifestyle). Set a reasonable initial goal and work toward meeting it.
- **Don't ignore the symptoms of depression.** Feelings of sadness or emptiness, loss of interest in ordinary or pleasurable activities, reduced energy, and eating and sleep disorders are just a few of depression's many warning signs. If they persist for more than 2 weeks, discuss these issues with your heart doctor. It may be that a psychologist working in collaboration with your physician would be beneficial.
- **Identify the sources of stress in your life and look for ways to reduce and manage them.** Seeing a professional like a psychologist to learn to manage stress is helpful not only for preventing heart disease, but also for speeding recovery from heart attacks when used along with structured exercise programs and other intensive lifestyle changes.
- **Enlist the support of friends, family, and work associates.** Talk with them about your condition and what they can do to help. Social support is particularly critical for overcoming feelings of depression and isolation during recovery from a heart attack.
- **If you feel overwhelmed by the challenge of managing the behaviors associated with heart disease, consult a qualified psychologist.** He or she can help develop personal strategies for setting and achieving reasonable health improvement

goals, as well as building on these successes to accomplish other more ambitious objectives. A psychologist can also help clarify the diagnosis of depression and work with the physician to devise a suitable treatment program.

The American Psychological Association Practice Directorate gratefully acknowledges the assistance of Sara Weiss, Ph.D., and Nancy Molitor, Ph.D., in developing this text.

Section 17.7

Depression and Human Immunodeficiency Virus/Acquired Immunodeficiency Syndrome

What Is Depression?

Depression is a mood disorder. It is more than sadness or grief. Depression is sadness or grief that is more intense and lasts longer than it should. It has various causes:

- events in your daily life
- chemical changes in the brain
- a side effect of medications
- several physical disorders

About 5% to 10% of the general population gets depressed. However, rates of depression in people with HIV are as high as 60%.

Being depressed is not a sign of weakness. It doesn't mean you're going crazy. You cannot "just get over it." Don't expect to be depressed because you are dealing with HIV!

Is Depression Important?

Depression can lead people to miss doses of their medication. It can increase high-risk behaviors that transmit HIV infection to others. Depression might cause some latent viral infections to become active. Overall, depression can make HIV disease progress faster. It also interferes with your ability to enjoy life.

Depression often gets overlooked. Also, many HIV specialists have not been trained to recognize depression. Depression can also be mistaken for signs of advancing HIV.

What Are the Signs of Depression?

Symptoms of depression vary from person to person. Most health care providers suspect depression if patients report feeling blue or having very little interest in daily activities. If these feelings go on for two weeks or longer, and the patient also has some of the following symptoms, they are probably depressed:

- Fatigue or feeling slow and sluggish
- Problems concentrating
- Problems sleeping
- Feeling guilty, worthless, or hopeless
- Decreased appetite or weight loss

What Causes Depression?

Some medications used to treat HIV can cause or worsen depression, especially efavirenz (Sustiva). Diseases such as anemia or diabetes can cause symptoms that look like depression. So can substance use, or low levels of testosterone, vitamin B6, or vitamin B12.

People who are infected with both HIV and hepatitis B or C are more likely to be depressed, especially if they are being treated with interferon. Other risk factors include:

- Being female
- Having a personal or family history of mental illness, alcohol, and substance abuse
- Not enough social support
- Not telling others you are HIV-positive
- Treatment failure (HIV or other)

Treatment for Depression

Depression can be treated with lifestyle changes, alternative therapies, and/or with medications. Many medications and therapies can interfere with your HIV treatment. Your health care provider can help you select the therapy or combination of therapies most appropriate for you. Do not try to self-medicate with alcohol or illegal drugs, as these can increase depression and create additional problems.

Lifestyle changes can improve depression for some people:

- Regular exercise
- Increased exposure to sunlight
- Stress management
- Counseling
- Improved sleep habits

Alternative Therapies

St. John's wort is widely used to treat depression. It interferes with some HIV medications. Do not take St. John's wort if you are taking antiretroviral medications (ARVs).

Valerian or melatonin can help improve your sleep. Supplements of vitamins B6 or B12 can help if you have a shortage.

Antidepressants

Some depression responds best to medication. Antidepressants can interact with some ARVs. They must be used under the supervision of a health care provider who is familiar with your HIV treatment. Ritonavir (in Norvir or Kaletra) and Indinavir (Crixivan) interact the most with antidepressants.

The most common antidepressants used are selective serotonin reuptake inhibitors, called SSRIs. They can cause loss of sexual desire and function, lack of appetite, headache, insomnia, fatigue, upset stomach, diarrhea, and restlessness or anxiety.

The tricyclics have more side effects than the SSRIs. They can also cause sedation, constipation, and erratic heart beat.

Some health care providers also use psychostimulants, the drugs used to treat attention deficit disorder.

A recent study showed that treatment with dehydroepiandrosterone (DHEA) can reduce depression in HIV patients.

A new depression treatment called vagus nerve stimulation (VNS) was approved by the U.S. Food and Drug Administration (FDA). A small generator about the size of a watch is implanted under the skin in the chest. It passes a signal to a part of the brain related to mood and anxiety.

The Bottom Line

Depression is a very common condition for people with HIV. Untreated depression can cause you to miss medication doses and lower your quality of life.

Depression is a "whole body" issue that can interfere with your physical health, thinking, feeling, and behavior.

Section 17.8

Depression and Parkinson Disease

"Combating Depression in Parkinson's Disease," by Matthew Menza, M.D. © 2004 Parkinson's Disease Foundation (www.pdf.org). Reprinted with permission.

Depression is one of the major, and most common, difficulties that faces people living with Parkinson's. Everyone feels sad from time to time and it is normal to experience sadness and stress when faced with a difficult medical illness such as Parkinson's disease. However, the sadness that is part of being human can become a significant problem if it crosses into the realm of clinical depression and is left untreated. People who are depressed often feel sad and don't enjoy life as they used to. They have little energy and struggle to get out of bed in the morning.

Other symptoms of depression include poor appetite, sleep disturbances, fatigue, feelings of guilt, self-criticism and worthlessness, irritability, and anxiety. The presence of these symptoms on most days for 2 weeks suggests a diagnosis of depression, and should be discussed with a physician.

At least 40 percent of people with PD experience clinical depression at some time during the illness. It tends to occur early in the illness and may wax and wane in severity. It causes personal suffering and also appears to accelerate problems with mobility and memory. A patient or caregiver may dismiss signs of depression because he or she assumes the Parkinson's disease itself is causing the problem, as if it is normal to be depressed. This can lead to feelings of helplessness and confusion, which may further exacerbate the problem.

What causes depression in PD? There is no clear answer but most specialists agree that it is probably a combination of living with the stress of a progressive chronic illness and changes in the neurochemistry of the brain that accompany Parkinson's. Depression early in the disease may be a reaction to an anticipated loss of ability and quality of life, while depression in later stages may actually be due to chemical deficiencies. Research suggests that there are PD-related chemical changes in the brain that may lead directly to clinical depression. Many of the areas of the brain that are affected in PD are also important in controlling mood. One of these is the area that produces serotonin, a brain chemical implicated in depression. In addition, the frontal lobe of the brain, which is important in controlling mood, is known to be under-active in PD.

There is no simple formula for treating depression in PD. It is, however, extremely important that the Parkinson's disease itself be optimally treated. Patients with uncontrolled "on-off" periods and freezing episodes are more prone to depression, so it is important to talk with your doctor about the best medications to control these symptoms. Furthermore, some other symptoms of PD—for example, poor sleep, constipation, and fatigue—should be treated to decrease the burden of living with the disease. Once detected, depression is often treatable using medication to help correct chemical imbalances.

Psychological treatments such as stress management and relaxation, as well as learning to cope with social relationships, can also be helpful—as can support groups. In addition, it is important to make efforts to increase activity and to exercise regularly. Exercise is an effective tool in helping both the symptoms of depression and PD.

Many medications are available for depression in PD. The selective "serotonin re-uptake inhibitors" (SSRIs)—which work by making serotonin available for use by the brain—are newer and safer medications of this class. Some common SSRIs are Paxil (paroxetine), Prozac (fluoxetine), and Zoloft (sertraline). These drugs generally have fewer side effects than older antidepressants like Elavil (amitriptyline) and Pamelor (nortriptyline), which can cause low blood pressure. If treatment is administered, remember that antidepressants generally take several weeks to lift symptoms of depression.

There remain many unanswered questions about the cause and the treatment of depression in patients with PD, and the problem is receiving increasing attention from the scientific community. In December 2003, the National Institute of Neurological Disorders and Stroke (NINDS) and the National Institute of Mental Health (NIMH) co-sponsored a conference to explore the mysteries of depression in Parkinson's. A major topic was the challenge of diagnosing depression in a context of similarities between PD symptoms and classic signs of depression. While the group agreed that the current diagnostic criteria for depression in Parkinson's are valid, it acknowledged that special care is required to distinguish depressive symptoms from PD symptoms.

Currently accepted rating scales for depression remain useful for screening PD patients for depression, and for measuring the severity of depression and its response to treatment. The conference ended with a consensus that awareness of depression in PD needs to be raised, along with exploration of the best ways to treat this illness in PD patients.

Finding better approaches to detect and treat depression in PD is already underway in several NIH [National Institutes of Health] clinical trials. Additional research is needed to understand not only the treatment of depression but also its effects on other aspects of life, including sleep, anxiety, memory, and concentration. If you (or a loved one) have PD and symptoms of depression, participating in a research study may help to bring solutions to this disabling problem.

Dr. Matthew Menza, of the Robert Wood Johnson Medical School, is now conducting the first National Institutes of Health-sponsored study of depression in patients with Parkinson's disease. He is a nationally known expert on the treatment of psychiatric problems in patients with PD. Dr. Menza is currently enrolling patients in an NIH sponsored study for research on depression in patients with Parkinson's disease. The study is being conducted at Robert Wood Johnson Medical School in Piscataway, NJ. If you are interested in finding out more about this study you can reach Dr. Menza, toll free 877-795-4673.

Section 17.9

Depression and Stroke

This section includes text excerpted from "Depression and Stroke," by the National Institute of Mental Health (NIMH, www.nimh.nih.gov), part of the National Institutes of Health, May 2002, reviewed and revised by David A. Cooke, M.D., January 10, 2009, and "Preventive Treatment May Help Head Off Depression Following a Stroke," by the NIMH, May 28, 2008.

Depression and Stroke

Depression can strike anyone, but people with serious illnesses such as stroke may be at greater risk. Appropriate diagnosis and treatment of depression may bring substantial benefits to persons recovering from a stroke by improving their medical status, enhancing their quality of life, and reducing their pain and disability. Treatment for depression also can shorten the rehabilitation process, lead to more rapid recovery and resumption of routine, and save health care costs (e.g., eliminate nursing home expenses).

Stroke can occur in all age groups and can happen even to fetuses still in the womb; but three quarters of strokes occur in people 65 years of age and over, making stroke a leading cause of disability in older persons. Of the 600,000 American men and women who experience a first or recurrent stroke each year, an estimated 10 to 27 percent experience major depression. An additional 15 to 40 percent experience some symptoms of depression within 2 months following a stroke. While disability caused by a stroke may give a person good reason to be depressed, the brain injury itself appears to be a major factor.

The average duration of major depression in people who have suffered a stroke is just under a year. Among the factors that affect the likelihood and severity of depression following a stroke are the location of the brain lesion, previous or family history of depression, and prestroke social functioning. Stroke survivors who are also depressed, particularly those with major depressive disorder, may be less compliant with rehabilitation, more irritable, and may experience personality change.

Despite the enormous advances in brain research in the past 20 years, depression often goes undiagnosed and untreated. Stroke survivors, their family members and friends, and even their physicians may misinterpret depressive symptoms as an inevitable reaction to the effects of a stroke. But depression is a separate illness that can and should be treated, even when a person is undergoing poststroke rehabilitation. Although depressive symptoms may overlap with poststroke symptoms, skilled health professionals will recognize the symptoms of depression and inquire about their duration and severity, diagnose the disorder, and suggest appropriate treatment.

Symptoms of Depression

- Persistent sad, anxious, or "empty" mood
- Feelings of hopelessness, pessimism
- Feelings of guilt, worthlessness, helplessness
- Loss of interest or pleasure in hobbies and activities that were once enjoyed, including sex
- Decreased energy, fatigue, being "slowed down"
- Difficulty concentrating, remembering, making decisions
- Insomnia, early-morning awakening, or oversleeping
- Appetite and/or weight changes
- Thoughts of death or suicide or suicide attempts
- Restlessness, irritability

If five or more of these symptoms are present every day for at least 2 weeks and interfere with routine daily activities such as work, self-care, and childcare or social life, seek an evaluation for depression.

Depression Facts

Depression is a serious medical condition that affects thoughts, feelings, and the ability to function in everyday life. Depression can occur at any age. NIMH-sponsored studies estimate that 6 percent of 9-to 17-year olds in the United States and almost 10 percent of American adults, or about 19 million people age 18 and older, experience some form of depression every year. Although available therapies alleviate symptoms in over 80 percent of those treated, less than half of people with depression get the help they need.

Depression results from abnormal functioning of the brain. The causes of depression are currently a matter of intense research. An interaction between genetic predisposition and life history appear to determine a person's level of risk. Episodes of depression may then be triggered by stress, difficult life events, side effects of medications, or other environmental factors. Whatever its origins, depression can limit the energy needed to keep focused on treatment for other disorders, such as a stroke.

Stroke Facts

A stroke occurs when the blood supply to part of the brain is suddenly interrupted or when a blood vessel in the brain bursts, spilling blood into the spaces surrounding brain cells. Symptoms of stroke appear suddenly and often there is more than one symptom at the same time:

- Sudden numbness or weakness of the face, arm, or leg, especially on one side of the body
- Sudden confusion, trouble talking, or understanding speech
- Sudden trouble seeing in one or both eyes
- Sudden trouble walking, dizziness, or loss of balance or coordination
- Sudden severe headache with no known cause

The most important risk factors for stroke are hypertension, heart disease, diabetes, and cigarette smoking. Others include heavy alcohol consumption, high blood cholesterol levels, illicit drug use, and genetic or congenital conditions, particularly vascular abnormalities.

Gender also plays a role in risk for stroke. Men have a higher risk for stroke, but since men do not live as long as women, women are generally older when they have strokes and are more likely to die from them. However, women's hormonal changes during pregnancy, childbirth and menopause increase their risk for stroke. The risk of stroke associated with pregnancy is greatest in the postpartum period—the 6 weeks following childbirth. Risk for stroke also varies among different ethnic and racial groups.

Although stroke is a disease of the brain, it can affect the entire body. Some of the disabilities that can result from a stroke include paralysis, cognitive deficits, speech problems, emotional difficulties, fatigue, and daily living problems. Many people require psychological or psychiatric help after a stroke. Depression, anxiety, frustration, and anger are common poststroke disabilities. Because stroke survivors often have complex rehabilitation needs, progress and recovery are unique for each person. Although a majority of functional abilities may be restored soon after a stroke, recovery is an ongoing process.

Get Treatment for Depression

Depression can affect mind, mood, body, and behavior. While there are many different treatments for depression, they must be carefully chosen by a trained professional based on the circumstances of the person and family. Prescription antidepressant medications are generally well-tolerated and safe for people recovering from a stroke. There are, however, possible interactions among some medications and side effects that require careful monitoring. Therefore, stroke survivors who develop depression, as well as people in treatment for depression who subsequently suffer a stroke, should make sure to tell any physician they visit about the full range of medications they are taking.

Specific types of psychotherapy, or "talk" therapy, also can relieve depression. Sometimes it is beneficial for family members of a stroke survivor to seek counseling as well.

Treatment for depression in stroke survivors should be managed by a mental health professional—for example, a psychiatrist, psychologist, or clinical social worker—who is in close communication with the physician providing the poststroke rehabilitation and treatment. This is especially important when antidepressant medication is prescribed, so that potentially harmful drug interactions can be avoided. In some cases, a mental health professional that specializes in treating individuals with depression and co-occurring physical illnesses such as a stroke may be available.

Recovery from depression takes time. Antidepressant medications can take several weeks to work and may need to be combined with ongoing psychotherapy. Not everyone responds to treatment in the same way. Prescriptions and dosing may need to be adjusted. No matter how severe a stroke, however, the person does not have to suffer from depression. Treatment can be effective.

Use of herbal supplements of any kind should be discussed with a physician before they are tried. For example, St. John's wort, an herbal remedy sold over-the-counter and promoted as a treatment for mild depression, has harmful interactions with a large number of other medications. Combining this herbal remedy with certain prescription medications can cause life-threatening or fatal side effects.

Remember, depression is a treatable disorder of the brain. Depression can be treated in addition to whatever other illnesses a person might have, including stroke. If you think you may be depressed or know someone who is, don't lose hope. Seek help for depression.

Preventive Treatment May Help Head off Depression following a Stroke

For the first time, researchers show that preventive treatment with an antidepressant medication or talk therapy can significantly reduce the risk or delay the start of depression following an acute stroke, according to a study funded by the National Institute of Mental Health (NIMH), part of the National Institutes of Health. These findings differ from past studies attempting to prevent poststroke depression. The study appears in the May 28, 2008, issue of the *Journal of the American Medical Association.*

"Poststroke depression can impede rehabilitation and recovery of functional skills, reduce quality of life, and may also shorten a person's lifespan," notes NIMH Director Thomas R. Insel, M.D. "Thus, early detection and intervention, in addition to preventive methods, are important components of poststroke treatment."

Robert G. Robinson, M.D., of the University of Iowa, and colleagues compared the effects of the antidepressant medication escitalopram (Lexapro) with placebo (sugar pill) in 117 adults, ages 50–90, who had suffered an acute stroke within the previous 3 months. Neither the participants nor the researchers knew who was receiving the medication or a placebo during the study. Another group of 59 adults were randomly selected to receive Problem Solving Therapy (PST), a talk therapy that helps people identify problems that interfere with daily living and contribute to depressive symptoms and then develop strategies to solve those problems. None of the participants had depression at the start of the study.

The researchers tested escitalopram because previous research had shown that it worked quickly and effectively and could be tolerated over the 12-month study period. They chose PST over other forms of talk therapy because it was developed for use in older people.

People who received either escitalopram or PST were less likely to develop depression (8.5 percent and 11.9 percent, respectively) than those who received the placebo (22.4 percent).

This is the first study of its kind to show some cases of poststroke depression can be prevented with intervention. In addition to the need for further studies, greater attention needs to be given to improving the early detection of and interventions for depression during standard stroke care, the researchers say.

Reference: Robinson RG, Jorge RE, Moser DJ, Acion L, Solodkin A, Small SL, Fonzetti P, Hegel M, Arndt S. Escitalopram and problem solving therapy for prevention of poststroke depression: A randomized trial. *JAMA*. 2008 May 28;299(20):2391–2400.

Section 17.10

Depression and Thyroid Problems

Excerpted from "Hypothyroidism In-Depth Report"

Background

The thyroid is a small, butterfly-shaped gland located in the front of the neck that produces hormones, notably thyroxine (T4) and triiodothyronine (T3), which stimulate vital processes in every part of the body. These thyroid hormones have a major impact on the following functions:

- Growth
- Use of energy and oxygen
- Heat production
- Fertility
- The use of vitamins, proteins, carbohydrates, fats, electrolytes, and water
- Immune regulation in the intestine

These hormones can also alter the actions of other hormones and drugs.

Hypothyroidism

Hypothyroidism occurs when thyroxine (T4) levels drop so low that body processes begin to slow down. Hypothyroidism was first diagnosed in the late nineteenth century when doctors observed that surgical removal of the thyroid resulted in the swelling of the hands, face, feet, and tissues around the eyes. They named this syndrome myxedema and correctly concluded that it was the outcome of the absence of substances, thyroid hormones, normally produced by the thyroid gland. Hypothyroidism is usually progressive and irreversible. Treatment, however, is nearly always completely successful and allows a patient to live a fully normal life.

Hypothyroidism is separated into either overt or subclinical disease. That diagnosis is determined on the basis of the TSH [thyroid-stimulating hormone] laboratory blood tests. The normal range of TSH concentration falls between 0.45–4.5 mU/L.

- Patients with mildly underactive (subclinical) thyroid have TSH levels of 4.5–10 mU/L.
- Patients with levels greater than 10 mU/L are considered to have overt hypothyroidism and should be treated with medication.

Subclinical, or mild, hypothyroidism (mildly underactive thyroid), also called early-stage hypothyroidism, is a condition in which thyrotropin (TSH) levels have started to increase in response to an early decline in T4 levels in the thyroid. However, blood tests for T4 are still normal. The patient may have mild symptoms (usually slight fatigue) or none at all. Mildly underactive thyroid is very common (affecting about 10 million Americans) and is a topic of considerable debate among professionals because it is not clear how to manage this condition.

Mildly underactive thyroid does not progress to the full-blown disorder in most people. Experts estimate that each year about 2–5% of people with subclinical thyroid go on to develop overt hypothyroidism. Other factors associated with a higher risk include being an older woman (up to 20% of women over age 60 have subclinical hypothyroidism), having a goiter (enlarged thyroid gland) or thyroid antibodies, or harboring immune factors that suggest an autoimmune condition.

Symptoms

Early symptoms and complaints: Early symptoms of hypothyroidism are subtle and, in older people, can be easily mistaken for symptoms of stress or aging. They include:

- Chronic fatigue
- Difficulty concentrating
- Sensitivity to cold
- Headache
- Muscle and joint aches
- Weight gain, despite diminished appetite
- Constipation
- Dry skin
- Early puberty
- Menstrual irregularities (either heavier-than-normal or lighter-than-normal bleeding)
- Milky discharge from the breasts (galactorrhea)

In premenopausal women, early symptoms can interfere with fertility. A history of miscarriage may be a sign of impending hypothyroidism. Studies suggest that even if thyroid levels are normal, women who have a history of miscarriages often have antithyroid antibodies during early pregnancy and are at risk for developing autoimmune thyroiditis over time.

Later symptoms: As free thyroxine levels fall over the following months, other symptoms may develop:

- Impaired mental activity, including concentration and memory, particularly in the elderly.
- Depression. Some experts believe that even mild thyroid failure may increase susceptibility to major depression.
- Muscle weakness, numbness, pain, and cramps. This can cause an unsteady gait.
- Muscle cramps are common, and carpal tunnel syndrome or symptoms similar to arthritis sometimes develop. In some cases, the arms and legs may feel numb.

- Numbness in the fingers.
- Hearing loss.
- Husky voice.
- Continuing weight gain and possible obesity, in spite of low appetite.
- Some people experience less sweating, and their skin becomes pale.
- Skin and hair changes. Skin becomes pale, rough, and dry. Patients may sweat less. Hair coarsens and even falls out. Nails become brittle.
- Snoring and obstructive sleep apnea (a condition in which in the soft palate in the throat collapses at intervals during sleep, thereby blocking the passage of air).

Effects of Hypothyroidism and Subclinical Hypothyroidism on the Mind

Depression: Depression is common in hypothyroidism and can be severe. Some psychiatrists suspect that even subclinical hypothyroidism may contribute to depression. The two disorders may have some common physiological basis. Adding thyroid hormones to antidepressants may hasten a depressed patient's recovery, even in some patients who have not been diagnosed with hypothyroidism. Hypothyroidism should be considered as a possible cause of any chronic depression, particularly in older women.

Mental and behavioral impairment: Untreated hypothyroidism can, over time, cause mental and behavioral impairment and, eventually, even dementia. Whether treatment can completely reverse problems in memory and concentration is uncertain, although many experts believe that only mental impairment in hypothyroidism that occurs at birth is permanent.

A 2006 study of nearly 6,000 people age 65 years and older concluded that subclinical hypothyroidism is not associated with depression, anxiety, or mental impairment in elderly patients.

Chapter 18

Bipolar Disorder and Its Treatment

Chapter Contents

Section 18.1

All about Bipolar Disorder

Excerpted from "Bipolar Disorder," a booklet by the National Institute of Mental Health (NIMH, www.nimh.nih.gov), part of the National Institutes of Health, January 2007.

Bipolar disorder, also known as manic-depressive illness, is a brain disorder that causes unusual shifts in a person's mood, energy, and ability to function. Different from the normal ups and downs that everyone goes through, the symptoms of bipolar disorder are severe. They can result in damaged relationships, poor job or school performance, and even suicide. But there is good news: bipolar disorder can be treated, and people with this illness can lead full and productive lives.

More than 5.7 million American adults, or about 2.6 percent of the population age 18 and older in any given year, have bipolar disorder. Bipolar disorder typically develops in late adolescence or early adulthood. However, some people have their first symptoms during childhood, and some develop them late in life. It is often not recognized as an illness, and people may suffer for years before it is properly diagnosed and treated. Like diabetes or heart disease, bipolar disorder is a long-term illness that must be carefully managed throughout a person's life.

What Are the Symptoms of Bipolar Disorder?

Bipolar disorder causes dramatic mood swings—from overly "high" and/or irritable to sad and hopeless, and then back again, often with periods of normal mood in between. Severe changes in energy and behavior go along with these changes in mood. The periods of highs and lows are called episodes of mania and depression.

Signs and symptoms of mania (or a manic episode) include:

- increased energy, activity, and restlessness;
- excessively "high," overly good, euphoric mood;
- extreme irritability;

- racing thoughts and talking very fast, jumping from one idea to another;
- distractibility, can't concentrate well;
- little sleep needed;
- unrealistic beliefs in one's abilities and powers;
- poor judgment;
- spending sprees;
- a lasting period of behavior that is different from usual;
- increased sexual drive;
- abuse of drugs, particularly cocaine, alcohol, and sleeping medications;
- provocative, intrusive, or aggressive behavior; and
- denial that anything is wrong.

A manic episode is diagnosed if elevated mood occurs with three or more of the other symptoms most of the day, nearly every day, for 1 week or longer. If the mood is irritable, four additional symptoms must be present.

Signs and symptoms of depression (or a depressive episode) include:

- lasting sad, anxious, or empty mood;
- feelings of hopelessness or pessimism;
- feelings of guilt, worthlessness, or helplessness;
- loss of interest or pleasure in activities once enjoyed, including sex;
- decreased energy, a feeling of fatigue or of being "slowed down";
- difficulty concentrating, remembering, making decisions;
- restlessness or irritability;
- sleeping too much, or can't sleep;
- change in appetite and/or unintended weight loss or gain;
- chronic pain or other persistent bodily symptoms that are not caused by physical illness or injury; and
- thoughts of death or suicide, or suicide attempts.

A depressive episode is diagnosed if five or more of these symptoms last most of the day, nearly every day, for a period of 2 weeks or longer.

A mild to moderate level of mania is called hypomania. Hypomania may feel good to the person who experiences it and may even be associated with good functioning and enhanced productivity. Thus even when family and friends learn to recognize the mood swings as possible bipolar disorder, the person may deny that anything is wrong. Without proper treatment, however, hypomania can become severe mania in some people or can switch into depression.

Sometimes, severe episodes of mania or depression include symptoms of psychosis (or psychotic symptoms). Common psychotic symptoms are hallucinations (hearing, seeing, or otherwise sensing the presence of things not actually there) and delusions (false, strongly held beliefs not influenced by logical reasoning or explained by a person's usual cultural concepts). Psychotic symptoms in bipolar disorder tend to reflect the extreme mood state at the time. For example, delusions of grandiosity, such as believing that one is the President or has special powers or wealth, may occur during mania; delusions of guilt or worthlessness, such as believing that one is ruined and penniless or has committed some terrible crime, may appear during depression. People with bipolar disorder who have these symptoms are sometimes incorrectly diagnosed as having schizophrenia, another severe mental illness.

It may be helpful to think of the various mood states in bipolar disorder as a spectrum or continuous range. At one end is severe depression, above which is moderate depression and then mild low mood, which many people call "the blues" when it is short-lived but is termed "dysthymia" when it is chronic. Then there is normal or balanced mood, above which comes hypomania (mild to moderate mania), and then severe mania.

In some people, however, symptoms of mania and depression may occur together in what is called a mixed bipolar state. Symptoms of a mixed state often include agitation, trouble sleeping, significant change in appetite, psychosis, and suicidal thinking. A person may have a very sad, hopeless mood while at the same time feeling extremely energized.

Bipolar disorder may appear to be a problem other than mental illness—for instance, alcohol or drug abuse, poor school or work performance, or strained interpersonal relationships. Such problems in fact may be signs of an underlying mood disorder.

Diagnosis of Bipolar Disorder

Descriptions offered by people with bipolar disorder give valuable insights into the various mood states associated with the illness:

Depression: I doubt completely my ability to do anything well. It seems as though my mind has slowed down and burned out to the point of being virtually useless . . . [I am] haunt[ed]...with the total, the desperate hopelessness of it all . . . Others say, "it's only temporary, it will pass, you will get over it," but of course they haven't any idea of how I feel, although they are certain they do. If I can't feel, move, think, or care, then what on earth is the point?

Hypomania: At first when I'm high, it's tremendous . . . ideas are fast . . . like shooting stars you follow until brighter ones appear . . . All shyness disappears, the right words and gestures are suddenly there . . . uninteresting people, things, become intensely interesting. Sensuality is pervasive, the desire to seduce and be seduced is irresistible. Your marrow is infused with unbelievable feelings of ease, power, well-being, omnipotence, euphoria . . . you can do anything . . . but, somewhere this changes.

Mania: The fast ideas become too fast and there are far too many . . . overwhelming confusion replaces clarity . . . you stop keeping up with it—memory goes. Infectious humor ceases to amuse. Your friends become frightened . . . everything is now against the grain . . . you are irritable, angry, frightened, uncontrollable, and trapped.

Suicide

Some people with bipolar disorder become suicidal. Anyone who is thinking about committing suicide needs immediate attention, preferably from a mental health professional or a physician. Anyone who talks about suicide should be taken seriously. Risk for suicide appears to be higher earlier in the course of the illness. Therefore, recognizing bipolar disorder early and learning how best to manage it may decrease the risk of death by suicide.

Signs and symptoms that may accompany suicidal feelings include:

- talking about feeling suicidal or wanting to die;
- feeling hopeless, that nothing will ever change or get better;
- feeling helpless, that nothing one does makes any difference;

- feeling like a burden to family and friends;
- abusing alcohol or drugs;
- putting affairs in order (e.g., organizing finances or giving away possessions to prepare for one's death);
- writing a suicide note; and
- putting oneself in harm's way, or in situations where there is a danger of being killed.

If you are feeling suicidal or know someone who is:

- call a doctor, emergency room, or 911 right away to get immediate help;
- make sure you, or the suicidal person, are not left alone; and
- make sure that access is prevented to large amounts of medication, weapons, or other items that could be used for self-harm.

While some suicide attempts are carefully planned over time, others are impulsive acts that have not been well thought out; thus, the final point above may be a valuable long-term strategy for people with bipolar disorder. Either way, it is important to understand that suicidal feelings and actions are symptoms of an illness that can be treated. With proper treatment, suicidal feelings can be overcome.

What Is the Course of Bipolar Disorder?

Episodes of mania and depression typically recur across the life span. Between episodes, most people with bipolar disorder are free of symptoms, but as many as one-third of people have some residual symptoms. A small percentage of people experience chronic unremitting symptoms despite treatment.

The classic form of the illness, which involves recurrent episodes of mania and depression, is called bipolar I disorder. Some people, however, never develop severe mania but instead experience milder episodes of hypomania that alternate with depression; this form of the illness is called bipolar II disorder. When four or more episodes of illness occur within a 12-month period, a person is said to have rapid-cycling bipolar disorder. Some people experience multiple episodes within a single week, or even within a single day. Rapid cycling tends to develop later in the course of illness and is more common among women than among men.

People with bipolar disorder can lead healthy and productive lives when the illness is effectively treated. Without treatment, however, the natural course of bipolar disorder tends to worsen. Over time a person may suffer more frequent (more rapid-cycling) and more severe manic and depressive episodes than those experienced when the illness first appeared. But in most cases, proper treatment can help reduce the frequency and severity of episodes and can help people with bipolar disorder maintain good quality of life.

Can Children and Adolescents Have Bipolar Disorder?

Both children and adolescents can develop bipolar disorder. It is more likely to affect the children of parents who have the illness.

Unlike many adults with bipolar disorder, whose episodes tend to be more clearly defined, children and young adolescents with the illness often experience very fast mood swings between depression and mania many times within a day. Children with mania are more likely to be irritable and prone to destructive tantrums than to be overly happy and elated. Mixed symptoms also are common in youths with bipolar disorder. Older adolescents who develop the illness may have more classic, adult-type episodes and symptoms.

Bipolar disorder in children and adolescents can be hard to tell apart from other problems that may occur in these age groups. For example, while irritability and aggressiveness can indicate bipolar disorder, they also can be symptoms of attention deficit hyperactivity disorder, conduct disorder, oppositional defiant disorder, or other types of mental disorders more common among adults such as major depression or schizophrenia. Drug abuse also may lead to such symptoms.

For any illness, however, effective treatment depends on appropriate diagnosis. Children or adolescents with emotional and behavioral symptoms should be carefully evaluated by a mental health professional. Any child or adolescent who has suicidal feelings, talks about suicide, or attempts suicide should be taken seriously and should receive immediate help from a mental health specialist.

What Causes Bipolar Disorder?

Scientists are learning about the possible causes of bipolar disorder through several kinds of studies. Most scientists now agree that there is no single cause for bipolar disorder—rather, many factors act together to produce the illness.

Because bipolar disorder tends to run in families, researchers have been searching for specific genes—the microscopic "building blocks" of DNA [deoxyribonucleic acid] inside all cells that influence how the body and mind work and grow—passed down through generations that may increase a person's chance of developing the illness. But genes are not the whole story. Studies of identical twins, who share all the same genes, indicate that both genes and other factors play a role in bipolar disorder. If bipolar disorder were caused entirely by genes, then the identical twin of someone with the illness would always develop the illness, and research has shown that this is not the case. But if one twin has bipolar disorder, the other twin is more likely to develop the illness than is another sibling.

In addition, findings from gene research suggest that bipolar disorder, like other mental illnesses, does not occur because of a single gene. It appears likely that many different genes act together, and in combination with other factors of the person or the person's environment, to cause bipolar disorder. Finding these genes, each of which contributes only a small amount toward the vulnerability to bipolar disorder, has been extremely difficult. But scientists expect that the advanced research tools now being used will lead to these discoveries and to new and better treatments for bipolar disorder.

Brain-imaging studies are helping scientists learn what goes wrong in the brain to produce bipolar disorder and other mental illnesses. New brain-imaging techniques allow researchers to take pictures of the living brain at work, to examine its structure and activity, without the need for surgery or other invasive procedures. These techniques include magnetic resonance imaging (MRI), positron emission tomography (PET), and functional magnetic resonance imaging (fMRI). There is evidence from imaging studies that the brains of people with bipolar disorder may differ from the brains of healthy individuals. As the differences are more clearly identified and defined through research, scientists will gain a better understanding of the underlying causes of the illness, and eventually may be able to predict which types of treatment will work most effectively.

How Is Bipolar Disorder Treated?

Most people with bipolar disorder—even those with the most severe forms—can achieve substantial stabilization of their mood swings and related symptoms with proper treatment. Because bipolar disorder is a recurrent illness, long-term preventive treatment is strongly recommended and almost always indicated. A strategy that combines medication and psychosocial treatment is optimal for managing the disorder over time.

In most cases, bipolar disorder is much better controlled if treatment is continuous than if it is on and off. But even when there are no breaks in treatment, mood changes can occur and should be reported immediately to your doctor. The doctor may be able to prevent a full-blown episode by making adjustments to the treatment plan. Working closely with the doctor and communicating openly about treatment concerns and options can make a difference in treatment effectiveness.

In addition, keeping a chart of daily mood symptoms, treatments, sleep patterns, and life events may help people with bipolar disorder and their families to better understand the illness. This chart also can help the doctor track and treat the illness most effectively.

Medications

Medications for bipolar disorder are prescribed by psychiatrists—medical doctors (M.D.) with expertise in the diagnosis and treatment of mental disorders. While primary care physicians who do not specialize in psychiatry also may prescribe these medications, it is recommended that people with bipolar disorder see a psychiatrist for treatment.

Medications known as "mood stabilizers" usually are prescribed to help control bipolar disorder. Several different types of mood stabilizers are available. In general, people with bipolar disorder continue treatment with mood stabilizers for extended periods of time (years). Other medications are added when necessary, typically for shorter periods, to treat episodes of mania or depression that break through despite the mood stabilizer.

- Lithium, the first mood-stabilizing medication approved by the U.S. Food and Drug Administration (FDA) for treatment of mania, is often very effective in controlling mania and preventing the recurrence of both manic and depressive episodes.
- Anticonvulsant medications, such as valproate (Depakote) or carbamazepine (Tegretol), also can have mood-stabilizing effects and may be especially useful for difficult-to-treat bipolar episodes. Valproate was FDA-approved in 1995 for treatment of mania.
- Newer anticonvulsant medications, including lamotrigine (Lamictal), gabapentin (Neurontin), and topiramate (Topamax), are being studied to determine how well they work in stabilizing mood cycles.

- Anticonvulsant medications may be combined with lithium, or with each other, for maximum effect.
- Children and adolescents with bipolar disorder generally are treated with lithium, but valproate and carbamazepine also are used. Researchers are evaluating the safety and efficacy of these and other psychotropic medications in children and adolescents. There is some evidence that valproate may lead to adverse hormone changes in teenage girls and polycystic ovary syndrome in women who began taking the medication before age 20. Therefore, young female patients taking valproate should be monitored carefully by a physician.
- Women with bipolar disorder who wish to conceive, or who become pregnant, face special challenges due to the possible harmful effects of existing mood stabilizing medications on the developing fetus and the nursing infant. Therefore, the benefits and risks of all available treatment options should be discussed with a clinician skilled in this area. New treatments with reduced risks during pregnancy and lactation are under study.
- Atypical antipsychotic medications, including clozapine (Clozaril), olanzapine (Zyprexa), risperidone (Risperdal), and ziprasidone (Geodon), can be used as possible treatments for bipolar disorder. Evidence suggests clozapine may be helpful as a mood stabilizer for people who do not respond to lithium or anticonvulsants. Other research has supported the efficacy of olanzapine for acute mania, an indication that has recently received FDA approval. Aripiprazole (Abilify) is another atypical antipsychotic medication used to treat the symptoms of schizophrenia and manic or mixed (manic and depressive) episodes of bipolar I disorder. Aripiprazole is in tablet and liquid form. An injectable form is used in the treatment of symptoms of agitation in schizophrenia and manic or mixed episodes of bipolar I disorder. Olanzapine may also help relieve psychotic depression.
- If insomnia is a problem, a high-potency benzodiazepine medication such as clonazepam (Klonopin) or lorazepam (Ativan) may be helpful to promote better sleep. However, since these medications may be habit-forming, they are best prescribed on a short-term basis. Other types of sedative medications, such as zolpidem (Ambien), are sometimes used instead.

- Changes to the treatment plan may be needed at various times during the course of bipolar disorder to manage the illness most effectively. A psychiatrist should guide any changes in type or dose of medication.
- Be sure to tell the psychiatrist about all other prescription drugs, over-the-counter medications, or natural supplements you may be taking. This is important because certain medications and supplements taken together may cause adverse reactions.
- To reduce the chance of relapse or of developing a new episode, it is important to stick to the treatment plan. Talk to your doctor if you have any concerns about the medications.

Thyroid Function

People with bipolar disorder often have abnormal thyroid gland function. Because too much or too little thyroid hormone alone can lead to mood and energy changes, it is important that thyroid levels are carefully monitored by a physician.

People with rapid cycling tend to have co-occurring thyroid problems and may need to take thyroid pills in addition to their medications for bipolar disorder. Also, lithium treatment may cause low thyroid levels in some people resulting in the need for thyroid supplementation.

Medication Side Effects

Before starting a new medication for bipolar disorder, always talk with your psychiatrist and/or pharmacist about possible side effects. Depending on the medication, side effects may include weight gain, nausea, tremor, reduced sexual drive or performance, anxiety, hair loss, movement problems, or dry mouth. Be sure to tell the doctor about all side effects you notice during treatment. He or she may be able to change the dose or offer a different medication to relieve them. Your medication should not be changed or stopped without the psychiatrist's guidance.

Psychosocial Treatments

As an addition to medication, psychosocial treatments—including certain forms of psychotherapy (or "talk" therapy)—are helpful in providing support, education, and guidance to people with bipolar disorder and their families. Studies have shown that psychosocial interventions can lead to increased mood stability, fewer hospitalizations, and improved functioning in several areas. A licensed psychologist, social worker, or counselor typically provides these therapies and often works together with the psychiatrist to monitor a patient's progress. The number, frequency, and type of sessions should be based on the treatment needs of each person.

Psychosocial interventions commonly used for bipolar disorder are cognitive behavioral therapy, psychoeducation, family therapy, and a newer technique, interpersonal and social rhythm therapy. NIMH researchers are studying how these interventions compare to one another when added to medication treatment for bipolar disorder.

- Cognitive behavioral therapy helps people with bipolar disorder learn to change inappropriate or negative thought patterns and behaviors associated with the illness.
- Psychoeducation involves teaching people with bipolar disorder about the illness and its treatment, and how to recognize signs of relapse so that early intervention can be sought before a full-blown illness episode occurs. Psychoeducation also may be helpful for family members.
- Family therapy uses strategies to reduce the level of distress within the family that may either contribute to or result from the ill person's symptoms.
- Interpersonal and social rhythm therapy helps people with bipolar disorder both to improve interpersonal relationships and to regularize their daily routines. Regular daily routines and sleep schedules may help protect against manic episodes.
- As with medication, it is important to follow the treatment plan for any psychosocial intervention to achieve the greatest benefit.

Other Treatments

- In situations where medication, psychosocial treatment, and the combination of these interventions prove ineffective, or work too slowly to relieve severe symptoms such as psychosis or suicidality, electroconvulsive therapy (ECT) may be considered. ECT may also be considered to treat acute episodes when medical conditions, including pregnancy, make the use of medications too risky. ECT is a highly effective treatment for severe depressive, manic, and/or mixed episodes. The possibility of long-lasting memory problems, although a concern in the past, has been significantly reduced with modern ECT techniques. However, the potential benefits and risks of ECT, and of available alternative interventions, should be carefully reviewed and discussed with individuals considering this treatment and, where appropriate, with family or friends.

- Herbal or natural supplements, such as St. John's wort (*Hypericum perforatum*), have not been well studied, and little is known about their effects on bipolar disorder. Because the FDA does not regulate their production, different brands of these supplements can contain different amounts of active ingredient. Before trying herbal or natural supplements, it is important to discuss them with your doctor. There is evidence that St. John's wort can reduce the effectiveness of certain medications. In addition, like prescription antidepressants, St. John's wort may cause a switch into mania in some individuals with bipolar disorder, especially if no mood stabilizer is being taken.
- Omega-3 fatty acids found in fish oil are being studied to determine their usefulness, alone and when added to conventional medications, for long-term treatment of bipolar disorder.

Do Other Illnesses Co-Occur with Bipolar Disorder?

Alcohol and drug abuse are very common among people with bipolar disorder. Research findings suggest that many factors may contribute to these substance abuse problems, including self-medication of symptoms, mood symptoms either brought on or perpetuated by substance abuse, and risk factors that may influence the occurrence of both bipolar disorder and substance use disorders. Treatment for co-occurring substance abuse, when present, is an important part of the overall treatment plan.

Anxiety disorders, such as post-traumatic stress disorder and obsessive-compulsive disorder, also may be common in people with bipolar disorder. Co-occurring anxiety disorders may respond to the treatments used for bipolar disorder, or they may require separate treatment.

Anyone with bipolar disorder should be under the care of a psychiatrist skilled in the diagnosis and treatment of this disease. Other mental health professionals, such as psychologists and psychiatric social workers, can assist in providing the person and family with additional approaches to treatment.

Help can be found at:

- university—or medical school—affiliated programs;
- hospital departments of psychiatry;
- private psychiatric offices and clinics;
- health maintenance organizations (HMOs);
- offices of family physicians, internists, and pediatricians; and
- public community mental health centers.

People with bipolar disorder may need help to get help.

- Often people with bipolar disorder do not realize how impaired they are, or they blame their problems on some cause other than mental illness.
- A person with bipolar disorder may need strong encouragement from family and friends to seek treatment. Family physicians can play an important role in providing referral to a mental health professional.
- Sometimes a family member or friend may need to take the person with bipolar disorder for proper mental health evaluation and treatment.
- A person who is in the midst of a severe episode may need to be hospitalized for his or her own protection and for much-needed treatment. There may be times when the person must be hospitalized against his or her wishes.
- Ongoing encouragement and support are needed after a person obtains treatment, because it may take a while to find the best treatment plan for each individual.
- In some cases, individuals with bipolar disorder may agree, when the disorder is under good control, to a preferred course of action in the event of a future manic or depressive relapse.
- Like other serious illnesses, bipolar disorder is also hard on spouses, family members, friends, and employers.
- Family members of someone with bipolar disorder often have to cope with the person's serious behavioral problems, such as wild spending sprees during mania or extreme withdrawal from others during depression, and the lasting consequences of these behaviors.

- Many people with bipolar disorder benefit from joining support groups such as those sponsored by the National Depressive and Manic Depressive Association (NDMDA), the National Alliance for the Mentally Ill (NAMI), and the National Mental Health Association (NMHA). Families and friends can also benefit from support groups offered by these organizations.

Some people with bipolar disorder receive medication and/or psychosocial therapy by volunteering to participate in clinical studies (clinical trials). Clinical studies involve the scientific investigation of illness and treatment of illness in humans. Clinical studies in mental health can yield information about the efficacy of a medication or a combination of treatments, the usefulness of a behavioral intervention or type of psychotherapy, the reliability of a diagnostic procedure, or the success of a prevention method. Clinical studies also guide scientists in learning how illness develops, progresses, lessens, and affects both mind and body. Millions of Americans diagnosed with mental illness lead healthy, productive lives because of information discovered through clinical studies. These studies are not always right for everyone, however. It is important for each individual to consider carefully the possible risks and benefits of a clinical study before making a decision to participate.

In recent years, NIMH has introduced a new generation of "real-world" clinical studies. They are called "real-world" studies for several reasons. Unlike traditional clinical trials, they offer multiple different treatments and treatment combinations. In addition, they aim to include large numbers of people with mental disorders living in communities throughout the United States and receiving treatment across a wide variety of settings. Individuals with more than one mental disorder, as well as those with co-occurring physical illnesses, are encouraged to consider participating in these new studies. The main goal of the real-world studies is to improve treatment strategies and outcomes for all people with these disorders. In addition to measuring improvement in illness symptoms, the studies will evaluate how treatments influence other important, real-world issues such as quality of life, ability to work, and social functioning. They also will assess the cost-effectiveness of different treatments and factors that affect how well people stay on their treatment plans.

The Systematic Treatment Enhancement Program for Bipolar Disorder (STEP-BD) completed data collection at the end of September 2005 for the largest-ever, "real-world" study of treatments for bipolar disorder. To learn more about STEP-BD or other clinical studies, see the Clinical Trials page on the NIMH website http://www.nimh.nih.gov, or visit the National Library of Medicine's clinical trials database http://www.clinicaltrials.gov.

Section 18.2

Cyclothymic Disorder: A Form of Bipolar Disorder

Alternative Names

Cyclothymia

Definition

Cyclothymic disorder is a mild form of bipolar disorder characterized by alternating episodes of mood swings from mild or moderate depression to hypomania, in which the person experiences elevated mood, euphoria, and excitement, but does not become disconnected from reality.

Causes

The cause of cyclothymic disorder is unknown. Although the changes in mood are irregular and abrupt, the severity of the mood swings is far less extreme than that seen with bipolar disorder (manic depressive illness). Unlike in bipolar disorder, periods of hypomania in cyclothymic disorder do not progress into actual mania. In actual mania, a person may lose control over his or her behavior and go on spending binges, engage in highly risky sexual or drug-taking behavior, and become detached from reality.

Hypomanic periods can be energizing and a source of productivity, but may cause some people to become impulsive and unconcerned about others' feelings, which can damage relationships. Because hypomania feels good, some people with cyclothymia do not want to treat it.

Symptoms

- Alternating episodes of hypomania and mild depression lasting for at least 2 years
- Persistent symptoms (less than 2 consecutive symptom-free months)

Exams and Tests

The person's own description of the behavior usually leads to diagnosis of the disorder.

Treatment

Cyclothymia can often be effectively treated with a combination of antimanic drugs, antidepressants, or psychotherapy.

Support Groups

The stress of illness may be eased by joining a support group whose members share common experiences and problems.

Outlook (Prognosis)

People may decline to seek treatment during their cheerful and uninhibited moods. Long-term therapy, however, is likely to be needed.

Possible Complications

Potential for progression to bipolar disorder.

When to Contact a Medical Professional

Call a mental health professional if you or your child experiences persistent alternating periods of depression and excitement that negatively affect work or social life.

Chapter 19

Seasonal Affective Disorder (SAD)

Chapter Contents

Section 19.1

What Is SAD?

Maggie started off her junior year of high school with great energy. She had no trouble keeping up with her schoolwork and was involved in several after-school activities. But after the Thanksgiving break, she began to have difficulty getting through her assigned reading and had to work harder to apply herself. She couldn't concentrate in class, and after school all she wanted to do was sleep.

Maggie's grades began to drop and she rarely felt like socializing. Even though Maggie was always punctual before, she began to have trouble getting up on time and was absent or late from school many days during the winter.

At first, Maggie's parents thought she was slacking off. They were upset with her, but figured it was just a phase—especially since her energy finally seemed to return in the spring. But when the same thing happened the following November, they took Maggie to the doctor, who diagnosed her with a type of depression called seasonal affective disorder.

What Is Seasonal Affective Disorder?

Seasonal affective disorder (SAD) is a form of depression that appears at the same time each year. With SAD, a person typically has symptoms of depression and unexplained fatigue as winter approaches and daylight hours become shorter. When spring returns and days become longer again, people with SAD experience relief from their symptoms, returning to their usual mood and energy level.

What Causes SAD?

Experts believe that, with SAD, depression is somehow triggered by the brain's response to decreased daylight exposure. No one really understands how and why this happens. Current theories about what causes SAD focus on the role that sunlight might play in the brain's production of key hormones.

Experts think that two specific chemicals in the brain, melatonin and serotonin may be involved in SAD. These two hormones help regulate a person's sleep-wake cycles, energy, and mood. Shorter days and longer hours of darkness in fall and winter may cause increased levels of melatonin and decreased levels of serotonin, creating the biological conditions for depression.

Melatonin is linked to sleep. The body produces this hormone in greater quantities when it's dark or when days are shorter. This increased production of melatonin can cause a person to feel sleepy and lethargic.

With serotonin, it's the reverse—serotonin production goes up when a person is exposed to sunlight, so it's likely that a person will have lower levels of serotonin during the winter when the days are shorter. Low levels of serotonin are associated with depression, whereas increasing the availability of serotonin helps to combat depression.

What Are the Symptoms of SAD?

Someone with SAD will show several particular changes from the way he or she normally feels and acts. These changes occur in a predictable seasonal pattern. The symptoms of SAD are the same as symptoms of depression, and a person with SAD may notice several or all of these symptoms:

Changes in mood: A person may feel sad or be in an irritable mood most of the time for at least 2 weeks during a specific time of year. During that time, a guy or girl may feel a sense of hopelessness or worthlessness. As part of the mood change that goes with SAD, people can be self-critical; they may also be more sensitive than usual to criticism and cry or get upset more often or more easily.

Lack of enjoyment: Someone with SAD may lose interest in things he or she normally likes to do and may seem unable to enjoy things as before. People with SAD can also feel like they no longer do certain tasks as well as they used to, and they may have feelings of dissatisfaction or guilt. A person with SAD may seem to lose interest in friends and may stop participating in social activities.

Low energy: Unusual tiredness or unexplained fatigue is also part of SAD and can cause people to feel low on energy.

Changes in sleep: A person may sleep much more than usual. Excessive sleeping can make it impossible for a student to get up and get ready for school in the morning.

Changes in eating: Changes in eating and appetite related to SAD may include cravings for simple carbohydrates (think comfort foods and sugary foods) and the tendency to overeat. Because of this change in eating, SAD can result in weight gain during the winter months.

Difficulty concentrating: SAD can affect concentration, too, interfering with a person's school performance and grades. A student may have more trouble than usual completing assignments on time or seem to lack his or her usual motivation. Someone with SAD may notice that his or her grades may drop, and teachers may comment that the student seems less motivated or is making less effort in school.

Less time socializing: People with SAD may spend less time with friends, in social activities, or in extracurricular activities.

The problems caused by SAD, such as lower-than-usual grades or less energy for socializing with friends, can affect self-esteem and leave a person feeling disappointed, isolated, and lonely—especially if he or she doesn't realize what's causing the changes in energy, mood, and motivation.

Like other forms of depression, the symptoms of SAD can be mild, severe, or anywhere in between. Milder symptoms interfere less with someone's ability to participate in everyday activities, but stronger symptoms can interfere much more. It's the seasonal pattern of SAD—the fact that symptoms occur only for a few months each winter (for at least 2 years in a row) but not during other seasons—that distinguishes SAD from other forms of depression.

Who Gets SAD?

SAD can affect adults, teens, and children. It's estimated that about 6 in every 100 people (6%) experience SAD.

The number of people with SAD varies from region to region. One study of SAD in the United States found the rates of SAD were seven times higher among people in New Hampshire than in Florida, suggesting that the farther people live from the equator, the more likely they are to develop SAD.

Interestingly, when people who get SAD travel to areas far south of the equator that have longer daylight hours during winter months, they do not get their seasonal symptoms. This supports the theory that SAD is related to light exposure.

Most people don't get seasonal depression (SAD), even if they live in areas where days are shorter during winter months. Experts don't fully understand why certain people are more likely to experience SAD than others. It may be that some people are more sensitive than others to variations in light, and therefore may experience more dramatic shifts in hormone production, depending on their exposure to light.

Like other forms of depression, females are about four times more likely than males to develop SAD. People with relatives who have experienced depression are also more likely to develop it. Individual biology, brain chemistry, family history, environment, and life experiences may also make certain individuals more prone to SAD and other forms of depression.

Researchers are continuing to investigate what leads to SAD, as well as why some people are more likely than others to experience it.

How Is SAD Diagnosed and Treated?

Doctors and mental health professionals make a diagnosis of SAD after a careful evaluation. A medical checkup is also important to make sure that symptoms aren't due to a medical condition that needs treatment. Tiredness, fatigue, and low energy could be a sign of another medical condition such as hypothyroidism, hypoglycemia, or mononucleosis. Other medical conditions can cause appetite changes, sleep changes, or extreme fatigue.

Once a person's been diagnosed with SAD, doctors may recommend one of several treatments:

Increased light exposure: Because the symptoms of SAD are triggered by lack of exposure to light, and they tend to go away on their own when available light increases, treatment for SAD often involves increased exposure to light during winter months. For someone with mild symptoms, it may be enough to spend more time outside during the daylight hours, perhaps by exercising outdoors or taking a daily walk. Full spectrum (daylight) light bulbs that fit in regular lamps can help bring a bit more daylight into your home in winter months and might help with mild symptoms.

Light therapy: Stronger symptoms of SAD may be treated with light therapy (also called phototherapy). Light therapy involves the use of a special light that simulates daylight. A special light box or panel is placed on a tabletop or desk, and the person sits in front of the light for a short period of time every day (45 minutes a day or so, usually in the morning). The person should occasionally glance at the light (the light has to be absorbed through the retinas in order to work), but not stare into it for long periods. Symptoms tend to improve within a few days in some cases or within a few weeks in others. Generally, doctors recommend the use of light therapy until enough sunlight is available outdoors.

Like any medical treatment, light treatment should only be used under the supervision of a doctor. People who have another type of depressive disorder, skin that's sensitive to light, or medical conditions that may make the eyes vulnerable to light damage should use light therapy with caution. The lights that are used for SAD phototherapy must filter out harmful UV rays. Tanning beds or booths should not be used to alleviate symptoms of SAD. Some mild side effects of phototherapy might include headache or eyestrain.

Talk therapy: Talk therapy (psychotherapy) is also used to treat people with SAD. Talk therapy focuses on revising the negative thoughts and feelings associated with depression and helps ease the sense of isolation or loneliness that people with depression often feel. The support and guidance of a professional therapist can be helpful for someone experiencing SAD. Talk therapy can also help someone to learn about and understand their condition as well as learn what to do to prevent or minimize future bouts of seasonal depression.

Medication: Doctors may also prescribe medications for teens with SAD. Antidepressant medications help to regulate the balance of serotonin and other neurotransmitters in the brain that affect mood and energy. Medications need to be prescribed and monitored by a doctor. If your doctor prescribes medication for SAD or another form of depression, be sure to let him or her know about any other medications or remedies you may be taking, including over-the-counter or herbal medicines. These can interfere with prescription medications.

Dealing with SAD

When symptoms of SAD first develop, it can be confusing, both for the person with SAD and family and friends. Some parents or teachers may mistakenly think that teens with SAD are slacking off or not trying their best. If you think you're experiencing some of the symptoms of SAD, talk to a parent, guidance counselor, or other trusted adult about what you're feeling.

If you've been diagnosed with SAD, there are a few things you can do to help:

- Follow your doctor's recommendations for treatment.
- Learn all you can about SAD and explain the condition to others so they can work with you.
- Get plenty of exercise, especially outdoors. Exercise can be a mood lifter.
- Spend time with friends and loved ones who understand what you're going through—they can help provide you with personal contact and a sense of connection.
- Be patient. Don't expect your symptoms to go away immediately.
- Ask for help with homework and other assignments if you need it.
- If you feel you can't concentrate on things, remember that it's part of the disorder and that things will get better again. Talk to your teachers and work out a plan to get your assignments done.
- Eat right. It may be hard, but avoiding simple carbohydrates and sugary snacks and concentrating on plenty of whole grains, vegetables, and fruits can help you feel better in the long term.
- Develop a sleep routine. Regular bedtimes can help you reap the mental health benefits of daytime light.

Depression in any form can be serious. If you think you have symptoms of any type of depression, talk to someone who can help you get treatment.

Section 19.2

Light and Melatonin Reduce SAD Symptoms

From "Properly Timed Light, Melatonin Lift Winter Depression by Syncing Rhythms," by the National Institute of Mental Health (NIMH, www.nimh.nih.gov), part of the National Institutes of Health, May 1, 2006.

Most seasonal affective disorder (SAD) symptoms stem from daily body rhythms that have gone out-of-sync with the sun, a NIMH-funded study has found. The researchers propose that most patients will respond best to a low dose of the light-sensitive hormone melatonin in the afternoon in addition to bright light in the morning. Rhythms that have lost their bearings due to winter's late dawn and early dusk accounted for 65 percent of SAD symptoms; realigning them explained 35 percent of melatonin's antidepressant effect in patients with delayed rhythms, the most common form of SAD, report NIMH grantee Alfred Lewy, M.D., Ph.D., and colleagues at the Oregon Health & Science University, online, April 28, 2006, in the *Proceedings of the National Academy of Sciences*.

SAD affects many people in northern latitudes in winter, especially young women, and is usually treated with bright light in the morning. The pineal gland, located in the middle of the brain, responds to darkness by secreting melatonin, which resets the brain's central clock and helps the light/dark cycle reset the sleep/wake cycle and other daily rhythms. Lewy and colleagues pinpointed how rhythms go astray in SAD and how they can be reset by taking melatonin supplements at the right time of day. The findings strengthen the case for daily rhythm mismatches as the cause of SAD.

The researchers tracked sleep, activity levels, melatonin rhythms, and depression symptoms of 68 SAD patients who took either low doses of melatonin or a placebo in the morning or afternoon for a winter month when they were most symptomatic. They had determined from healthy subjects that a person's rhythms are synchronized when the interval between the time the pineal gland begins secreting melatonin and the middle of sleep is about 6 hours.

Seventy-one percent of the SAD patients had intervals shorter than 6 hours, indicating that their rhythms were delayed due to the later winter dawn. Taking melatonin capsules in the afternoon lengthened their intervals, bringing their rhythms back toward normal. The closer their intervals approached the ideal 6 hours, the more their mood improved on depression rating scales, supporting the hypothesized link between out-of-sync rhythms and SAD.

"SAD may be the first psychiatric disorder in which a physiological marker correlates with symptom severity before, and in the course of, treatment in the same patients," explained Lewy, referring to patients' rhythm shifts towards the 6 hour interval in response to melatonin.

Taking melatonin at the correct time of day—afternoon for patients with short intervals and morning for the 29 percent of patients with long intervals—more than doubled their improvement in depression scores, compared to taking a placebo or the hormone at the incorrect time. While the study was not designed to test the efficacy of melatonin treatment, the researchers suggest that its clinical benefit "appears to be substantial, although not as robust as light treatment." They propose that the 6-hour interval index may be useful for analyzing the circadian components of non-seasonal depression and other sleep and psychiatric disorders.

Also participating in the study were: Bryan Lefler, Jonathan Emens, Oregon Health and Science University, and Vance Bauer, Kaiser Permanente Northwest Center for Health Research.

Lewy AJ, Lefler BJ, Emens JS, Bauer VK. The circadian basis of winter depression. *Proc Natl Acad Sci U S A.* 2006 Apr 28.

Chapter 20

Premenstrual Syndrome and Premenstrual Dysphoric Disorder

Chapter Contents

Section 20.1

Premenstrual Syndrome

From the Office of Women's Health (www.womenshealth.gov), part of the U.S. Department of Health and Human Services, January 2007.

What is premenstrual syndrome (PMS)?

Premenstrual syndrome (PMS) is a group of symptoms linked to the menstrual cycle. PMS symptoms occur in the week or 2 weeks before your period (menstruation or monthly bleeding). The symptoms usually go away after your period starts. PMS can affect menstruating women of any age. It is also different for each woman. PMS may be just a monthly bother or it may be so severe that it makes it hard to even get through the day. Monthly periods stop during menopause, bringing an end to PMS.

What causes PMS?

The causes of PMS are not clear. It is linked to the changing hormones during the menstrual cycle. Some women may be affected more than others by changing hormone levels during the menstrual cycle. Stress and emotional problems do not seem to cause PMS, but they may make it worse.

Diagnosis of PMS is usually based on your symptoms, when they occur, and how much they affect your life.

What are the symptoms of PMS?

PMS often includes both physical and emotional symptoms. Common symptoms are:

- acne;
- breast swelling and tenderness;
- feeling tired;
- having trouble sleeping;

- upset stomach, bloating, constipation, or diarrhea;
- headache or backache;
- appetite changes or food cravings;
- joint or muscle pain;
- trouble concentrating or remembering;
- tension, irritability, mood swings, or crying spells; and
- anxiety or depression.

Symptoms vary from one woman to another. If you think you have PMS, keep track of which symptoms you have and how severe they are for a few months. You can use a calendar to write down the symptoms you have each day or you can use a form to track your symptoms. If you go to the doctor for your PMS, take this form with you.

How common is PMS?

Estimates of the percentage of women affected by PMS vary widely. According to the American College of Obstetricians and Gynecologists, at least 85 percent of menstruating women have at least one PMS symptom as part of their monthly cycle. Most of these women have symptoms that are fairly mild and do not need treatment. Some women (about 3 to 8 percent of menstruating women) have a more severe form of PMS, called premenstrual dysphoric disorder (PMDD).

PMS occurs more often in women who:

- are between their late 20s and early 40s;
- have at least one child;
- have a family history of depression; or
- have a past medical history of either postpartum depression or a mood disorder.

What is the treatment for PMS?

Many things have been tried to ease the symptoms of PMS. No treatment works for every woman, so you may need to try different ones to see what works. If your PMS is not so bad that you need to see a doctor, some lifestyle changes may help you feel better. Below are some lifestyle changes that may help ease your symptoms.

- Take a multivitamin every day that includes 400 micrograms of folic acid. A calcium supplement with vitamin D can help keep bones strong and may help ease some PMS symptoms.
- Exercise regularly.
- Eat healthy foods, including fruits, vegetables, and whole grains.
- Avoid salt, sugary foods, caffeine, and alcohol, especially when you are having PMS symptoms.
- Get enough sleep. Try to get 8 hours of sleep each night.
- Find healthy ways to cope with stress. Talk to your friends, exercise, or write in a journal.
- Don't smoke.

Over-the-counter pain relievers such as ibuprofen, aspirin, or naproxen may help ease cramps, headaches, backaches, and breast tenderness.

In more severe cases of PMS, prescription medicines may be used to ease symptoms. One approach has been to use drugs such as birth control pills to stop ovulation from occurring. Women on the pill report fewer PMS symptoms, such as cramps and headaches, as well as lighter periods.

What is premenstrual dysphoric disorder (PMDD)?

There is evidence that a brain chemical called serotonin plays a role in a severe form of PMS, called premenstrual dysphoric disorder (PMDD). The main symptoms, which can be disabling, include:

- feelings of sadness or despair, or possibly suicidal thoughts;
- feelings of tension or anxiety;
- panic attacks;
- mood swings, crying;
- lasting irritability or anger that affects other people;
- disinterest in daily activities and relationships;
- trouble thinking or focusing;
- tiredness or low energy;

- food cravings or binge eating;
- having trouble sleeping;
- feeling out of control;
- physical symptoms, such as bloating, breast tenderness, headaches; and
- and joint or muscle pain.

You must have five or more of these symptoms to be diagnosed with PMDD. Symptoms occur during the week before your period and go away after bleeding starts.

Making some lifestyle changes may help ease PMDD symptoms.

Antidepressants called selective serotonin reuptake inhibitors (SSRIs) that change serotonin levels in the brain have also been shown to help some women with PMDD. The Food and Drug Administration (FDA) has approved three medications for the treatment of PMDD:

- sertraline (Zoloft®);
- fluoxetine (Sarafem®); and
- paroxetine HCI (Paxil CR®).

Individual counseling, group counseling, and stress management may also help relieve symptoms.

Section 20.2

Premenstrual Dysphoric Disorder

Definition

Premenstrual dysphoric disorder (PMDD) is a condition marked by severe depression, irritability, and tension before menstruation. These symptoms are more severe than those seen with premenstrual syndrome (PMS).

Causes

The causes of PMS and PMDD have not been identified, although social, cultural, biological, and psychological factors all appear to be involved. Researchers estimate that PMDD affects between 3% and 8% of women in their reproductive years.

Major depression is very common with PMDD, although PMDD can occur in women who do not have a history of major depression.

Studies have found that women who have seasonal affective disorder (SAD), a form of depression characterized by annual episodes of depression during fall or winter that improve in the spring or summer, are likely to also have PMDD.

Symptoms

The symptoms of PMDD are similar to those of PMS, but they are generally more severe and debilitating. Symptoms occur during the last week of most menstrual cycles and usually improve within a few days after the period starts.

Five or more of the following symptoms must be present:

- Feeling of sadness or hopelessness, possible suicidal thoughts
- Feelings of tension or anxiety
- Panic attacks

- Mood swings marked by periods of teariness
- Persistent irritability or anger that affects other people
- Disinterest in daily activities and relationships
- Trouble concentrating
- Fatigue or low energy
- Food cravings or binge eating
- Sleep disturbances
- Feeling out of control
- Physical symptoms, such as bloating, breast tenderness, headaches, and joint or muscle pain

Exams and Tests

There are no physical examination findings or lab tests specific to the diagnosis of PMDD. A complete history, physical examination (including a pelvic exam), and psychiatric evaluation should be conducted to rule out other potential conditions.

Keeping a calendar or diary of symptoms can help women identify the most troublesome symptoms and the times they are likely to occur. This information may help the health care provider diagnose PMDD and determine the appropriate treatment.

Treatment

Women with PMDD may be helped by the following:

- Regular exercise 3–5 times per week
- Adequate rest
- A balanced diet (with increased whole grains, vegetables, fruit, and decreased or no salt, sugar, alcohol, and caffeine)

In addition, it is important to keep a diary or calendar to record the type, severity, and duration of symptoms.

Selective serotonin-reuptake inhibitors (SSRIs) are antidepressant drugs that can treat PMDD. SSRIs include fluoxetine (Prozac, Sarafem), sertraline (Zoloft), paroxetine (Paxil), fluvoxamine (Luvox), and citalopram (Celexa).

Nutritional supplements—such as vitamin B6, calcium, and magnesium—may be recommended. Pain relievers such as aspirin or ibuprofen may be prescribed for headache, backache, menstrual cramping, and breast tenderness. Diuretics may be useful for women who have significant weight gain due to fluid retention.

Outlook (Prognosis)

After proper diagnosis and treatment, most women with PMDD find that their symptoms go away or drop to tolerable levels.

Possible Complications

PMDD symptoms may become severe enough that they interfere with a woman's daily life. Women with depression may have worse symptoms during the second half of their cycle and may require medication adjustments.

As many as 10% of women who report PMS symptoms, particularly those with PMDD, have had suicidal thoughts. The incidence of suicide in women with depression is significantly higher during the latter half of the menstrual cycle.

PMDD may be associated with eating disorders and smoking.

When to Contact a Medical Professional

Call 911 immediately if you are having suicidal thoughts.

Call for an appointment with your health care provider if:

- PMS symptoms do not improve with self-treatment
- PMS symptoms are interfering with your daily life

Part Three

Anxiety Disorders

Chapter 21

What Are Anxiety Disorders?

Anxiety disorders affect about 40 million American adults age 18 years and older (about 18%) in a given year, causing them to be filled with fearfulness and uncertainty. Unlike the relatively mild, brief anxiety caused by a stressful event (such as speaking in public or a first date), anxiety disorders last at least 6 months and can get worse if they are not treated. Anxiety disorders commonly occur along with other mental or physical illnesses, including alcohol or substance abuse, which may mask anxiety symptoms or make them worse. In some cases, these other illnesses need to be treated before a person will respond to treatment for the anxiety disorder.

Effective therapies for anxiety disorders are available, and research is uncovering new treatments that can help most people with anxiety disorders lead productive, fulfilling lives. If you think you have an anxiety disorder, you should seek information and treatment right away.

Panic Disorder

Each anxiety disorder has different symptoms, but all the symptoms cluster around excessive, irrational fear and dread. Panic disorder is a real illness that can be successfully treated. It is characterized by sudden attacks of terror, usually accompanied by a pounding heart,

---

Excerpted from the booklet "Anxiety Disorders," by the National Institute of Mental Health (NIMH, www.nimh.nih.gov), part of the National Institutes of Health, 2007.

sweatiness, weakness, faintness, or dizziness. During these attacks, people with panic disorder may flush or feel chilled; their hands may tingle or feel numb; and they may experience nausea, chest pain, or smothering sensations. Panic attacks usually produce a sense of unreality, a fear of impending doom, or a fear of losing control.

A fear of one's own unexplained physical symptoms is also a symptom of panic disorder. People having panic attacks sometimes believe they are having heart attacks, losing their minds, or on the verge of death. They can't predict when or where an attack will occur, and between episodes many worry intensely and dread the next attack.

Panic attacks can occur at any time, even during sleep. An attack usually peaks within 10 minutes, but some symptoms may last much longer. Panic disorder affects about 6 million American adults and is twice as common in women as men. Panic attacks often begin in late adolescence or early adulthood, but not everyone who experiences panic attacks will develop panic disorder. Many people have just one attack and never have another. The tendency to develop panic attacks appears to be inherited.

People who have full-blown, repeated panic attacks can become very disabled by their condition and should seek treatment before they start to avoid places or situations where panic attacks have occurred. For example, if a panic attack happened in an elevator, someone with panic disorder may develop a fear of elevators that could affect the choice of a job or an apartment, and restrict where that person can seek medical attention or enjoy entertainment.

Some people's lives become so restricted that they avoid normal activities, such as grocery shopping or driving. About one-third become housebound or are able to confront a feared situation only when accompanied by a spouse or other trusted person. When the condition progresses this far, it is called agoraphobia, or fear of open spaces.

Early treatment can often prevent agoraphobia, but people with panic disorder may sometimes go from doctor to doctor for years and visit the emergency room repeatedly before someone correctly diagnoses their condition. This is unfortunate, because panic disorder is one of the most treatable of all the anxiety disorders, responding in most cases to certain kinds of medication or certain kinds of cognitive psychotherapy, which help change thinking patterns that lead to fear and anxiety.

Panic disorder is often accompanied by other serious problems, such as depression, drug abuse, or alcoholism. These conditions need to be treated separately. Symptoms of depression include feelings of sadness or hopelessness, changes in appetite or sleep patterns, low energy, and difficulty concentrating. Most people with depression can be effectively treated with antidepressant medications, certain types of psychotherapy, or a combination of the two.

Obsessive-Compulsive Disorder (OCD)

People with obsessive-compulsive disorder (OCD) have persistent, upsetting thoughts (obsessions) and use rituals (compulsions) to control the anxiety these thoughts produce. Most of the time, the rituals end up controlling them.

For example, if people are obsessed with germs or dirt, they may develop a compulsion to wash their hands over and over again. If they develop an obsession with intruders, they may lock and relock their doors many times before going to bed. Being afraid of social embarrassment may prompt people with OCD to comb their hair compulsively in front of a mirror—sometimes they get "caught" in the mirror and can't move away from it. Performing such rituals is not pleasurable. At best, it produces temporary relief from the anxiety created by obsessive thoughts.

Other common rituals are a need to repeatedly check things, touch things (especially in a particular sequence),or count things. Some common obsessions include having frequent thoughts of violence and harming loved ones, persistently thinking about performing sexual acts the person dislikes, or having thoughts that are prohibited by religious beliefs. People with OCD may also be preoccupied with order and symmetry, have difficulty throwing things out (so they accumulate), or hoard unneeded items.

Healthy people also have rituals, such as checking to see if the stove is off several times before leaving the house. The difference is that people with OCD perform their rituals even though doing so interferes with daily life and they find the repetition distressing. Although most adults with OCD recognize that what they are doing is senseless, some adults and most children may not realize that their behavior is out of the ordinary.

OCD affects about 2.2 million American adults, and the problem can be accompanied by eating disorders, other anxiety disorders, or depression. It strikes men and women in roughly equal numbers and usually appears in childhood, adolescence, or early adulthood. One third of adults with OCD develop symptoms as children, and research indicates that OCD might run in families.

The course of the disease is quite varied. Symptoms may come and go, ease over time, or get worse. If OCD becomes severe, it can keep a person from working or carrying out normal responsibilities at home. People with OCD may try to help themselves by avoiding situations that trigger their obsessions, or they may use alcohol or drugs to calm themselves. OCD usually responds well to treatment with certain medications and/or exposure-based psychotherapy, in which people face situations that cause fear or anxiety and become less sensitive (desensitized) to them. NIMH is supporting research into new treatment approaches for people whose OCD does not respond well to the usual therapies. These approaches include combination and augmentation (add-on) treatments, as well as modern techniques such as deep brain stimulation.

Posttraumatic Stress Disorder (PTSD)

Posttraumatic stress disorder (PTSD) develops after a terrifying ordeal that involved physical harm or the threat of physical harm. The person who develops PTSD may have been the one who was harmed, the harm may have happened to a loved one, or the person may have witnessed a harmful event that happened to loved ones or strangers.

PTSD was first brought to public attention in relation to war veterans, but it can result from a variety of traumatic incidents, such as mugging, rape, torture, being kidnapped or held captive, child abuse, car accidents, train wrecks, plane crashes, bombings, or natural disasters such as floods or earthquakes.

People with PTSD may startle easily, become emotionally numb (especially in relation to people with whom they used to be close), lose interest in things they used to enjoy, have trouble feeling affectionate, be irritable, become more aggressive, or even become violent. They avoid situations that remind them of the original incident, and anniversaries of the incident are often very difficult. PTSD symptoms seem to be worse if the event that triggered them was deliberately initiated by another person, as in a mugging or a kidnapping.

Most people with PTSD repeatedly relive the trauma in their thoughts during the day and in nightmares when they sleep. These are called flashbacks. Flashbacks may consist of images, sounds, smells, or feelings, and are often triggered by ordinary occurrences, such as a door slamming or a car backfiring on the street. A person having a flashback may lose touch with reality and believe that the traumatic incident is happening all over again.

Not every traumatized person develops full-blown or even minor PTSD. Symptoms usually begin within 3 months of the incident but occasionally emerge years afterward. They must last more than a month to be considered PTSD. The course of the illness varies. Some people recover within 6 months, while others have symptoms that last much longer. In some people, the condition becomes chronic.

PTSD affects about 7.7 million American adults, but it can occur at any age, including childhood. Women are more likely to develop PTSD than men, and there is some evidence that susceptibility to the disorder may run in families. PTSD is often accompanied by depression, substance abuse, or one or more of the other anxiety disorders. Certain kinds of medication and certain kinds of psychotherapy usually treat the symptoms of PTSD very effectively.

Social Phobia (Social Anxiety Disorder)

Social phobia, also called social anxiety disorder, is diagnosed when people become overwhelmingly anxious and excessively self-conscious in everyday social situations. People with social phobia have an intense, persistent, and chronic fear of being watched and judged by others and of doing things that will embarrass them. They can worry for days or weeks before a dreaded situation. This fear may become so severe that it interferes with work, school, and other ordinary activities, and can make it hard to make and keep friends.

While many people with social phobia realize that their fears about being with people are excessive or unreasonable, they are unable to overcome them. Even if they manage to confront their fears and be around others, they are usually very anxious beforehand, are intensely uncomfortable throughout the encounter, and worry about how they were judged for hours afterward.

Social phobia can be limited to one situation (such as talking to people, eating or drinking, or writing on a blackboard in front of others) or may be so broad (such as in generalized social phobia) that the person experiences anxiety around almost anyone other than the family.

Physical symptoms that often accompany social phobia include blushing, profuse sweating, trembling, nausea, and difficulty talking. When these symptoms occur, people with PTSD feel as though all eyes are focused on them.

Social phobia affects about 15 million American adults. Women and men are equally likely to develop the disorder, which usually begins in childhood or early adolescence. There is some evidence that genetic factors are involved. Social phobia is often accompanied by other anxiety disorders or depression, and substance abuse may develop if people try to self-medicate their anxiety.

Social phobia can be successfully treated with certain kinds of psychotherapy or medications.

Specific Phobias

A specific phobia is an intense, irrational fear of something that actually poses little or no threat. Some of the more common specific phobias are heights, escalators, tunnels, highway driving, closed-in places, water, flying, dogs, spiders, and injuries involving blood. People with specific phobias may be able to ski the world's tallest mountains with ease but be unable to go above the fifth floor of an office building. While adults with phobias realize that these fears are irrational, they often find that facing, or even thinking about facing, the feared object or situation brings on a panic attack or severe anxiety.

Specific phobias affect around 19.2 million American adults and are twice as common in women as men. They usually appear in childhood or adolescence and tend to persist into adulthood. The causes of specific phobias are not well understood, but there is some evidence that the tendency to develop them may run in families.

If the feared situation or feared object is easy to avoid, people with specific phobias may not seek help; but if avoidance interferes with their careers or their personal lives, it can become disabling and treatment is usually pursued.

Specific phobias respond very well to carefully targeted psychotherapy.

Generalized Anxiety Disorder (GAD)

People with generalized anxiety disorder (GAD) go through the day filled with exaggerated worry and tension, even though there is little or nothing to provoke it. They anticipate disaster and are overly concerned about health issues, money, family problems, or difficulties at work. Sometimes just the thought of getting through the day produces anxiety.

GAD is diagnosed when a person worries excessively about a variety of everyday problems for at least 6 months. People with GAD can't seem to get rid of their concerns, even though they usually realize that their anxiety is more intense than the situation warrants. They can't relax, startle easily, and have difficulty concentrating. Often they have trouble falling asleep or staying asleep. Physical symptoms that often accompany the anxiety include fatigue, headaches, muscle tension, muscle aches, difficulty swallowing, trembling, twitching, irritability, sweating, nausea, lightheadedness, having to go to the bathroom frequently, feeling out of breath, and hot flashes.

When their anxiety level is mild, people with GAD can function socially and hold down a job. Although they don't avoid certain situations as a result of their disorder, people with GAD can have difficulty carrying out the simplest daily activities if their anxiety is severe.

GAD affects about 6.8 million American adults, including twice as many women as men. The disorder develops gradually and can begin at any point in the life cycle, although the years of highest risk are between childhood and middle age. There is evidence that genes play a modest role in the disorder.

Other anxiety disorders, depression, or substance abuse often accompany GAD, which rarely occurs alone. GAD is commonly treated with medication or cognitive-behavioral therapy, but co-occurring conditions must also be treated using the appropriate therapies.

Treatment of Anxiety Disorders

In general, anxiety disorders are treated with medication, specific types of psychotherapy, or both. Treatment choices depend on the problem and the person's preference. Before treatment begins, a doctor must conduct a careful diagnostic evaluation to determine whether a person's symptoms are caused by an anxiety disorder or a physical problem. If an anxiety disorder is diagnosed, the type of disorder or the combination of disorders that are present must be identified, as well as any coexisting conditions, such as depression or substance abuse. Sometimes alcoholism, depression, or other coexisting conditions have such a strong effect on the individual that treating the anxiety disorder must wait until the coexisting conditions are brought under control.

People with anxiety disorders who have already received treatment should tell their current doctor about that treatment in detail. If they received medication, they should tell their doctor what medication was used, what the dosage was at the beginning of treatment, whether the dosage was increased or decreased while they were under treatment, what side effects occurred, and whether the treatment helped them become less anxious. If they received psychotherapy, they should describe the type of therapy, how often they attended sessions, and whether the therapy was useful.

Often people believe that they have "failed" at treatment or that the treatment didn't work for them when, in fact, it was not given for an adequate length of time or was administered incorrectly. Sometimes people must try several different treatments or combinations of treatment before they find the one that works for them.

Medication

Medication will not cure anxiety disorders, but it can keep them under control while the person receives psychotherapy. Medication must be prescribed by physicians, usually psychiatrists, who can either offer psychotherapy themselves or work as a team with psychologists, social workers, or counselors who provide psychotherapy. The principal medications used for anxiety disorders are antidepressants, anti-anxiety drugs, and beta-blockers to control some of the physical symptoms. With proper treatment, many people with anxiety disorders can lead normal, fulfilling lives.

Antidepressants: Antidepressants were developed to treat depression but are also effective for anxiety disorders. Although these medications begin to alter brain chemistry after the very first dose, their full effect requires a series of changes to occur; it is usually about 4 to 6 weeks before symptoms start to fade. It is important to continue taking these medications long enough to let them work.

- **SSRIs:** Some of the newest antidepressants are called selective serotonin reuptake inhibitors, or SSRIs. SSRIs alter the levels of the neurotransmitter serotonin in the brain, which, like other neurotransmitters, helps brain cells communicate with one another. Fluoxetine (Prozac®), sertraline (Zoloft®), escitalopram (Lexapro®), paroxetine (Paxil®), and citalopram (Celexa®) are some of the SSRIs commonly prescribed for panic disorder, OCD, PTSD, and social phobia. SSRIs are also used to treat panic disorder when it occurs in combination with OCD, social phobia, or depression. Venlafaxine (Effexor®), a drug closely related to the SSRIs, is used to treat GAD. These medications are started at low doses and gradually increased until they have a beneficial effect. SSRIs have fewer side effects than older antidepressants, but they sometimes produce slight nausea or jitters when people first start to take them. These symptoms fade with time. Some people also experience sexual dysfunction with SSRIs, which may be helped by adjusting the dosage or switching to another SSRI.
- **Tricyclics:** Tricyclics are older than SSRIs and work as well as SSRIs for anxiety disorders other than OCD. They are also started at low doses that are gradually increased. They sometimes cause

dizziness, drowsiness, dry mouth, and weight gain, which can usually be corrected by changing the dosage or switching to another tricyclic medication. Tricyclics include imipramine (Tofranil®), which is prescribed for panic disorder and GAD, and clomipramine (Anafranil®), which is the only tricyclic antidepressant useful for treating OCD.

- **MAOIs:** Monoamine oxidase inhibitors (MAOIs) are the oldest class of antidepressant medications. The MAOIs most commonly prescribed for anxiety disorders are phenelzine (Nardil®), followed by tranylcypromine (Parnate®), and isocarboxazid (Marplan®), which are useful in treating panic disorder and social phobia. People who take MAOIs cannot eat a variety of foods and beverages (including cheese and red wine) that contain tyramine or take certain medications, including some types of birth control pills, pain relievers (such as Advil®, Motrin®, or Tylenol®), cold and allergy medications, and herbal supplements; these substances can interact with MAOIs to cause dangerous increases in blood pressure. The development of a new MAOI skin patch may help lessen these risks. MAOIs can also react with SSRIs to produce a serious condition called "serotonin syndrome," which can cause confusion, hallucinations, increased sweating, muscle stiffness, seizures, changes in blood pressure or heart rhythm, and other potentially life-threatening conditions.

Anti-anxiety drugs: High-potency benzodiazepines combat anxiety and have few side effects other than drowsiness. Because people can get used to them and may need higher and higher doses to get the same effect, benzodiazepines are generally prescribed for short periods of time, especially for people who have abused drugs or alcohol and who become dependent on medication easily. One exception to this rule is people with panic disorder, who can take benzodiazepines for up to a year without harm. Clonazepam (Klonopin®) is used for social phobia and GAD, lorazepam (Ativan®) is helpful for panic disorder, and alprazolam (Xanax®) is useful for both panic disorder and GAD.

Some people experience withdrawal symptoms if they stop taking benzodiazepines abruptly instead of tapering off, and anxiety can return once the medication is stopped. These potential problems have led some physicians to shy away from using these drugs or to use them in inadequate doses.

Buspirone (BuSpar®), an azapirone, is a newer anti-anxiety medication used to treat GAD. Possible side effects include dizziness, headaches, and nausea. Unlike benzodiazepines, buspirone must be taken consistently for at least 2 weeks to achieve an anti-anxiety effect.

Beta-blockers: Beta-blockers, such as propranolol (Inderal®), which is used to treat heart conditions, can prevent the physical symptoms that accompany certain anxiety disorders, particularly social phobia. When a feared situation can be predicted (such as giving a speech), a doctor may prescribe a beta-blocker to keep physical symptoms of anxiety under control.

Taking Medication

Before taking medication for an anxiety disorder:

- Ask your doctor to tell you about the effects and side effects of the drug.
- Tell your doctor about any alternative therapies or over-the-counter medications you are using.
- Ask your doctor when and how the medication should be stopped. Some drugs can't be stopped abruptly but must be tapered off slowly under a doctor's supervision.
- Work with your doctor to determine which medication is right for you and what dosage is best.
- Be aware that some medications are effective only if they are taken regularly and that symptoms may recur if the medication is stopped.

Psychotherapy

Psychotherapy involves talking with a trained mental health professional, such as a psychiatrist, psychologist, social worker, or counselor, to discover what caused an anxiety disorder and how to deal with its symptoms.

Cognitive-behavioral therapy: Cognitive-behavioral therapy (CBT) is very useful in treating anxiety disorders. The cognitive part helps people change the thinking patterns that support their fears, and the behavioral part helps people change the way they react to anxiety-provoking situations.

For example, CBT can help people with panic disorder learn that their panic attacks are not really heart attacks and help people with social phobia learn how to overcome the belief that others are always watching and judging them. When people are ready to confront their fears, they are shown how to use exposure techniques to desensitize themselves to situations that trigger their anxieties.

People with OCD who fear dirt and germs are encouraged to get their hands dirty and wait increasing amounts of time before washing them. The therapist helps the person cope with the anxiety that waiting produces; after the exercise has been repeated a number of times, the anxiety diminishes. People with social phobia may be encouraged to spend time in feared social situations without giving in to the temptation to flee and to make small social blunders and observe how people respond to them. Since the response is usually far less harsh than the person fears, these anxieties are lessened.

People with PTSD may be supported through recalling their traumatic event in a safe situation, which helps reduce the fear it produces. CBT therapists also teach deep breathing and other types of exercises to relieve anxiety and encourage relaxation.

Exposure-based behavioral therapy has been used for many years to treat specific phobias. The person gradually encounters the object or situation that is feared, perhaps at first only through pictures or tapes, then later face-to-face. Often the therapist will accompany the person to a feared situation to provide support and guidance.

CBT is undertaken when people decide they are ready for it and with their permission and cooperation. To be effective, the therapy must be directed at the person's specific anxieties and must be tailored to his or her needs. There are no side effects other than the discomfort of temporarily increased anxiety.

CBT or behavioral therapy often lasts about 12 weeks. It may be conducted individually or with a group of people who have similar problems. Group therapy is particularly effective for social phobia. Often "homework" is assigned for participants to complete between sessions. There is some evidence that the benefits of CBT last longer than those of medication for people with panic disorder, and the same may be true for OCD, PTSD, and social phobia. If a disorder recurs at a later date, the same therapy can be used to treat it successfully a second time.

Medication can be combined with psychotherapy for specific anxiety disorders, and this is the best treatment approach for many people.

How to Get Help for Anxiety Disorders

If you think you have an anxiety disorder, the first person you should see is your family doctor. A physician can determine whether the symptoms that alarm you are due to an anxiety disorder, another medical condition, or both.

If an anxiety disorder is diagnosed, the next step is usually seeing a mental health professional. The practitioners who are most helpful with anxiety disorders are those who have training in cognitive behavioral therapy and/or behavioral therapy, and who are open to using medication if it is needed.

You should feel comfortable talking with the mental health professional you choose. If you do not, you should seek help elsewhere. Once you find a mental health professional with whom you are comfortable, the two of you should work as a team and make a plan to treat your anxiety disorder together.

Remember that once you start on medication, it is important not to stop taking it abruptly. Certain drugs must be tapered off under the supervision of a doctor or bad reactions can occur. Make sure you talk to the doctor who prescribed your medication before you stop taking it. If you are having trouble with side effects, it's possible that they can be eliminated by adjusting how much medication you take and when you take it.

Most insurance plans, including health maintenance organizations (HMOs), will cover treatment for anxiety disorders. Check with your insurance company and find out. If you don't have insurance, the Health and Human Services division of your county government may offer mental health care at a public mental health center that charges people according to how much they are able to pay. If you are on public assistance, you may be able to get care through your state Medicaid plan.

Ways to Make Treatment More Effective

Many people with anxiety disorders benefit from joining a self-help or support group and sharing their problems and achievements with others. Internet chat rooms can also be useful in this regard, but any advice received over the Internet should be used with caution, as Internet acquaintances have usually never seen each other and false identities are common. Talking with a trusted friend or member of the clergy can also provide support, but it is not a substitute for care from a mental health professional.

Stress management techniques and meditation can help people with anxiety disorders calm themselves and may enhance the effects of therapy. There is preliminary evidence that aerobic exercise may have a calming effect. Since caffeine, certain illicit drugs, and even some over-the-counter cold medications can aggravate the symptoms of anxiety disorders, they should be avoided. Check with your physician or pharmacist before taking any additional medications.

The family is very important in the recovery of a person with an anxiety disorder. Ideally, the family should be supportive but not help perpetuate their loved one's symptoms. Family members should not trivialize the disorder or demand improvement without treatment. If your family is doing either of these things, you may want to show them this information so they can become educated allies and help you succeed in therapy.

The Role of Research in Improving the Understanding and Treatment of Anxiety Disorders

NIMH supports research into the causes, diagnosis, prevention, and treatment of anxiety disorders and other mental illnesses. Scientists are looking at what role genes play in the development of these disorders and are also investigating the effects of environmental factors such as pollution, physical and psychological stress, and diet. In addition, studies are being conducted on the "natural history" (what course the illness takes without treatment) of a variety of individual anxiety disorders, combinations of anxiety disorders, and anxiety disorders that are accompanied by other mental illnesses such as depression.

Scientists currently think that, like heart disease and type 1 diabetes, mental illnesses are complex and probably result from a combination of genetic, environmental, psychological, and developmental factors. For instance, although NIMH-sponsored studies of twins and families suggest that genetics play a role in the development of some anxiety disorders, problems such as PTSD are triggered by trauma. Genetic studies may help explain why some people exposed to trauma develop PTSD and others do not.

Several parts of the brain are key actors in the production of fear and anxiety. Using brain imaging technology and neurochemical techniques, scientists have discovered that the amygdala and the hippocampus play significant roles in most anxiety disorders.

The amygdala is an almond-shaped structure deep in the brain that is believed to be a communications hub between the parts of the brain that process incoming sensory signals and the parts that interpret these signals. It can alert the rest of the brain that a threat is present and trigger a fear or anxiety response. It appears that emotional memories are stored in the central part of the amygdala and may play a role in anxiety disorders involving very distinct fears, such as fears of dogs, spiders, or flying.

The hippocampus is the part of the brain that encodes threatening events into memories. Studies have shown that the hippocampus appears to be smaller in some people who were victims of child abuse or who served in military combat. Research will determine what causes this reduction in size and what role it plays in the flashbacks, deficits in explicit memory, and fragmented memories of the traumatic event that are common in PTSD.

By learning more about how the brain creates fear and anxiety, scientists may be able to devise better treatments for anxiety disorders. For example, if specific neurotransmitters are found to play an important role in fear, drugs may be developed that will block them and decrease fear responses; if enough is learned about how the brain generates new cells throughout the lifecycle, it may be possible to stimulate the growth of new neurons in the hippocampus in people with PTSD.

Current research at NIMH on anxiety disorders includes studies that address how well medication and behavioral therapies work in the treatment of OCD, and the safety and effectiveness of medications for children and adolescents who have a combination of anxiety disorders and attention deficit hyperactivity disorder.

Chapter 22

Generalized Anxiety Disorder

People with anxiety disorders feel extremely fearful and unsure. Most people feel anxious about something for a short time now and again, but people with anxiety disorders feel this way most of the time. Their fears and worries make it hard for them to do everyday tasks. About 18% of American adults have anxiety disorders. Children also may have them.

Treatment is available for people with anxiety disorders. Researchers are also looking for new treatments that will help relieve symptoms.

This information is about one kind of anxiety disorder called generalized anxiety disorder, or GAD.

Generalized Anxiety Disorder

All of us worry about things like health, money, or family problems at one time or another. But people with GAD are extremely worried about these and many other things, even when there is little or no reason to worry about them.

They may be very anxious about just getting through the day. They think things will always go badly. At times, worrying keeps people with GAD from doing everyday tasks.

This is a list of common symptoms. People with GAD:

From "Generalized Anxiety Disorder," a booklet by the National Institute of Mental Health (NIMH, www.nimh.nih.gov), part of the National Institutes of Health, 2007.

- worry very much about everyday things for at least 6 months, even if there is little or no reason to worry about them;
- can't control their constant worries;
- know that they worry much more than they should;
- can't relax;
- have a hard time concentrating;
- are easily startled; and
- have trouble falling asleep or staying asleep.

Common body symptoms are:

- feeling tired for no reason;
- headaches;
- muscle tension and aches;
- having a hard time swallowing;
- trembling or twitching;
- being irritable;
- sweating;
- nausea;
- feeling lightheaded;
- feeling out of breath;
- having to go to the bathroom a lot; and
- hot flashes.

When Does GAD Start?

GAD develops slowly. It often starts during the time between childhood and middle age. Symptoms may get better or worse at different times, and often are worse during times of stress.

People with GAD may visit a doctor many times before they find out they have this disorder. They ask their doctors to help them with the signs of GAD, such as headaches or trouble falling asleep, but don't always get the help they need right away. It may take doctors some time to be sure that a person has GAD instead of something else. The first step is to go to a doctor to talk about symptoms.

Is There Help?

There is help for people with GAD. The first step is to go to a doctor or health clinic to talk about symptoms. People who think they have GAD may want to bring this information to the doctor, to help them talk about the symptoms in it. The doctor will do an exam to make sure that another physical problem isn't causing the symptoms. The doctor may make a referral to a mental health specialist.

Doctors may prescribe medication to help relieve GAD. It's important to know that some of these medicines may take a few weeks to start working. In most states only a medical doctor (a family doctor or psychiatrist) can prescribe medications.

The kinds of medicines used to treat GAD are listed in the following text. Some are used to treat other problems, such as depression, but also are helpful for GAD:

- antidepressants,
- anti-anxiety medicines, and
- beta blockers.

Doctors also may ask people with GAD to go to therapy with a licensed social worker, psychologist, or psychiatrist. This treatment can help people with GAD feel less anxious and fearful.

There is no cure for GAD yet, but treatments can give relief to people who have it and help them live a more normal life. If you know someone with signs of GAD, talk to him or her about seeing a doctor. Offer to go along for support.

Who Pays for Treatment?

Most insurance plans cover treatment for anxiety disorders. People who are going to have treatment should check with their own insurance companies to find out about coverage. For people who don't have insurance, local city or county governments may offer treatment at a clinic or health center, where the cost is based on income. Medicaid plans also may pay for GAD treatment.

Why Do People Get GAD?

GAD sometimes runs in families, but no one knows for sure why some people have it, while others don't. When chemicals in the brain are not at a certain level it can cause a person to have GAD. That is why medications often help with the symptoms because they help the brain chemicals stay at the correct levels.

To improve treatment, scientists are studying how well different medicines and therapies work. In one kind of research, people with GAD choose to take part in a clinical trial to help doctors find out what treatments work best for most people, or what works best for different symptoms. Usually, the treatment is free. Scientists are learning more about how the brain works so that they can discover new treatments.

Chapter 23

Panic Disorder

People with panic disorder have sudden and repeated attacks of fear that last for several minutes, but sometimes symptoms may last longer. These are called panic attacks. Panic attacks are characterized by a fear of certain disaster or a fear of losing control. A person may also have a strong physical reaction. It may feel like having a heart attack. Panic attacks can occur at any time, and many people worry about and dread the possibility of having another attack.

A person with panic disorder may become discouraged and feel ashamed because he or she cannot carry out normal routines like going to the grocery store, or driving. Having panic disorder can also interfere with school or work.

What are the symptoms of panic disorder?

People with panic disorder have:

- sudden and repeated attacks of fear;
- a feeling of being out of control during a panic attack;
- a feeling that things are not real;
- an intense worry about when the next attack will happen;

From "When Fear Overwhelms: Panic Disorder," by the National Institute of Mental Health (NIMH, www.nimh.nih.gov), part of the National Institutes of Health, 2008.

- a fear or avoidance of places where panic attacks have occurred in the past; and
- physical symptoms including:
  - pounding heart;
  - sweating;
  - weakness, faintness, or dizziness;
  - feeling a hot flush or a cold chill;
  - tingly or numb hands;
  - chest pain; and
  - feeling nauseous or stomach pain.

When does panic disorder start?

Panic disorder often begins in the late teens or early adulthood. More women than men have panic disorder. But not everyone who experiences panic attacks will develop panic disorder.

Is there help?

There is help for people with panic disorder. In fact, it is one of the most treatable anxiety disorders. First, a person should visit a doctor or health care provider to discuss the symptoms or feelings he or she is having. The list of symptoms in this text can be a useful guide when talking with the doctor. The doctor will do an examination to make sure that another physical problem is not causing the symptoms. The doctor may make a referral to a specialist such as a psychiatrist, psychologist or licensed social worker.

Medications can help reduce the severity and frequency of panic attacks, but they may take several weeks to start working. A doctor can prescribe medications. Different types of medications are used to treat panic disorder. They are antidepressants, anti-anxiety drugs, and beta blockers. These same medications are used to treat other types of disorders as well.

Psychotherapy, or "talk therapy" with a specialist can help people learn to control the symptoms of a panic attack. Therapy can be with a licensed social worker, counselor, psychologist or psychiatrist. There is no cure for panic disorder, but most people can live a normal life when they receive treatment with medicine and/or therapy.

If you know someone with symptoms of panic disorder, talk to him or her about seeing a doctor. Offer to go with your friend to the doctor's appointment for support.

Who pays for treatment?

Most insurance plans cover treatment for anxiety disorders. Check with your insurance company to find out. If you do not have insurance, the health or human services agency of your city or county government may offer care at a clinic or health center where payment is usually based on a person's income. If you receive Medicaid, the plan you are in may pay for treatment.

Why do people get panic disorder?

Panic disorder sometimes runs in families, but no one knows for sure why some people have it, while others don't. When chemicals in the brain are not at a certain level it can cause a person to have panic disorder. That is why medications often help with symptoms because they help the brain chemicals stay at the correct levels.

To improve treatment, scientists are studying how well different medicines and therapies work. In one kind of research, people with panic disorder choose to take part in a clinical trial to help doctors find out what treatments work best for most people, or what works best for different symptoms. Usually, the treatment is free. Scientists are learning more about how the brain works so that they can discover new treatments.

Chapter 24

Specific Phobias

Chapter Contents

Section 24.1

What Are Specific Phobias?

"Specific Phobias," from the Anxiety Disorders Association of America (ADAA, www.adaa.org), © 2008. Reprinted with permission.

About Anxiety Disorders

Anxiety is a normal part of living. It's the body's way of telling us something isn't right. It keeps us from harm's way and prepares us to act quickly in the face of danger. However, for some people, anxiety is persistent, irrational, and overwhelming. It may get in the way of day-to-day activities or even make them impossible. This may be a sign of an anxiety disorder.

The term "anxiety disorders" describes a group of conditions including generalized anxiety disorder (GAD), obsessive-compulsive disorder (OCD), panic disorder, posttraumatic stress disorder (PTSD), social anxiety disorder (SAD), and specific phobias. For information on all of the anxiety disorders, visit www.adaa.org.

Table 24.1. What's the difference between normal anxiety and a phobia?

Normal Anxiety	Phobia
Feeling queasy while climbing a tall ladder	Refusing to attend your best friend's wedding because it's on the 25th floor of a hotel
Worrying about taking off in an airplane during a lightning storm	Turning down a big promotion because it involves air travel
Feeling anxious around your neighbor's pit bull	Avoiding visiting your neighbors for fear of seeing a dog

What Is a Phobia?

We all have things that frighten us or make us uneasy. New places, insects, driving over high bridges, or creaky elevators. And although we sometimes try to avoid things that make us uncomfortable, we generally manage to control our fears and carry on with daily activities. Some people, however, have very strong, irrational, involuntary fear reactions that lead them to avoid common everyday places, situations, or objects even though they logically know there isn't any danger. The fear doesn't make any sense, but it seems nothing can stop it. When confronted with the feared situation, they may even have a panic attack, the abrupt onset of intense fear that makes people feel as if they are having a heart attack, or will lose control and die.

People who experience these seemingly out-of-control fears have a phobia. There are three types of phobias—agoraphobia, social phobia (also known as social anxiety disorder), and specific phobias. This text focuses on specific phobias. For information about agoraphobia and social phobia go to www.adaa.org.

What Is a Specific Phobia?

People with a specific phobia have an excessive and unreasonable fear in the presence of or anticipation of a specific object, place, or situation. Common specific phobias include animals, insects, heights, thunder, driving, public transportation, flying, dental or medical procedures, and elevators. Although the person with a phobia realizes that the fear is irrational, even thinking about it can cause extreme anxiety.

How Can Specific Phobias Affect Your Life?

The impact of a phobia on one's life depends on how easy it is to avoid the feared object, place, or situation. Since individuals do whatever they can to avoid the uncomfortable and often terrifying feelings of phobic anxiety, phobias can disrupt daily routines, limit work efficiency, reduce self-esteem, and place a strain on relationships.

What Causes Specific Phobias?

Specific phobias are the most common type of anxiety disorder, affecting 19 million American adults. Most phobias seem to come out of the blue, usually arising in childhood or early adulthood. Scientists believe that phobias can be traced to a combination of genetic tendencies, brain chemistry, and other biological, psychological, and environmental factors.

What Treatments Are Available?

Most individuals who seek treatment for phobias and other anxiety disorders see significant improvement and enjoy a better quality of life. A variety of treatment options exists, including cognitive-behavioral therapy, exposure therapy, anxiety management, relaxation techniques, and medications. One or a combination of these may be recommended. Details about these treatments are available on the ADAA website at www.adaa.org.

It is important to remember that there is no single "right" treatment. What works for one person may or may not be the best choice for someone else. A course of treatment should be tailored to individual needs. Ask your doctor to explain why a particular type of treatment is being recommended, what other options are available, and what you need to do to fully participate in your recovery.

How Can ADAA Help You?

Suffering from a specific phobia or any anxiety disorder can interfere with many aspects of your life. You may feel alone, embarrassed, or frightened. ADAA can provide the resources that will help you and your loved ones better understand your condition, connect you with a community of people who know what you are experiencing, and assist you in finding local mental health professionals. Visit the ADAA website at www.adaa.org to locate mental health professionals who treat phobias and other anxiety disorders in your area, as well as local support groups. Learn about the causes, symptoms, and best treatments for all of the anxiety disorders, review questions to ask a therapist or doctor, and find helpful materials for family and loved ones. ADAA is here to help you make good decisions so that you can get on with your life.

Take Five and Manage Your Anxiety

Whether you have normal anxiety or an anxiety disorder, these strategies will help you cope:

1. Exercise. Go for a walk or jog. Do yoga. Dance. Just get moving!

2. Talk to someone—spouse, significant other, friend, child, or doctor.
3. Keep a daily journal. Become aware of what triggers your anxiety.
4. Eat a balanced diet. Don't skip meals. Avoid caffeine, which can trigger anxiety symptoms.
5. Contact ADAA at www.adaa.org. Let us help you help yourself.

Specific Phobias Self-Test

If you think you might have a specific phobia, take the test below. Answer "yes" or "no" to the questions and discuss the results with your doctor.

Are you troubled by . . .

- Fear of places or situations where getting help or escape might be difficult, such as in a crowd or on a bridge?
- Shortness of breath or a racing heart for no apparent reason when confronting certain situations?
- Persistent and unreasonable fear of an object or situation, such as flying, heights, animals, blood, etc.?
- Being unable to travel alone?
- Fears that continue despite causing problems for you or your loved ones?
- Fear that interferes with your daily life?

Having more than one illness at the same time can make it difficult to diagnose and treat the different conditions. Conditions that sometimes complicate anxiety disorders include depression and substance abuse, among others. The following information will help your health care professional in evaluating you for a specific phobia.

In the last year, have you experienced . . .

- Changes in sleeping or eating habits?
- Feeling sad or depressed more days than not?
- A disinterest in life more days than not?
- A feeling of worthlessness or guilt more days than not?

During the last year, has the use of alcohol or drugs . . .

- Resulted in failure with work or school, or difficulties with your family?
- Placed you in a dangerous situation, such as driving under the influence?
- Gotten you arrested?
- Continued despite causing problems for you or your loved ones?

Section 24.2

Agoraphobia

Definition

Agoraphobia is fear of being in places where help might not be available, and is usually manifested by fear of crowds, bridges, or of being outside alone.

Causes

Agoraphobia often accompanies another anxiety disorder, such as panic disorder or a specific phobia.

If it occurs with panic disorder, the onset is usually in the 20s, and women are affected more often than men. People with this disorder may become housebound for years, which is likely to hurt social and interpersonal relationships.

Symptoms

- Fear of being alone
- Fear of losing control in a public place

- Fear of being in places where escape might be difficult
- Becoming housebound for prolonged periods of time
- Feelings of detachment or estrangement from others
- Feelings of helplessness
- Dependence on others
- Feeling that the body is unreal
- Feeling that the environment is unreal
- Anxiety or panic attack (acute severe anxiety)
- Unusual temper or agitation with trembling or twitching

Additional symptoms that may occur:

- Lightheadedness, near fainting
- Dizziness
- Excessive sweating
- Skin flushing
- Breathing difficulty
- Chest pain
- Heartbeat sensations
- Nausea and vomiting
- Numbness and tingling
- Abdominal distress that occurs when upset
- Confused or disordered thoughts
    - Intense fear of going crazy
    - Intense fear of dying

Exams and Tests

The individual may have a history of phobias, or family, friends, or the affected person may tell the health care provider about agoraphobic behavior.

The individual may sweat, have a rapid pulse (heart rate), or have high blood pressure.

Treatment

The goal of treatment is to help the phobic person function effectively. The success of treatment usually depends upon the severity of the phobia.

Systematic desensitization is a technique used to treat phobias. The person is asked to relax, then imagine the things that cause the anxiety, working from the least fearful to the most fearful. Graded real-life exposure has also been used with success to help people overcome their fears.

Antianxiety and antidepressive medications are often used to help relieve the symptoms associated with phobias.

Outlook (Prognosis)

Phobias tend to be chronic, but respond well to treatment.

Possible Complications

Some phobias may affect job performance or social functioning.

When to Contact a Medical Professional

Call for an appointment with your health care provider if symptoms suggestive of agoraphobia develop.

Prevention

As with other panic disorders, prevention may not be possible. Early intervention may reduce the severity of the condition.

Chapter 25

Social Phobia (Social Anxiety Disorder)

Social phobia is a strong fear of being judged by others and of being embarrassed. This fear can be so strong that it gets in the way of going to work or school or doing other everyday things.

People with social phobia are afraid of doing common things in front of other people; for example, they might be afraid to sign a check in front of a cashier at the grocery store, or they might be afraid to eat or drink in front of other people. All of us have been a little bit nervous, at one time or another, about things like meeting new people or giving a speech. But people with social phobia worry about these and other things for weeks before they happen.

Most of the people who have social phobia know that they shouldn't be as afraid as they are, but they can't control their fear. Sometimes, they end up staying away from places or events where they think they might have to do something that will embarrass them. That can keep them from doing the everyday tasks of living and from enjoying times with family and friends.

Most people who have social phobia know they shouldn't be as afraid as they are, but they can't control their fear.

This is a list of common symptoms. People with social phobia:

- are very anxious about being with other people.
- are very self-conscious in front of other people; that is, they are very worried about how they themselves will act.

Excerpted from a booklet by the National Institute of Mental Health (NIMH, www.nimh.nih.gov), part of the National Institutes of Health, 2007.

- are very afraid of being embarrassed in front of other people.
- are very afraid that other people will judge them.
- worry for days or weeks before an event where other people will be.
- stay away from places where there are other people.
- have a hard time making friends and keeping friends.
- may have body symptoms when they are with other people, such as:
    - blushing,
    - heavy sweating,
    - trembling,
    - nausea, and
    - having a hard time talking.

When does social phobia start?

Social phobia usually starts during the child or teen years, usually at about age 13. A doctor can tell that a person has social phobia if the person has had symptoms for at least 6 months. Without treatment, social phobia can last for many years or a lifetime.

Is there help?

There is help for people with social phobia. The first step is to go to a doctor or health clinic to talk about symptoms. The doctor will do an exam to make sure that another physical problem isn't causing the symptoms. The doctor may make a referral to a mental health specialist.

Doctors may prescribe medication to help relieve social phobia. It's important to know that some of these medicines may take a few weeks to start working. In most states only a medical doctor (a family doctor or psychiatrist) can prescribe medications.

Treatment can help people with social phobia feel less anxious and fearful.

The kinds of medicines used to treat social phobia are listed below. Some of these medicines are used to treat other problems, such as depression, but also are helpful for social phobia:

- antidepressants,
- anti-anxiety medicines, and
- beta blockers.

Doctors also may ask people with social phobia to go to therapy with a licensed social worker, psychologist, or psychiatrist. This treatment can help people with social phobia feel less anxious and fearful.

There is no cure for social phobia yet, but treatments can give relief to people who have it and help them live a more normal life. If you know someone with signs of social phobia, talk to him or her about seeing a doctor. Offer to go along for support.

Who pays for treatment?

Most insurance plans cover treatment for anxiety disorders. People who are going to have treatment should check with their own insurance companies to find out about coverage. For people who don't have insurance, local city or county governments may offer treatment at a clinic or health center, where the cost is based on income. Medicaid plans also may pay for social phobia treatment.

Why do people get social phobia?

Social phobia sometimes runs in families, but no one knows for sure why some people have it, while others don't. When chemicals in the brain are not at a certain level it can cause a person to have social phobia. That is why medications often help with the symptoms because they help the brain chemicals stay at the correct levels.

To improve treatment, scientists are studying how well different medicines and therapies work. In one kind of research, people with social phobia choose to take part in a clinical trial to help doctors find out what treatments work best for most people, or what works best for different symptoms. Usually, the treatment is free. Scientists are learning more about how the brain works so that they can discover new treatments.

Chapter 26

Reactions to Trauma

Chapter Contents

Section 26.1

Acute Stress Disorder: Initial Reaction to Trauma

Excerpted from "Acute Stress Disorder: A Brief Description," by Laura E. Gibson, Ph.D., published by the National Center for Posttraumatic Stress Disorder (NCPTSD, www.ncptsd.va.gov), part of the Veterans Administration, 2003. Reviewed by David A. Cooke, M.D., January 23, 2009.

What is acute stress disorder?

Acute stress disorder (ASD) is a psychiatric diagnosis that can be given to individuals in the first month following a traumatic event. The symptoms that define ASD overlap with those for PTSD [posttraumatic stress disorder], although there are a greater number of dissociative symptoms for ASD, such as not knowing where you are or feeling as if you are outside of your body.

How common is ASD?

Because ASD is a relatively new diagnosis, research on the disorder is in the early stages. Rates range from 6% to 33% depending on the type of trauma:

- **Motor vehicle accidents:** Rates of ASD range from approximately 13% to 21%.
- **Typhoon:** A study of survivors of a typhoon yielded an ASD rate of 7%.
- **Industrial accident:** One study found a rate of 6% in survivors of an industrial accident.
- **Violent assault:** A rate of 19% was found in survivors of violent assault, and a rate of 13% was found among a mixed group consisting of survivors of assaults, burns, and industrial accidents. A recent study of victims of robbery and assault found that 25% met criteria for ASD, and a study of victims of a mass shooting found that 33% met criteria for ASD.

Who is at risk for ASD as a result of trauma?

A few studies have examined factors that place individuals at risk for developing ASD.

One study found that individuals who (1) had experienced other traumatic events, (2) had PTSD previously, and (3) had prior psychological problems were all more likely to develop ASD as the result of a new traumatic stressor.

A study of motor vehicle accident survivors found that those individuals (1) with depression symptoms, (2) who had previous mental heath treatment, and (3) who had been in other motor vehicle accidents were more likely to have more severe ASD.

A final study suggests that people who dissociate when confronted with traumatic stressors may be more likely to develop ASD.

How predictive of PTSD is ASD?

A diagnosis of ASD appears to be a strong predictor of subsequent PTSD. In one study, more than three quarters of the individuals who were in motor vehicle accidents and met criteria for ASD went on to develop PTSD. This finding is consistent with other studies that found that over 80% of people with ASD developed PTSD by the time they were assessed 6 months later.

Are there effective treatments for ASD?

Cognitive-behavioral interventions: At present, cognitive-behavioral interventions during the acute aftermath of trauma exposure have yielded the most consistently positive results in terms of preventing subsequent posttraumatic psychopathology.

Psychological debriefing: Psychological debriefing is an early intervention that was originally developed for rescue workers but has been widely applied in the acute aftermath of potentially traumatic events. It has received much attention in the wake of 9/11. However, there is little evidence to support the continued use of debriefing with acutely traumatized individuals.

Section 26.2

Understanding Posttraumatic Stress Disorder (PTSD)

From "What Is Posttraumatic Stress Disorder?" by the National Center for Posttraumatic Stress Disorder (www.ncptsd.va.gov), part of the Veterans Administration, November 30, 2007.

Posttraumatic stress disorder (PTSD) is an anxiety disorder that can occur after you have been through a traumatic event. A traumatic event is something horrible and scary that you see or that happens to you. During this type of event, you think that your life or others' lives are in danger. You may feel afraid or feel that you have no control over what is happening.

Anyone who has gone through a life-threatening event can develop PTSD. These events can include:

- combat or military exposure;
- child sexual or physical abuse;
- terrorist attacks;
- sexual or physical assault;
- serious accidents, such as a car wreck; and
- natural disasters, such as a fire, tornado, hurricane, flood, or earthquake.

After the event, you may feel scared, confused, or angry. If these feelings don't go away or they get worse, you may have PTSD. These symptoms may disrupt your life, making it hard to continue with your daily activities.

How Does PTSD Develop?

All people with PTSD have lived through a traumatic event that caused them to fear for their lives, see horrible things, and feel helpless.

Strong emotions caused by the event create changes in the brain that may result in PTSD.

Most people who go through a traumatic event have some symptoms at the beginning. Yet only some will develop PTSD. It isn't clear why some people develop PTSD and others don't. How likely you are to get PTSD depends on many things. These include:

- how intense the trauma was or how long it lasted;
- if you lost someone you were close to or were hurt;
- how close you were to the event;
- how strong your reaction was;
- how much you felt in control of events; and
- how much help and support you got after the event.

Many people who develop PTSD get better at some time. But about 1 out of 3 people with PTSD may continue to have some symptoms. Even if you continue to have symptoms, treatment can help you cope. Your symptoms don't have to interfere with your everyday activities, work, and relationships.

What Are the Symptoms of PTSD?

Symptoms of posttraumatic stress disorder (PTSD) can be terrifying. They may disrupt your life and make it hard to continue with your daily activities. It may be hard just to get through the day.

PTSD symptoms usually start soon after the traumatic event, but they may not happen until months or years later. They also may come and go over many years. If the symptoms last longer than 4 weeks, cause you great distress, or interfere with your work or home life, you probably have PTSD.

There are four types of symptoms: reliving the event, avoidance, numbing, and feeling keyed up.

Reliving the event (also called re-experiencing symptoms): Bad memories of the traumatic event can come back at any time. You may feel the same fear and horror you did when the event took place. You may have nightmares. You even may feel like you're going through the event again. This is called a flashback. Sometimes there is a trigger: a sound or sight that causes you to relive the event. Triggers might include:

- hearing a car backfire, which can bring back memories of gunfire and war for a combat veteran;
- seeing a car accident, which can remind a crash survivor of his or her own accident; or
- seeing a news report of a sexual assault, which may bring back memories of assault for a woman who was raped.

Avoiding situations that remind you of the event: You may try to avoid situations or people that trigger memories of the traumatic event. You may even avoid talking or thinking about the event.

- A person who was in an earthquake may avoid watching television shows or movies in which there are earthquakes.
- A person who was robbed at gunpoint while ordering at a hamburger drive-in may avoid fast-food restaurants.
- Some people may keep very busy or avoid seeking help. This keeps them from having to think or talk about the event.

Feeling numb: You may find it hard to express your feelings. This is another way to avoid memories.

- You may not have positive or loving feelings toward other people and may stay away from relationships.
- You may not be interested in activities you used to enjoy.
- You may forget about parts of the traumatic event or not be able to talk about them.

Feeling keyed up (also called hyperarousal): You may be jittery, or always alert and on the lookout for danger. This is known as hyperarousal. It can cause you to:

- suddenly become angry or irritable;
- have a hard time sleeping;
- have trouble concentrating;
- fear for your safety and always feel on guard; and
- be very startled when someone surprises you.

What Are Other Common Problems?

People with PTSD may also have other problems. These include:

- drinking or drug problems;
- feelings of hopelessness, shame, or despair;
- employment problems;
- relationships problems including divorce and violence; and
- physical symptoms.

Can Children Have PTSD?

Children can have PTSD, too. They may have the symptoms described above or other symptoms depending on how old they are. As children get older their symptoms are more like those of adults.

- Young children may become upset if their parents are not close by, have trouble sleeping, or suddenly have trouble with toilet training or going to the bathroom.
- Children who are in the first few years of elementary school (ages 6 to 9) may act out the trauma through play, drawings, or stories. They may complain of physical problems or become more irritable or aggressive. They also may develop fears and anxiety that don't seem to be caused by the traumatic event.

What Treatments Are Available?

When you have PTSD, dealing with the past can be hard. Instead of telling others how you feel, you may keep your feelings bottled up. But treatment can help you get better.

There are good treatments available for PTSD. Cognitive-behavioral therapy (CBT) is one type of counseling. It appears to be the most effective type of counseling for PTSD. There are different types of cognitive behavioral therapies such as cognitive therapy and exposure therapy. A similar kind of therapy called EMDR, or eye movement desensitization and reprocessing, is also used for PTSD. Medications can be effective, too. A type of drug known as a selective serotonin reuptake inhibitor (SSRI), which is also used for depression, is effective for PTSD.

Section 26.3

PTSD Research

From "Posttraumatic Stress Disorder Research Fact Sheet," by the National Institute of Mental Health (NIMH, www.nimh.nih.gov), part of the National Institutes of Health, June 26, 2008.

Posttraumatic stress disorder (PTSD) is an anxiety disorder that some people develop after seeing or living through an event that caused or threatened serious harm or death. Symptoms include flashbacks or bad dreams, emotional numbness, intense guilt or worry, angry outbursts, feeling "on edge," or avoiding thoughts and situations that remind them of the trauma. In PTSD, these symptoms last at least one month.

Research on Possible Risk Factors for PTSD

Currently, many scientists are focusing on genes that play a role in creating fear memories. Understanding how fear memories are created may help to refine or find new interventions for reducing the symptoms of PTSD. For example, PTSD researchers have pinpointed genes that make:

- Stathmin, a protein needed to form fear memories. In one study, mice that did not make stathmin were less likely than normal mice to "freeze," a natural, protective response to danger, after being exposed to a fearful experience. They also showed less innate fear by exploring open spaces more willingly than normal mice.
- GRP (gastrin-releasing peptide), a signaling chemical in the brain released during emotional events. In mice, GRP seems to help control the fear response, and lack of GRP may lead to the creation of greater and more lasting memories of fear.

Researchers have also found a version of the 5-HTTLPR [serotonin-transporter-linked polymorphic region] gene, which controls levels of serotonin—a brain chemical related to mood-that appears to fuel the fear response. Like other mental disorders, it is likely that many genes with small effects are at work in PTSD.

Studying parts of the brain involved in dealing with fear and stress also helps researchers to better understand possible causes of PTSD. One such brain structure is the amygdala, known for its role in emotion, learning, and memory. The amygdala appears to be active in fear acquisition, or learning to fear an event (such as touching a hot stove), as well as in the early stages of fear extinction, or learning not to fear.

Storing extinction memories and dampening the original fear response appears to involve the prefrontal cortex (PFC) area of the brain, involved in tasks such as decision-making, problem-solving, and judgment. Certain areas of the PFC play slightly different roles. For example, when it deems a source of stress controllable, the medial PFC suppresses the amygdala, an alarm center deep in the brainstem, and controls the stress response. The ventromedial PFC helps sustain long-term extinction of fearful memories, and the size of this brain area may affect its ability to do so.

Individual differences in these genes or brain areas may only set the stage for PTSD without actually causing symptoms. Environmental factors, such as childhood trauma, head injury, or a history of mental illness, may further increase a person's risk by affecting the early growth of the brain. Also, personality and cognitive factors, such as optimism and the tendency to view challenges in a positive or negative way, as well as social factors, such as the availability and use of social support, appear to influence how people adjust to trauma. More research may show what combinations of these or perhaps other factors could be used someday to predict who will develop PTSD following a traumatic event.

Research on Treating PTSD

Currently, people with PTSD may be treated with psychotherapy ("talk" therapy), medications, or a combination of the two.

Psychotherapy

Cognitive behavioral therapy (CBT) teaches different ways of thinking and reacting to the frightening events that trigger PTSD symptoms and can help bring those symptoms under control. There are several types of CBT, including:

- exposure therapy—uses mental imagery, writing, or visiting the scene of a trauma to help survivors face and gain control of overwhelming fear and distress;

- cognitive restructuring—encourages survivors to talk about upsetting (often incorrect) thoughts about the trauma, question those thoughts, and replace them with more balanced and correct ones;
- stress inoculation training—teaches anxiety reduction techniques and coping skills to reduce PTSD symptoms, and helps correct inaccurate thoughts related to the trauma.

NIMH is currently studying how the brain responds to CBT compared to sertraline (Zoloft), one of the two medications recommended and approved by the U.S. Food and Drug Administration (FDA) for treating PTSD. This research may help clarify why some people respond well to medication and others to psychotherapy.

Medications

In a small study, NIMH researchers recently found that for people already taking a bedtime dose of the medication prazosin (Minipress), adding a daytime dose helped to reduce overall PTSD symptom severity, as well as stressful responses to trauma reminders.

Another medication of interest is D-cycloserine (Seromycin), which boosts the activity of a brain chemical called NMDA [N-methyl d-aspartate], which is needed for fear extinction. In a study of 28 people with a fear of heights, scientists found that those treated with D-cycloserine before exposure therapy showed reduced fear during the therapy sessions compared to those who did not receive the drug. Researchers are currently studying the effects of using D-cycloserine with therapy to treat PTSD.

Propranolol (Inderal), a type of medicine called a beta-blocker, is also being studied to see if it may help reduce stress following a traumatic event and interrupt the creation of fearful memories. Early studies have successfully reduced or seemingly prevented PTSD in small numbers of trauma victims.

Treatment after Mass Trauma

NIMH researchers are testing creative approaches to making CBT widely available, such as with internet-based self-help therapy and telephone-assisted therapy. Less formal treatments for those experiencing acute stress reactions are also being explored to reduce chances of developing full blown PTSD.

For example, in one preliminary study, researchers created a self-help website using concepts of stress inoculation training. People with PTSD first met face-to-face with a therapist. After this meeting, participants could log onto the website to find more information about PTSD and ways to cope, and their therapists could also log on to give advice or coaching as needed. Overall, the scientists found delivering therapy this way to be a promising method for reaching a large number of people suffering with PTSD symptoms.

Researchers are also working to improve methods of screening, providing early treatment, and tracking mass trauma survivors; and approaches for guiding survivors through self-evaluation/screening and prompting referral to mental health care providers based on need.

The Next Steps for PTSD Research

In the last decade, rapid progress in research on the mental and biological foundations of PTSD has lead scientists to focus on prevention as a realistic and important goal.

For example, NIMH-funded researchers are exploring new and orphan medications thought to target underlying causes of PTSD in an effort to prevent the disorder. Other research is attempting to enhance cognitive, personality, and social protective factors and to minimize risk factors to ward off full-blown PTSD after trauma. Still other research is attempting to identify what factors determine whether someone with PTSD will respond well to one type of intervention or another, aiming to develop more personalized, effective, and efficient treatments.

As gene research and brain imaging technologies continue to improve, scientists are more likely to be able to pinpoint when and where in the brain PTSD begins. This understanding may then lead to better targeted treatments to suit each person's own needs or even prevent the disorder before it causes harm.

Chapter 27

Obsessive-Compulsive Disorder (OCD)

Everyone double-checks things sometimes—for example, checking the stove before leaving the house, to make sure it's turned off. But people with OCD feel the need to check things over and over, or have certain thoughts or perform routines and rituals over and over. The thoughts and rituals of OCD cause distress and get in the way of daily life.

The repeated, upsetting thoughts of OCD are called obsessions. To try to control them, people with OCD repeat rituals or behaviors, which are called compulsions. People with OCD can't control these thoughts and rituals.

Examples of obsessions are fear of germs, of being hurt or of hurting others, and troubling religious or sexual thoughts. Examples of compulsions are repeatedly counting things, cleaning things, washing the body or parts of it, or putting things in a certain order, when these actions are not needed, and checking things over and over.

People with OCD have these thoughts and do these rituals for at least an hour on most days, often longer. The reason OCD gets in the way of their lives is that they can't stop the thoughts or rituals, so they sometimes miss school, work, or meetings with friends, for example.

From "When Unwanted Thoughts Take Over: Obsessive-Compulsive Disorder," by the National Institute of Mental Health (NIMH, www.nimh.nih.gov), part of the National Institutes of Health, 2006.

What are the symptoms of OCD?

People with OCD:

- have repeated thoughts or images about many different things, such as fear of germs, dirt, or intruders; violence; hurting loved ones; sexual acts; conflicts with religious beliefs; or being overly neat.
- do the same rituals over and over such as washing hands, locking and unlocking doors, counting, keeping unneeded items, or repeating the same steps again and again.
- have unwanted thoughts and behaviors they can't control.
- don't get pleasure from the behaviors or rituals, but get brief relief from the anxiety the thoughts cause.
- spend at least an hour a day on the thoughts and rituals, which cause distress and get in the way of daily life

When does OCD start?

For many people, OCD starts during childhood or the teen years. Most people are diagnosed at about age 19. Symptoms of OCD may come and go and be better or worse at different times.

Is there help?

There is help for people with OCD. The first step is to go to a doctor or health clinic to talk about symptoms. People who think they have OCD may want to bring this information to the doctor, to help them talk about the symptoms in it. The doctor will do an exam to make sure that another physical problem isn't causing the symptoms. The doctor may make a referral to a mental health specialist.

Doctors may prescribe medication to help relieve OCD. It's important to know that some of these medicines may take a few weeks to start working. Medications can be prescribed by M.D.s (usually a psychiatrist) and in some states also by clinical psychologists, psychiatric nurse practitioners, and advanced psychiatric nurse specialists. Check with your state's licensing agency for specifics.

The kinds of medicines used to treat OCD are listed below. Some of these medicines are used to treat other problems, such as depression, but also are helpful for OCD:

- antidepressants;
- antianxiety medicines; and
- beta-blockers.

Doctors also may ask people with OCD to go to therapy with a licensed social worker, psychologist, or psychiatrist. This treatment can help people with OCD feel less anxious and fearful.

There is no cure for OCD yet, but treatments can give relief to people who have it and help them live a more normal life. If you know someone with signs of OCD, talk to him or her about seeing a doctor. Offer to go along for support.

Who pays for treatment?

Most insurance plans cover treatment for anxiety disorders. People who are going to have treatment should check with their own insurance companies to find out about coverage. For people who don't have insurance, local city or county governments may offer treatment at a clinic or health center, where the cost is based on income. Medicaid plans also may pay for OCD treatment.

Why do people get OCD?

OCD sometimes runs in families, but no one knows for sure why some people have it, while others don't. When chemicals in the brain are not at a certain level it may result in OCD. Medications can often help the brain chemicals stay at the correct levels.

To improve treatment, scientists are studying how well different medicines and therapies work. In one kind of research, people with OCD choose to take part in a clinical trial to help doctors find out what treatments work best for most people, or what works best for different symptoms. Usually, the treatment is free. Scientists are learning more about how the brain works, so that they can discover new treatments.

Chapter 28

Treating Anxiety Disorders

Chapter Contents

Section 28.1

Treatment Options

"Guide to Treatment," from the Anxiety Disorders Association of America (ADAA, www.adaa.org), © 2008. Reprinted with permission.

Anxiety disorders are real, serious, and treatable. Experts believe that anxiety disorders are caused by a combination of biological and environmental factors, much like other disorders, such as heart disease and diabetes.

The vast majority of people with an anxiety disorder can be helped with professional care. Success of treatment varies among people. Some may respond to treatment after a few months, while others may need more than a year. Treatment is sometimes complicated by the fact that people very often have more than one anxiety disorder or suffer from depression or substance abuse. This is why treatment must be tailored to the individual.

Although treatment is individualized, several standard approaches have proved effective. Therapists will use one or a combination of these therapies.

Treatment Options

Cognitive-Behavioral Therapy (CBT)

Many therapists use a combination of cognitive and behavior therapies, often referred to as CBT. In this type of therapy the patient is actively involved in his or her own recovery, has a sense of control, and learns skills that are useful throughout life. CBT focuses on identifying, understanding, and modifying thinking and behavior patterns. When a person changes thinking and behavior, emotional changes usually follow. Because CBT teaches skills for handling anxiety, patients who learn and practice the skills can use them when needed.

Cognitive therapy: The goal of cognitive therapy is to change unwanted and disturbing thought patterns. The individual examines his or her feelings and learns to separate realistic from unrealistic thoughts.

Behavior therapy: The goal of behavior therapy is to modify and gain control over unwanted behavior. The individual learns to cope with difficult situations, often through controlled exposure to them.

Relaxation

Techniques for relaxing help people develop the ability to cope more effectively with the stresses and physical symptoms that contribute to anxiety. Common techniques are breathing retraining and exercise.

Medication

Medicines can be very useful in the treatment of anxiety disorders, and it is often used in conjunction with one or more therapies listed above. Sometimes antidepressants or anxiolytics (antianxiety medications) are prescribed to alleviate severe symptoms so that other forms of therapy can be effective. Depending on the person, medication may be either a short-term or long-term treatment option.

Choosing a Therapist

Anxiety disorders can be treated by a wide range of mental health professionals, including, psychiatrists, psychologists, clinical social workers, and psychiatric nurses. Primary care physicians are increasingly aware of the problems of anxiety disorders and depression, making these diagnoses more frequently. A primary care physician may prescribe medication or refer a patient to a mental health provider.

Finding the right therapist can be tricky, because satisfactory credentials are not the only factors to take into consideration. It is important to feel comfortable, so speak to the therapist, either on the phone or in the office, and don't be embarrassed if you feel uncomfortable and would rather see someone else.

Questions to Ask

A therapist should be willing to answer any questions you may have about methods, training, and fees. Here are some questions you may want to ask a therapist during a consultation:

- What training and experience do you have in treating anxiety disorders?
- What is your basic approach to treatment?

- Can you prescribe medication or refer me to someone who can, if that proves necessary?
- How long is the course of treatment?
- How frequent are treatment sessions and how long do they last?
- Do you include family members in therapy?
- Will you or a staff member go to the home of a phobic person, if necessary?
- What is your fee schedule, and do you have a sliding scale for varying financial circumstances?
- What kinds of health insurance do you accept?

If a therapist is reluctant to answer your questions, or if you do not feel comfortable, see someone else.

Section 28.2

Medications for Anxiety Disorders

"Treating Anxiety Disorders With Medications," from the Anxiety Disorders Association of America (ADAA, www.adaa.org), © 2008. Reprinted with permission.

If you are suffering from an anxiety disorder, you may face the issue of taking medication. Because excessive worry is a hallmark of anxiety disorders, it is not uncommon for this issue to become a focus of worry. And because excessive worry is often associated with procrastination and difficulty with decision-making, the task of deciding about the use of medication in treatment may become even more difficult. Medication treatment of anxiety is generally safe and effective. However, it often takes time and patience to find the drug that works best for you. Read on to learn more information to help you decide.

The first line of treatment for an anxiety disorder is often cognitive-behavioral therapy, or CBT. This is a well-established, highly effective, and lasting treatment. But some people find that excessively high levels of anxiety make them unable to get the most out of such treatment. They may avoid treatment sessions or feel unable to complete homework assigned by the therapist. In this case, medication may help overall levels of anxiety and allow full participation in CBT. Those without access to CBT or those who have not had a satisfactory response to it may benefit from medication treatment, too.

Considering Medication

Have a discussion with your doctor about medication if you are suffering from significant insomnia, which is frequently associated with generalized anxiety disorder, or GAD. Distressed by repetitive and excessive worry, people with GAD usually focus on the day's activities, such as what was left undone, what went wrong, what needs to be done tomorrow, and the like. People describe this condition as a difficulty turning their mind off, and they often have difficulty falling asleep. Improving sleep has been shown to reduce anxiety and depressive symptoms, and it can often be achieved with medication treatment.

Depression often complicates chronic anxiety. Don't ignore depressive symptoms such as a sad mood, bouts of tearfulness, low self-esteem, and feelings of guilt or hopelessness. Medication is often helpful in reducing symptoms of anxiety and alleviating those of depression. Most drugs used to treat anxiety come from the antidepressant class of medication, so they can be used to treat both conditions effectively.

Variety of Medications

Four major classes of medications are used in the treatment of anxiety disorders:

- benzodiazepines
- tricyclic antidepressants
- selective serotonin reuptake inhibitors (SSRIs)
- serotonin-norepinephrine reuptake inhibitors (SNRIs)

Benzodiazepines

Introduced in the 1960s, the benzodiazepines (such as alprazolam, clonazepam, diazepam, and lorazepam) are frequently used for short-term management of anxiety, such as for minor medical procedures.

They are highly effective in promoting relaxation and reducing muscular tension and other physical symptoms of anxiety. Long-term use may require increased doses to achieve the same effect, which may lead to problems related to tolerance and dependence. And abrupt discontinuation may result in significant withdrawal symptoms, including rebound anxiety and insomnia.

Tricyclic Antidepressants

Concerns about long-term use of the benzodiazepines led many doctors to favor the tricyclic antidepressants such as amitriptyline, imipramine, and nortriptyline. Although effective in the treatment of anxiety, they can cause significant side effects, including orthostatic hypotension (drop in blood pressure on standing), constipation, urinary retention, dry mouth, and blurry vision.

SSRIs

The introduction of the first selective serotonin reuptake inhibitor, or SSRI, for the treatment of depression in the 1980s led to testing this medication class for treating anxiety disorders. SSRIs relieve symptoms by blocking the reabsorption, or reuptake, of serotonin by certain nerve cells in the brain. This leaves more serotonin available, which enhances neurotransmission—the sending of nerve impulses—and improves mood. SSRIs are "selective" because they affect only serotonin, not other neurotransmitters. The SSRIs quickly gained popularity with doctors and patients because they generally produced fewer side effects, especially when compared with tricyclic antidepressants. However, common side effects include insomnia or sleepiness, sexual dysfunction, and weight gain. Included in the SSRI class are citalopram, escitalopram, fluoxetine, paroxetine, and sertraline. They are considered an effective treatment for all anxiety disorders, although the treatment of obsessive-compulsive disorder, or OCD, typically requires higher doses.

SNRIs

The serotonin-norepinephrine reuptake inhibitor, or SNRI, class is notable for a dual mechanism of action: increasing the levels of the neurotransmitters serotonin and norepinephrine by inhibiting their reabsorption into cells in the brain. Included in this class are venlafaxine and duloxetine. As with other medications, side effects may occur, including stomach upset, insomnia, headache, sexual dysfunction, and minor increase in blood pressure. These medications are considered as effective as SSRIs, so they are also considered a first-line treatment, particularly for the treatment of generalized anxiety disorder.

Additional Options

Beyond those mentioned above there are additional medications used in the treatment of anxiety disorders. Buspirone is commonly used to treat generalized anxiety disorder. Although it takes more time than the benzodiazepines to achieve an anti-anxiety effect (typically three to four weeks), it has not been associated with tolerance or dependency problems. Some psychiatrists are now prescribing the newest class of antipsychotics, known as "second-generation" or "atypical" antipsychotics, at low doses in the treatment of anxiety. This group includes aripiprazole, olanzapine, paliperidone, quetiapine, risperidone, and ziprasidone. These medications may be especially effective in treating ruminative worry and in aiding sleep.

Making a Decision

If you and your doctor have decided on medication as a treatment option, you have many choices. Work with your doctor to find the medication that's right for you. With patience and persistence, you will find a treatment that will help alleviate your anxiety symptoms.

Dr. Justine Kent is an Adjunct Assistant Professor of Psychiatry at Columbia University's College of Physicians & Surgeons.

Part Four

Eating, Impulse Control, and Addiction Disorders

Chapter 29

Understanding Eating and Body Image Disorders

Chapter Contents

Section 29.1

What Are Eating Disorders?

From the booklet "Eating Disorders," by the National Institute of Mental Health (NIMH, www.nimh.nih.gov), part of the National Institutes of Health, 2007.

What Are Eating Disorders?

An eating disorder is marked by extremes. It is present when a person experiences severe disturbances in eating behavior, such as extreme reduction of food intake or extreme overeating, or feelings of extreme distress or concern about body weight or shape. A person with an eating disorder may have started out just eating smaller or larger amounts of food than usual, but at some point, the urge to eat less or more spirals out of control.

Eating disorders are very complex, and despite scientific research to understand them, the biological, behavioral and social underpinnings of these illnesses remain elusive.

The two main types of eating disorders are anorexia nervosa and bulimia nervosa. A third category is "eating disorders not otherwise specified (EDNOS)," which includes several variations of eating disorders. Most of these disorders are similar to anorexia or bulimia but with slightly different characteristics. Binge eating disorder, which has received increasing research and media attention in recent years, is one type of EDNOS.

Eating disorders frequently appear during adolescence or young adulthood, but some reports indicate that they can develop during childhood or later in adulthood. Women and girls are much more likely than males to develop an eating disorder. Men and boys account for an estimated 5 to 15 percent of patients with anorexia or bulimia and an estimated 35 percent of those with binge eating disorder.

Eating disorders are real, treatable medical illnesses with complex underlying psychological and biological causes. They frequently coexist with other psychiatric disorders such as depression, substance abuse, or anxiety disorders. People with eating disorders also can suffer from numerous other physical health complications, such as heart conditions or kidney failure, which can lead to death.

Eating disorders are treatable diseases. Psychological and medicinal treatments are effective for many eating disorders. However, in more chronic cases, specific treatments have not yet been identified.

In these cases, treatment plans often are tailored to the patient's individual needs that may include medical care and monitoring; medications; nutritional counseling; and individual, group and/or family psychotherapy. Some patients may also need to be hospitalized to treat malnutrition or to gain weight, or for other reasons.

Anorexia Nervosa

Anorexia nervosa is characterized by emaciation, a relentless pursuit of thinness and unwillingness to maintain a normal or healthy weight, a distortion of body image and intense fear of gaining weight, a lack of menstruation among girls and women, and extremely disturbed eating behavior. Some people with anorexia lose weight by dieting and exercising excessively; others lose weight by self-induced vomiting, or misusing laxatives, diuretics, or enemas.

Many people with anorexia see themselves as overweight, even when they are starved or are clearly malnourished. Eating, food, and weight control become obsessions. A person with anorexia typically weighs herself or himself repeatedly, portions food carefully, and eats only very small quantities of only certain foods.

Some who have anorexia recover with treatment after only one episode. Others get well but have relapses. Still others have a more chronic form of anorexia, in which their health deteriorates over many years as they battle the illness.

According to some studies, people with anorexia are up to ten times more likely to die as a result of their illness compared to those without the disorder. The most common complications that lead to death are cardiac arrest, and electrolyte and fluid imbalances. Suicide also can result.

Many people with anorexia also have coexisting psychiatric and physical illnesses, including depression, anxiety, obsessive behavior, substance abuse, cardiovascular and neurological complications, and impaired physical development.

Other symptoms may develop over time, including:

- thinning of the bones (osteopenia or osteoporosis)
- brittle hair and nails

- dry and yellowish skin
- growth of fine hair over body (e.g., lanugo)
- mild anemia, and muscle weakness and loss
- severe constipation
- low blood pressure, slowed breathing, and pulse
- drop in internal body temperature, causing a person to feel cold all the time
- lethargy

Treating anorexia involves three components:

1. restoring the person to a healthy weight;
2. treating the psychological issues related to the eating disorder; and
3. reducing or eliminating behaviors or thoughts that lead to disordered eating, and preventing relapse.

Some research suggests that the use of medications, such as antidepressants, antipsychotics, or mood stabilizers, may be modestly effective in treating patients with anorexia by helping to resolve mood and anxiety symptoms that often co-exist with anorexia. Recent studies, however, have suggested that antidepressants may not be effective in preventing some patients with anorexia from relapsing. In addition, no medication has shown to be effective during the critical first phase of restoring a patient to healthy weight. Overall, it is unclear if and how medications can help patients conquer anorexia, but research is ongoing.

Different forms of psychotherapy, including individual, group, and family-based, can help address the psychological reasons for the illness. Some studies suggest that family-based therapies in which parents assume responsibility for feeding their afflicted adolescent are the most effective in helping a person with anorexia gain weight and improve eating habits and moods. Shown to be effective in case studies and clinical trials, this particular approach is discussed in some guidelines and studies for treating eating disorders in younger, nonchronic patients.

Others have noted that a combined approach of medical attention and supportive psychotherapy designed specifically for anorexia patients is more effective than just psychotherapy. But the effectiveness of a treatment depends on the person involved and his or her situation. Unfortunately, no specific psychotherapy appears to be consistently effective for treating adults with anorexia. However, research into novel treatment and prevention approaches is showing some promise. One study suggests that an online intervention program may prevent some at-risk women from developing an eating disorder.

Bulimia Nervosa

Bulimia nervosa is characterized by recurrent and frequent episodes of eating unusually large amounts of food (e.g., binge eating), and feeling a lack of control over the eating. This binge eating is followed by a type of behavior that compensates for the binge, such as purging (e.g., vomiting, excessive use of laxatives or diuretics), fasting, and/or excessive exercise.

Unlike anorexia, people with bulimia can fall within the normal range for their age and weight. But like people with anorexia, they often fear gaining weight, want desperately to lose weight, and are intensely unhappy with their body size and shape. Usually, bulimic behavior is done secretly, because it is often accompanied by feelings of disgust or shame. The binging and purging cycle usually repeats several times a week.

Similar to anorexia, people with bulimia often have coexisting psychological illnesses, such as depression, anxiety, and/or substance abuse problems. Many physical conditions result from the purging aspect of the illness, including electrolyte imbalances, gastrointestinal problems, and oral and tooth-related problems.

Other symptoms include:

- chronically inflamed and sore throat
- swollen glands in the neck and below the jaw
- worn tooth enamel and increasingly sensitive and decaying teeth as a result of exposure to stomach acids
- gastroesophageal reflux disorder
- intestinal distress and irritation from laxative abuse
- kidney problems from diuretic abuse
- severe dehydration from purging of fluids

As with anorexia, treatment for bulimia often involves a combination of options and depends on the needs of the individual.

To reduce or eliminate binge and purge behavior, a patient may undergo nutritional counseling and psychotherapy, especially cognitive behavioral therapy (CBT), or be prescribed medication. Some antidepressants, such as fluoxetine (Prozac), which is the only medication approved by the U.S. Food and Drug Administration for treating bulimia, may help patients who also have depression and/or anxiety. It also appears to help reduce binge eating and purging behavior, reduces the chance of relapse, and improves eating attitudes.

CBT that has been tailored to treat bulimia also has shown to be effective in changing binging and purging behavior, and eating attitudes. Therapy may be individually oriented or group-based.

Binge Eating Disorder

Binge eating disorder is characterized by recurrent binge eating episodes during which a person feels a loss of control over his or her eating. Unlike bulimia, binge eating episodes are not followed by purging, excessive exercise or fasting. As a result, people with binge eating disorder often are overweight or obese. They also experience guilt, shame and/or distress about the binge eating, which can lead to more binge eating.

Obese people with binge eating disorder often have coexisting psychological illnesses including anxiety, depression, and personality disorders. In addition, links between obesity and cardiovascular disease and hypertension are well documented.

Treatment options for binge eating disorder are similar to those used to treat bulimia. Fluoxetine and other antidepressants may reduce binge eating episodes and help alleviate depression in some patients. Patients with binge eating disorder also may be prescribed appetite suppressants.

Psychotherapy, especially CBT, is also used to treat the underlying psychological issues associated with binge eating, in an individual or group environment.

Warnings on Antidepressants

Despite the relative safety and popularity of selective serotonin reuptake inhibitors (SSRIs) and other antidepressants, some studies have suggested that they may have unintentional effects on some people, especially adolescents and young adults. In 2004, after a thorough review of data, the Food and Drug Administration (FDA) adopted a "black box" warning label on all antidepressant medications to alert the public about the potential increased risk of suicidal thinking or attempts in children and adolescents taking antidepressants. In 2007, the FDA proposed that makers of all antidepressant medications extend the warning to include young adults up through age 24. A "black box" warning is the most serious type of warning on prescription drug labeling. The warning emphasizes that children, adolescents, and young adults taking antidepressants should be closely monitored, especially during the initial weeks of treatment, for any worsening depression, suicidal thinking or behavior, or any unusual changes in behavior such as sleeplessness, agitation, or withdrawal from normal social situations. However, results of a comprehensive review of pediatric trials conducted between 1988 and 2006 suggested that the benefits of antidepressant medications likely outweigh their risks to children and adolescents with major depression and anxiety disorders. The study was partially funded by the National Institute of Mental Health.

How Are Men and Boys Affected?

Although eating disorders primarily affect women and girls, boys and men are also vulnerable. One in four preadolescent cases of anorexia occurs in boys, and binge eating disorder affects females and males about equally.

Like females who have eating disorders, males with the illness have a warped sense of body image and often have muscle dysmorphia, a type of disorder that is characterized by an extreme concern with becoming more muscular. Some boys with the disorder want to lose weight, while others want to gain weight or "bulk up." Boys who think they are too small are at a greater risk for using steroids or other dangerous drugs to increase muscle mass.

Boys with eating disorders exhibit the same types of emotional, physical, and behavioral signs and symptoms as girls, but for a variety of reasons, boys are less likely to be diagnosed with what is often considered a stereotypically "female" disorder.

How Are We Working to Better Understand and Treat Eating Disorders?

Researchers are unsure of the underlying causes and nature of eating disorders. Unlike a neurological disorder, which generally can be pinpointed to a specific lesion on the brain, an eating disorder likely involves abnormal activity distributed across brain systems. With increased recognition that mental disorders are brain disorders, more researchers are using tools from both modern neuroscience and modern psychology to better understand eating disorders.

One approach involves the study of the human genes. With the publication of the human genome sequence in 2003, mental health researchers are studying the various combinations of genes to determine if any DNA variations are associated with the risk of developing a mental disorder. Neuroimaging, such as the use of magnetic resonance imaging (MRI), may also lead to a better understanding of eating disorders.

Neuroimaging already is used to identify abnormal brain activity in patients with schizophrenia, obsessive-compulsive disorder, and depression. It may also help researchers better understand how people with eating disorders process information, regardless of whether they have recovered or are still in the throes of their illness.

Conducting behavioral or psychological research on eating disorders is even more complex and challenging. As a result, few studies of treatments for eating disorders have been conducted in the past. New studies currently underway, however, are aiming to remedy the lack of information available about treatment.

Researchers also are working to define the basic processes of the disorders, which should help identify better treatments.

For example, is anorexia the result of skewed body image, self esteem problems, obsessive thoughts, compulsive behavior, or a combination of these? Can it be predicted or identified as a risk factor before drastic weight loss occurs, and therefore avoided?

These and other questions may be answered in the future as scientists and doctors think of eating disorders as medical illnesses with certain biological causes. Researchers are studying behavioral questions, along with genetic and brain systems information, to understand risk factors, identify biological markers, and develop medications that can target specific pathways that control eating behavior. Finally, neuroimaging and genetic studies may also provide clues for how each person may respond to specific treatments.

Section 29.2

Binge Eating Disorder

From the Office of Women's Health (www.womenshealth.gov), part of the U.S. Department of Health and Human Services, January 2005.

What is binge eating disorder?

People with binge eating disorder often eat an unusually large amount of food and feel out of control during the binges. People with binge eating disorder also may:

- eat more quickly than usual during binge episodes;
- eat until they are uncomfortably full;
- eat when they are not hungry;
- eat alone because of embarrassment; and
- feel disgusted, depressed, or guilty after overeating.

What causes binge eating disorder?

No one knows for sure what causes binge eating disorder. Researchers are looking at the following factors that may affect binge eating:

- **Depression:** As many as half of all people with binge eating disorder are depressed or have been depressed in the past.
- **Dieting:** Some people binge after skipping meals, not eating enough food each day, or avoiding certain kinds of food.
- **Coping skills:** Studies suggest that people with binge eating may have trouble handling some of their emotions. Many people who are binge eaters say that being angry, sad, bored, worried, or stressed can cause them to binge eat.
- **Biology:** Researchers are looking into how brain chemicals and metabolism (the way the body uses calories) affect binge eating disorder. Research also suggests that genes may be involved in

binge eating, since the disorder often occurs in several members of the same family.

Certain behaviors and emotional problems are more common in people with binge eating disorder. These include abusing alcohol, acting quickly without thinking (impulsive behavior), and not feeling in charge of themselves.

What are the health consequences of binge eating disorder?

People with binge eating disorder are usually very upset by their binge eating and may become depressed. Research has shown that people with binge eating disorder report more health problems, stress, trouble sleeping, and suicidal thoughts than people without an eating disorder. People with binge eating disorder often feel badly about themselves and may miss work, school, or social activities to binge eat.

People with binge eating disorder may gain weight. Weight gain can lead to obesity, and obesity raises the risk for these health problems:

- type 2 diabetes;
- high blood pressure;
- high cholesterol;
- gallbladder disease;
- heart disease; and
- certain types of cancer.

What is the treatment for binge eating disorder?

People with binge eating disorder should get help from a health care provider, such as a psychiatrist, psychologist, or clinical social worker. There are several different ways to treat binge eating disorder:

- Cognitive-behavioral therapy teaches people how to keep track of their eating and change their unhealthy eating habits. It teaches them how to cope with stressful situations. It also helps them feel better about their body shape and weight.
- Interpersonal psychotherapy helps people look at their relationships with friends and family and make changes in problem areas.
- Drug therapy, such as antidepressants, may be helpful for some people.

Other treatments include dialectical behavior therapy, which helps people regulate their emotions; drug therapy with the anti-seizure medication topiramate; exercise in combination with cognitive-behavioral therapy; and support groups.

Many people with binge eating disorder also have a problem with obesity. There are treatments for obesity, like weight loss surgery (gastrointestinal surgery), but these treatments will not treat the underlying problem of binge eating disorder.

Section 29.3

Body Dysmorphic Disorder

"Body Dysmorphic Disorder," November 2007, reprinted with permission from www.kidshealth.org. Copyright ©2007 The Nemours Foundation. This information was provided by KidsHealth, one of the largest resources online for medically reviewed health information written for parents, kids, and teens. For more articles like this one, visit www.KidsHealth.org, or www.TeensHealth.org.

We all spend time in front of the mirror—dressing, grooming, or checking our appearance. This is especially true for teens, who are undergoing rapid growth and appearance changes, and taking new interest in the way they look. How they feel about their appearance is important, since body image can be such a big part of self-esteem during the teen years.

As a parent, you want to teach that there's much more to people than appearance. You want your teen's self-image to include personality, character, abilities, and his or her unique strengths and interests. Parents want their teens to appreciate and care for their bodies, and to take pride in how they look.

But feeling satisfied isn't always easy. Many kids who have positive body images become self-conscious or self-critical as they enter the teen years. It's not uncommon for teens to express dissatisfaction about their appearance or to compare themselves with their friends, celebrities, or people they see in the media. Ads for everything from makeup and clothing to hair products and toothpaste send messages that a person needs to look a certain way to be happy. It's hard not to be influenced by that.

While many teens feel dissatisfied with some aspect of their appearance, usually these concerns aren't consuming and don't cause extreme distress. They don't constantly occupy their thoughts or torment them and keep them from thinking about other things.

But for some teens, concerns about appearance become quite extreme and upsetting. They become so focused on imagined or minor imperfections that they can't seem to stop checking or obsessing about their appearance.

If your teen is constantly preoccupied and upset about body imperfections or appearance flaws, it may be a sign of body dysmorphic disorder.

What Is Body Dysmorphic Disorder?

Body dysmorphic disorder (BDD) is a condition that involves obsessions, which are distressing thoughts that repeatedly intrude into a person's awareness. With BDD, the distressing thoughts are about appearance flaws. Teens who have BDD might focus on what they perceive as a facial flaw, but they can also worry about other body parts, such as short legs or breast size or body shape. Just as people with eating disorders obsess about their weight, teens who have BDD worry about an aspect of their appearance. They may worry that their hair is thin, their face is scarred, their eyes aren't exactly the same size, their nose is too big, or their lips are too thin.

The disorder has been called "imagined ugliness" because the appearance flaws usually are so small that others consider them minor or don't even notice them. But for a person with BDD, the concerns feel very real because the obsessive thoughts distort and magnify any tiny imperfection. Because of the distorted body image caused by the disorder, a person may believe that he or she is too horribly ugly or disfigured to be seen.

Besides obsessions, BDD also involves compulsions. A compulsion is something a person does to try to relieve the tension caused by the obsessive thoughts. For example, a girl with obsessive thoughts that her nose is horribly ugly might constantly feel the need to check her appearance in the mirror, apply makeup, or ask someone many times a day whether her nose looks ugly.

Compulsions can provide temporary relief from the distress, so someone with BDD can feel a strong or irresistible urge to keep doing them. Someone might repeat compulsions almost constantly, and they can take up a lot of time and energy. They can feel like the only way to escape the bad feelings caused by the bad thoughts. Some people who have BDD also might do things to avoid the bad thoughts, like trying not to be seen by others, staying home, covering up, not participating in class, not socializing, or even refusing to look in mirrors.

With BDD, the pattern of obsessive thoughts, compulsive actions, and avoidance efforts gets so strong it feels impossible to control. Someone with BDD does not want to be preoccupied with the thoughts and behaviors, but might feel powerless to break the pattern. Even though the checking, fixing, asking, and avoiding seem to relieve terrible feelings, the relief is just temporary. In reality, the more a person avoids things or performs compulsions, the stronger the obsessions, compulsions, and avoidance become. After a while, it takes more and more compulsive behavior to relieve the distress caused by the bad thoughts.

What Causes BDD?

Although the exact cause of BDD is unclear, it is believed to be related to problems with serotonin, one of the brain's chemical neurotransmitters. Poor regulation of serotonin is also involved in other conditions, including obsessive-compulsive disorder (OCD), depression, and some eating disorders. If family members have experienced problems with OCD, anxiety or depression, or eating disorders, a person may be genetically prone to similar conditions. Compulsive behaviors contribute to the problem, too, by creating learned "habits" that reinforce symptoms and can cause them to worsen over time.

Cultural messages can also contribute to BDD. They reinforce a person's concerns about appearance. Criticism or unkind teasing about appearance may also contribute to BDD. But while these might harm a person's body image, alone they usually do not cause BDD.

How common is BDD? It's hard to know because few people with BDD are willing to talk about their concerns or seek help. But while it's very common for people to feel somewhat dissatisfied with their looks, true BDD, where it becomes a consuming part of everyday life, is rather uncommon. It usually begins in the teen years and, if untreated, can continue into adulthood.

The Impact of BDD

Sometimes people with BDD feel ashamed and keep their concerns secret. They may think that others would consider them vain or superficial, or become annoyed or irritated with the obsessions and compulsions about appearance.

It may be difficult to understand what your teen is going through, so he or she may feel misunderstood, unfairly judged, or alone.

The obsessions of BDD can disrupt daily life. Someone struggling with BDD might seem tense and distressed about appearance almost all the time and find it hard to stay focused on other things. A teen with BDD may keep a hand over the face for the entire school year, trying to hide a flaw, or might measure or examine the "flawed" body part repeatedly or spend lots of money and time on makeup to cover the problem.

A teen with has BDD may avoid going to school, quit a part-time job, or just stay at home all the time. BDD can lead to depression and, in severe cases, suicidal thoughts. A teen with BDD may ask to see a dermatologist or a plastic surgeon to correct a seeming appearance flaw. But with BDD, whatever the fix or treatment, obsession with appearance will continue.

Treating BDD

If you're concerned that your son or daughter has BDD, talk to a doctor or mental health professional. A careful assessment can help to clarify what's causing the distress and whether BDD is behind it. Many times, people with BDD are so focused on appearance that they (and those who love them) believe the answer is about correcting the appearance. If someone you love has BDD, you probably already know that no amount of reassurance seems to quiet the distress for long.

The problem with BDD lies in the obsessions and compulsions, which distort body image and make those who have it feel ugly. It's hard for them to see that, because they believe that what they perceive is truly there. Sometimes the most challenging part is helping someone accept a new idea of what might help.

BDD can be treated by an experienced mental health professional. Usually, treatment involves a particular type of talk therapy called cognitive-behavioral therapy, which focuses on the thoughts, feelings, and behaviors, and helps to correct the pattern behind the body image distortion and distress.

A therapist can help someone examine and change his or her faulty beliefs, resist compulsive behaviors, and face stressful situations that trigger appearance concerns. Sometimes, but not always, medication is used with the therapy. The treatment takes time, hard work, and patience. Support from family members can help a great deal.

It is often useful for parents to be involved in some aspects of the treatment, too, especially if a parent has been participating in the teen's compulsions by providing repeated reassurance. Parents in this situation need to know how to best respond to their teen's anxiety, distress, and requests for reassurance.

It's also helpful to tell the therapist about any family members who have experienced other conditions that involve obsessions and compulsions, anxiety disorders, or depression. If a parent is dealing with BDD, OCD, depression, or another related condition, it's important to mention this and for the parent to get treatment too. If a teen with BDD is also dealing with depression, anxiety, feeling isolated or alone, or dealing with difficult life situations, the therapy also can address those issues.

Getting Help for BDD

Body dysmorphic disorder, like other obsessions, can interfere with your teen's life—robbing it of pleasure and draining his or her energy.

It's not always easy to find the help you may need for your family. Your doctor, health care network, or community mental health center can direct you to local resources. Your son or daughter might resist your offer to see a mental health professional, so you might need to be persistent.

Though living with a person who's dealing with BDD can be frustrating and difficult, avoid blame, anger, or guilt. BDD is no one's fault. But with help and time, relief is possible. An experienced psychologist or psychiatrist who is knowledgeable about BDD can help break the grip of the disorder.

Chapter 30

Anorexia Nervosa

What is anorexia nervosa?

A person with anorexia nervosa, often called anorexia, has an intense fear of gaining weight. Someone with anorexia thinks about food a lot and limits the food she or he eats, even though she or he is too thin. Anorexia is more than just a problem with food. It's a way of using food or starving oneself to feel more in control of life and to ease tension, anger, and anxiety. Most people with anorexia are female. An anorexic:

- has a low body weight for her or his height;
- resists keeping a normal body weight;
- has an intense fear of gaining weight;
- thinks she or he is fat even when very thin; and/or
- misses three (menstrual) periods in a row—for girls/women who have started having their periods.

Who becomes anorexic?

While anorexia mostly affects girls and women (90–95 percent), it can also affect boys and men. It was once thought that women of color

---

From the Office of Women's Health (www.womenshealth.gov), part of the U.S. Department of Health and Human Services, September 2006.

were shielded from eating disorders by their cultures, which tend to be more accepting of different body sizes. Sadly, research shows that as African American, Latina, Asian/Pacific Islander, and American Indian and Alaska Native women are more exposed to images of thin women, they also become more likely to develop eating disorders.

What causes anorexia?

There is no single known cause of anorexia. But some things may play a part:

- **Culture:** Women in the United States are under constant pressure to fit a certain ideal of beauty. Seeing images of flawless, thin females everywhere makes it hard for women to feel good about their bodies. More and more, men are also feeling pressure to have a perfect body.
- **Families:** If you have a mother or sister with anorexia, you are more likely to develop the disorder. Parents who think looks are important, diet themselves, or criticize their children's bodies are more likely to have a child with anorexia.
- **Life changes or stressful events:** Traumatic events like rape, as well as stressful things like starting a new job, can lead to the onset of anorexia.
- **Personality traits:** Someone with anorexia may not like her or himself, hate the way she or he looks, or feel hopeless. She or he often sets hard-to-reach goals for her or himself and tries to be perfect in every way.
- **Biology:** Genes, hormones, and chemicals in the brain may be factors in developing anorexia.

What are signs of anorexia?

Someone with anorexia may look very thin. She or he may use extreme measures to lose weight by:

- making her or himself throw up;
- taking pills to urinate or have a bowel movement;
- taking diet pills;
- not eating or eating very little;
- exercising a lot, even in bad weather or when hurt or tired;

- weighing food and counting calories; or
- moving food around the plate instead of eating it.

Someone with anorexia may also have a distorted body image, shown by thinking she or he is fat, wearing baggy clothes, weighing her or himself many times a day, and fearing weight gain.

Anorexia can also cause someone to not act like her or himself. She or he may talk about weight and food all the time, not eat in front of others, be moody or sad, or not want to go out with friends.

What happens to your body with anorexia?

With anorexia, your body doesn't get the energy from foods that it needs, so it slows down. See Figure 30.1.

Can someone with anorexia get better?

Yes. Someone with anorexia can get better. A health care team of doctors, nutritionists, and therapists will help the patient get better. They will help her or him learn healthy eating patterns, cope with thoughts and feelings, and gain weight. With outpatient care, the patient receives treatment through visits with members of their health care team. Some patients may need "partial hospitalization." This means that the person goes to the hospital during the day for treatment, but lives at home. Sometimes, the patient goes to a hospital and stays there for treatment. After leaving the hospital, the patient continues to get help from her or his health care team.

Individual counseling can also help someone with anorexia. If the patient is young, counseling may involve the whole family, too. Support groups may also be a part of treatment. In support groups, patients and families meet and share what they've been through.

Often, eating disorders happen along with mental health problems such as depression and anxiety. These problems are treated along with the anorexia. Treatment may include medicines that fix hormone imbalances that play a role in these disorders.

Can women who had anorexia in the past still get pregnant?

It depends. When a woman has active anorexia, meaning she currently has anorexia, she does not get her period and usually does not ovulate. This makes it hard to get pregnant. Women who have recovered from anorexia and are at a healthy weight have a better chance

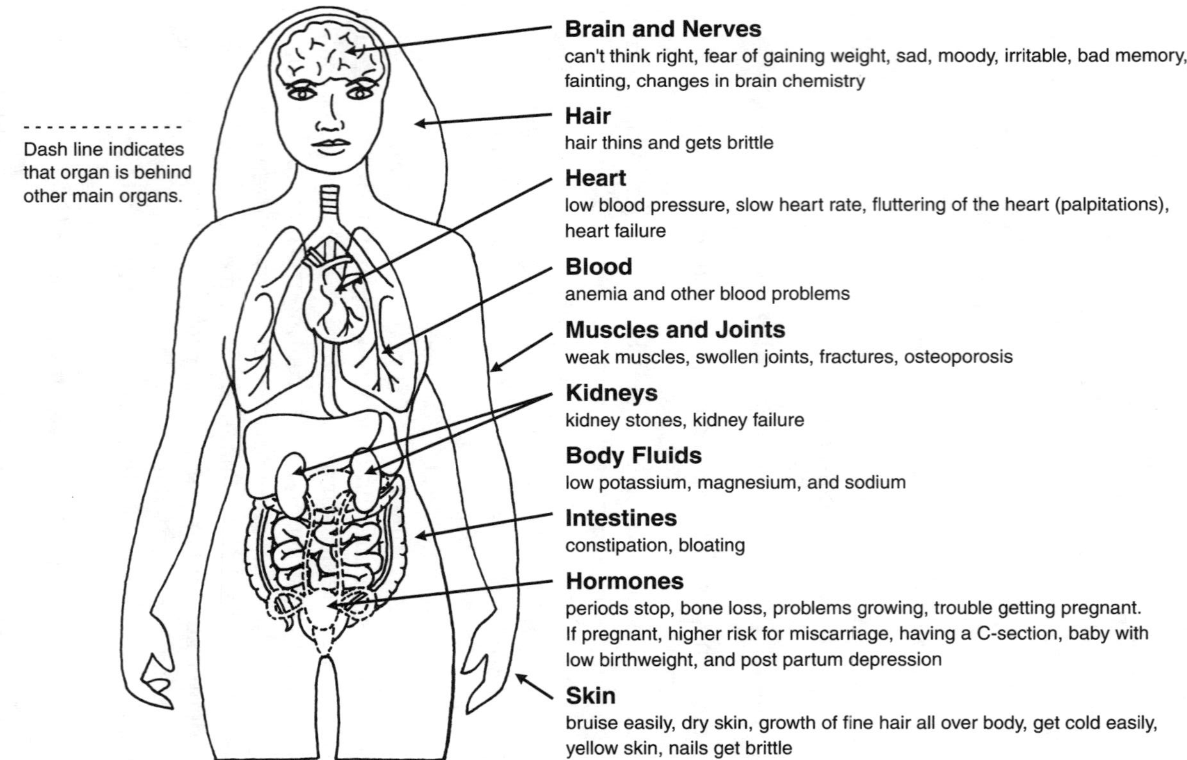

***Figure 30.1.** What happens to the body when a person has anorexia.*

of getting pregnant. If you're having a hard time getting pregnant, see your doctor.

Can anorexia hurt a baby when the mother is pregnant?

Yes. Women who have anorexia while they are pregnant are more likely to lose the baby. If a woman with anorexia doesn't lose the baby, she is more likely to have the baby early, deliver by C-section [Cesarean section], and have depression after the baby is born.

What should I do if I think someone I know has anorexia?

If someone you know is showing signs of anorexia, you may be able to help.

1. Set a time to talk. Set aside a time to talk privately with your friend. Make sure you talk in a quiet place where you won't be distracted.
2. Tell your friend about your concerns. Be honest. Tell your friend about your worries about her or his not eating or over exercising. Tell your friend you are concerned and that you think these things may be a sign of a problem that needs professional help.
3. Ask your friend to talk to a professional. Your friend can talk to a counselor or doctor who knows about eating issues. Offer to help your friend find a counselor or doctor and make an appointment, and offer to go with her or him to the appointment.
4. Avoid conflicts. If your friend won't admit that she or he has a problem, don't push. Be sure to tell your friend you are always there to listen if she or he wants to talk.
5. Don't place shame, blame, or guilt on your friend. Don't say, "You just need to eat." Instead, say things like, "I'm concerned about you because you won't eat breakfast or lunch." Or, "It makes me afraid to hear you throwing up."
6. Don't give simple solutions. Don't say, "If you'd just stop, then things would be fine!"
7. Let your friend know that you will always be there no matter what.

Chapter 31

Bulimia Nervosa

What is bulimia?

Bulimia nervosa is a type of eating disorder. It is often called just bulimia. A person with bulimia eats a lot of food in a short amount of time. This is called binging. The person may fear gaining weight after a binge. Binging also can cause feelings of shame and guilt. So, the person tries to "undo" the binge by getting rid of the food. This is called purging. Purging might be done by:

- making yourself throw up;
- taking laxatives—pills or liquids that speed up the movement of food through your body and lead to a bowel movement;
- exercising a lot;
- eating very little or not at all; and
- taking water pills to urinate.

Who becomes bulimic?

Many people think that only young, upper-class, white females get eating disorders. It is true that many more women than men have bulimia. In fact, 9 out of 10 people with bulimia are women. But bulimia can affect anyone: Men, older women, and women of color can

From the Office of Women's Health (www.womenshealth.gov), part of the U.S. Department of Health and Human Services, January 2007.

become bulimic. It was once thought that women of color were protected from eating disorders by their cultures. These cultures tend to be more accepting of all body sizes. But research shows that as women of color are more exposed to images of thin women, they are more likely to get eating disorders. African-American, Latina, Asian/Pacific Islander, and American Indian and Alaska Native women can become bulimic.

What causes bulimia?

Bulimia is more than just a problem with food. A binge can be set off by dieting or stress. Painful emotions, like anger or sadness, also can bring on binging. Purging is how people with bulimia try to gain control and to ease stress and anxiety. There is no single known cause of bulimia. But these factors might play a role:

- **Culture:** Women in the United States are under constant pressure to be very thin. This "ideal" is not realistic for most women. But seeing images of flawless, thin females everywhere can make it hard for women to feel good about their bodies. More and more, men are also feeling pressure to have a perfect body.
- **Families:** It is likely that bulimia runs in families. Many people with bulimia have sisters or mothers with bulimia. Parents who think looks are important, diet themselves, or judge their children's bodies are more likely to have a child with bulimia.
- **Life changes or stressful events:** Traumatic events like rape can lead to bulimia. So can stressful events like being teased about body size.
- **Psychology:** Having low self-esteem is common in people with bulimia. People with bulimia have higher rates of depression. They may have problems expressing anger and feelings. They might be moody or feel like they can't control impulsive behaviors.
- **Biology:** Genes, hormones, and chemicals in the brain may be factors in getting bulimia.

What are signs of bulimia?

A person with bulimia may be thin, overweight, or normal weight. This makes it hard to know if someone has bulimia. But there are warning signs to look out for. Someone with bulimia may do extreme things to lose weight, such as:

- using diet pills, or taking pills to urinate or have a bowel movement;
- going to the bathroom all the time after eating (to throw up); or
- exercising too much, even when hurt or tired.

Someone with bulimia may show signs of throwing up, such as:

- swollen cheeks or jaw area;
- rough skin on knuckles (if using fingers to make one throw up);
- teeth that look clear; and
- broken blood vessels in the eyes.

Someone with bulimia often thinks she or he is fat, even if this is not true. The person might hate his or her body. Or worry a lot about gaining weight. Bulimia can cause someone to not seem like him or herself. The person might be moody or sad. Someone with bulimia might not want to go out with friends.

What happens to someone who has bulimia?

Bulimia can hurt your body. Look at Figure 31.1 to find out how bulimia harms your health.

Can someone with bulimia get better?

Yes. Someone with bulimia can get better with the help of a health care team. A doctor will provide medical care. A nutritionist can teach healthy eating patterns. A therapist can help the patient learn new ways to cope with thoughts and feelings.

Therapy is an important part of any treatment plan. It might be alone, with family members, or in a group. Medicines can help some people with bulimia. These include medicines used to treat depression. Medicines work best when used with therapy.

Chances of getting better are greatest when bulimia is found out and treated early.

Can a woman who once had bulimia but is now better get pregnant?

Active bulimia can cause a woman to miss her period sometimes. Or, she may never get her period. If this happens, she usually does

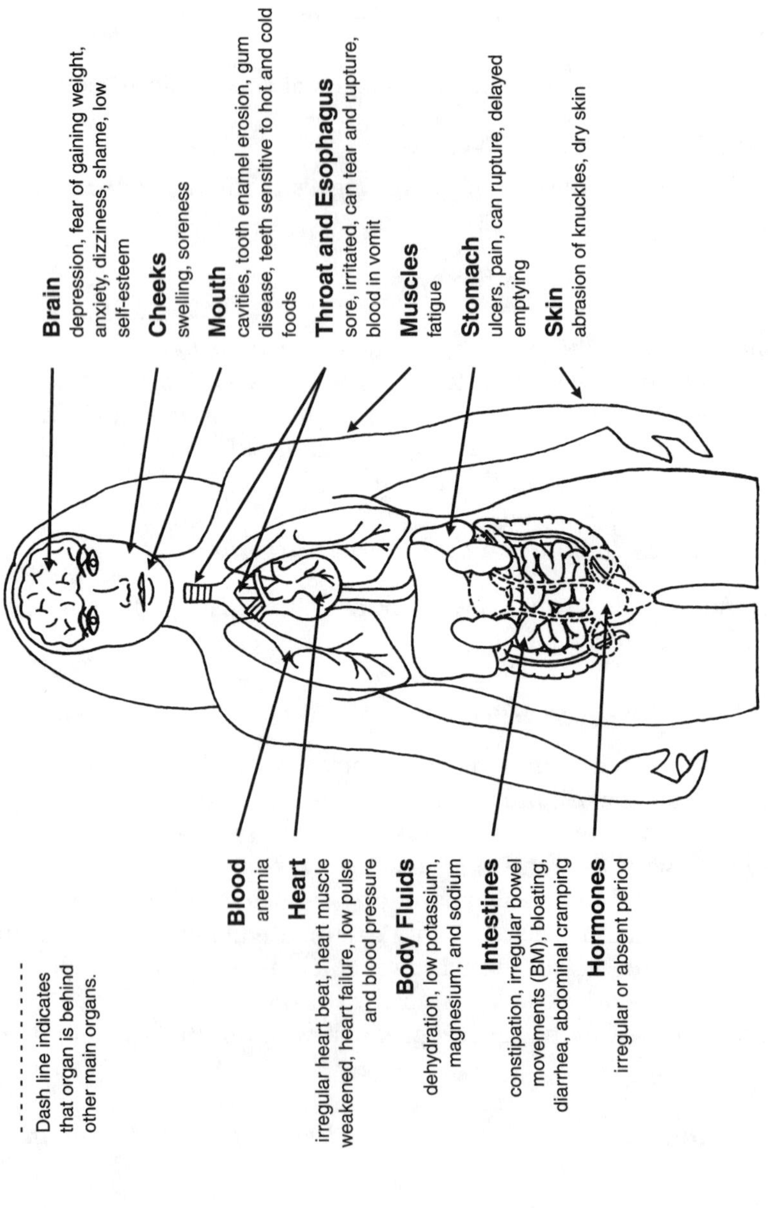

Dash line indicates that organ is behind other main organs.

Brain
depression, fear of gaining weight, anxiety, dizziness, shame, low self-esteem

Cheeks
swelling, soreness

Mouth
cavities, tooth enamel erosion, gum disease, teeth sensitive to hot and cold foods

Throat and Esophagus
sore, irritated, can tear and rupture, blood in vomit

Muscles
fatigue

Stomach
ulcers, pain, can rupture, delayed emptying

Skin
abrasion of knuckles, dry skin

Blood
anemia

Heart
irregular heart beat, heart muscle weakened, heart failure, low pulse and blood pressure

Body Fluids
dehydration, low potassium, magnesium, and sodium

Intestines
constipation, irregular bowel movements (BM), bloating, diarrhea, abdominal cramping

Hormones
irregular or absent period

Figure 31.1. *What happens to the body in a person with bulimia.*

not ovulate. This makes it hard to get pregnant. Women who have recovered from bulimia have a better chance of getting pregnant once their monthly cycle is normal. If you're having a hard time getting pregnant, see your doctor.

How does bulimia affect pregnancy?

If a woman with active bulimia gets pregnant, these problems may result:

- miscarriage;
- high blood pressure in the mother;
- baby isn't born alive;
- baby tries to come out with feet or bottom first;
- birth by C-section [Cesarean section];
- baby is born early;
- low birth weight;
- birth defects, such as blindness or mental retardation;
- problems breastfeeding; and
- depression in the mother after the baby is born.

What should I do if I think someone I know has bulimia?

If someone you know is showing signs of bulimia, you may be able to help.

- Set a time to talk. Find a time to talk alone with your friend.
- Make sure you talk in a quiet place where you won't be bothered.
- Tell your friend about your concerns. Be honest. Tell your friend that you are worried about her or his not eating or exercising too much. Tell your friend that you think these things may be a sign of a problem that needs professional help.
- Ask your friend to talk to a professional. Your friend can talk to a counselor or doctor who knows about eating issues. Offer to help your friend find a counselor or doctor and to make an appointment.

- Offer to go with her or him to the appointment.
- Avoid conflicts. If your friend won't admit that she or he has a problem, don't push. Be sure to tell your friend you are always there to listen if he or she wants to talk.
- Don't place shame, blame, or guilt on your friend. Don't say, "You just need to eat." Instead, say things like, "I'm concerned about you because you won't eat breakfast or lunch." Or, "It scares me to hear you throwing up."
- Don't give simple solutions. Don't say, "If you'd just stop, then things would be fine!"
- Let your friend know that you will always be there no matter what.

Chapter 32

Compulsive Exercise

Melissa has been a track fanatic since she was 12 years old. She has run the mile in meets in junior high and high school, constantly improving her times and winning several medals. Best of all, Melissa truly loves her sport.

Recently, however, Melissa's parents have noticed a change in their daughter. She used to return tired but happy from practice and relax with her family, but now she's hardly home for 15 minutes before she heads out for another run on her own. On many days, she gets up to run before school. When she's unable to squeeze in extra runs, she becomes irritable and anxious. And she no longer talks about how much fun track is, just how many miles she has to run today and how many more she should run tomorrow.

Melissa is living proof that even though exercise has many positive benefits, too much can be harmful. Teens, like Melissa, who exercise compulsively are at risk for both physical and psychological problems.

What Is Compulsive Exercise?

Compulsive exercise (also called obligatory exercise and anorexia athletica) is best defined by an exercise addict's frame of mind: He or

---

she no longer chooses to exercise but feels compelled to do so and struggles with guilt and anxiety if he or she doesn't work out. Injury, illness, an outing with friends, bad weather—none of these will deter those who compulsively exercise. In a sense, exercising takes over a compulsive exerciser's life because he or she plans life around it. Of course, it's nearly impossible to draw a clear line dividing a healthy amount of exercise from too much. The government's 2005 dietary guidelines, published by the U.S. Department of Agriculture (USDA) and the U.S. Department of Health and Human Services (HHS), recommend at least 60 minutes of physical activity for kids and teens on most—if not all—days of the week.

Experts say that repeatedly exercising beyond the requirements for good health is an indicator of compulsive behavior, but because different amounts of exercise are appropriate for different people, this definition covers a range of activity levels. However, several workouts a day, every day, is overdoing it for almost anyone.

Much like with eating disorders, many people who engage in compulsive exercise do so to feel more in control of their lives, and the majority of them are female. They often define their self-worth through their athletic performance and try to deal with emotions like anger or depression by pushing their bodies to the limit. In sticking to a rigorous workout schedule, they seek a sense of power to help them cope with low self-esteem.

Although compulsive exercising doesn't have to accompany an eating disorder, the two often go hand in hand. In anorexia nervosa, the excessive workouts usually begin as a means to control weight and become more and more extreme. As the person's rate of activity increases, the amount he or she eats may also decrease. A person with bulimia may also use exercise as a way to compensate for binge eating.

Compulsive exercise behavior can also grow out of student athletes' demanding practice schedules and their quest to excel. Pressure, both external (from coaches, peers, or parents) and internal, can drive the athlete to go too far to be the best. He or she ends up believing that just one more workout will make the difference between first and second place . . . then keeps adding more workouts.

Eventually, compulsive exercising can breed other compulsive behavior, from strict dieting to obsessive thoughts about perceived flaws. Exercise addicts may keep detailed journals about their exercise schedules and obsess about improving themselves. Unfortunately, these behaviors often compound each other, trapping the person in a downward spiral of negative thinking and low self-esteem.

Why Is Exercising Too Much a Bad Thing?

We all know that regular exercise is an important part of a healthy lifestyle. But few people realize that too much can cause physical and psychological harm:

- Excessive exercise can damage tendons, ligaments, bones, cartilage, and joints, and when minor injuries aren't allowed to heal, they often result in long-term damage. Instead of building muscle, too much exercise actually destroys muscle mass, especially if the body isn't getting enough nutrition, forcing it to break down muscle for energy.
- Girls who exercise compulsively may disrupt the balance of hormones in their bodies. This can change their menstrual cycles (some girls lose their periods altogether, a condition known as amenorrhea) and increase the risk of premature bone loss (a condition known as osteoporosis). And of course, working their bodies so hard leads to exhaustion and constant fatigue.
- An even more serious risk is the stress that excessive exercise can place on the heart, particularly when someone is also engaging in unhealthy weight loss behaviors such as restricting intake, vomiting, and using diet pills or supplements. In extreme cases, the combination of anorexia and compulsive exercise can be fatal.
- Psychologically, exercise addicts are often plagued by anxiety and depression. They may have a negative image of themselves and feel worthless. Their social and academic lives may suffer as they withdraw from friends and family to fixate on exercise. Even if they want to succeed in school or in relationships, working out always comes first, so they end up skipping homework or missing out on time spent with friends.

Warning Signs

A child may be exercising compulsively if he or she:

- won't skip a workout, even if tired, sick, or injured
- doesn't enjoy exercise sessions, but feels obligated to do them
- seems anxious or guilty when missing even one workout
- does miss one workout and exercises twice as long the next time

- is constantly preoccupied with his or her weight and exercise routine
- doesn't like to sit still or relax because of worry that not enough calories are being burnt
- has lost a significant amount of weight
- exercises more after eating more
- skips seeing friends, gives up activities, and abandons responsibilities to make more time for exercise
- seems to base self-worth on the number of workouts completed and the effort put into training
- is never satisfied with his or her own physical achievements

It's important, too, to recognize the types of athletes who are more prone to compulsive exercise because their sports place a particular emphasis on being thin. Ice skaters, gymnasts, wrestlers, and dancers can feel even more pressure than most athletes to keep their weight down and their body toned. Runners also frequently fall into a cycle of obsessive workouts.

Getting Professional Help

If you recognize two or more warning signs of compulsive exercise in your child, call your doctor to discuss your concerns. After evaluating your child, the doctor may recommend medical treatment and/or other therapy. Because compulsive exercise is so often linked to an eating disorder, a community agency that focuses on treating these disorders might be able to offer advice or referrals. Extreme cases may require hospitalization to get a child's weight back up to a safe range.

Treating a compulsion to exercise is never a quick-fix process—it may take several months or even years. But with time and effort, kids can get back on the road to good health. Therapy can help improve self-esteem and body image, as well as teach them how to deal with emotions. Sessions with a nutritionist can help develop healthy eating habits. Once they know what to watch out for, kids will be better equipped to steer clear of unsafe exercise and eating patterns.

Ways to Help at Home

Parents can do a lot to help a child overcome a compulsion to exercise:

- Involve kids in preparing nutritious meals.
- Combine activity and fun by going for a hike or a bike ride together as a family.
- Be a good body-image role model. In other words, don't fixate on your own physical flaws, as that just teaches kids that it's normal to dislike what they see in the mirror.
- Never criticize another family member's weight or body shape, even if you're just kidding around. Such remarks might seem harmless, but they can leave a lasting impression on kids or teens struggling to define and accept themselves.
- Examine whether you're putting too much pressure on your kids to excel, particularly in a sport (because some teens turn to exercise to cope with pressure). Take a look at where kids might be feeling too much pressure. Help them put it in perspective and find other ways to cope.

Most important, just be there with constant support. Point out all of your child's great qualities that have nothing to do with how much he or she works out—small daily doses of encouragement and praise can help improve self-esteem. If you teach kids to be proud of the challenges they've faced and not just the first-place ribbons they've won, they will likely be much happier and healthier kids now and in the long run.

Chapter 33

Impulse Control Disorders

Chapter Contents

Section 33.1

What Are Impulse Control Disorders?

From "Impulse Control Disorders," © 2003 Queensland Health (www.health.qld.gov.au). Reprinted with permission. Reviewed by David A. Cooke, M.D., January 23, 2009. Dr. Cooke is not affiliated with Queensland Health.

What Is an Addiction or Impulse Control Disorder?

When someone has an impulse control disorder (ICD) it means that they experience irresistible urges to carry out a particular behaviour which will result in feelings of relief or pleasure. Afterwards they may experience a period of guilt or remorse. Common behaviours include abusing drugs or alcohol, gambling, stealing, excessive anger, and setting things alight. When these behaviours become part of day to day life despite the consequences, they also become known as addictions.

What Are the Causes of ICDs?

The causes of ICDs and addiction are numerous. Some people may have a genetic predisposition to it, which would make them particularly prone to developing the behaviour. For example trichotillomania may be a neurological disorder not just a bad habit. Biological and physiological explanations are also given whereby behaviours are the result of chemical reactions in the body. Upbringing, a developmental disorder, or learning disability may also be responsible. These factors together with any number of social and environmental features and significant life events can all have an impact on the occurrence of an ICD or addiction.

What Treatment Is Available?

Counselling and psychotherapy involves working with a therapist on developing inner strengths, capabilities, resources, and potential.

Cognitive behaviour therapy that focuses on:

- The introduction of a 'reward' scheme to provide a greater incentive to discontinue the behaviour, or towards increasing positive behaviours such as attending support groups and making steps to find employment.
- Working to resolve ambivalence and help people to recognise the greater benefits in changing behaviour as opposed to the benefits in maintaining old behaviour patterns. It focuses on increasing the use of internal resources.
- Learning to recognise personal 'high-risk' situations and applying specific coping skills and strategies to avoid continuing the behaviour. Self-efficacy and confidence are boosted as a result.
- It is well understood how the environment can affect a person's desire to continue negative behaviour patterns thus individual environments can be assessed and modified to minimise this desire and make it more rewarding to maintain abstinence.
- Joining a self-help group. This enables individuals to talk to each other about their experiences and provide mutual support.
- Enlisting and using the support of family and friends.

Section 33.2

Compulsive Gambling

From "Impulse Control Disorders," © 2003 Queensland Health (www.health .qld.gov.au). Reprinted with permission. Reviewed by David A. Cooke, M.D., January 23, 2009. Dr. Cooke is not affiliated with Queensland Health.

Pathological gambling is one of the most common disorders. It affects 1-3 per cent of the adult population and typically begins in adolescence. The process to addiction is slow and is likely to increase during times of stress and anxiety. These people have a preoccupation with gambling to the extent that family life and work are affected. They are excited by the thrill more than the financial gain. These individuals can be restless and irritated if attempts are made to cut down. They will often lie to family members about debt and may steal or extort money.

The personalities of these people are competitive, easily bored, energetic, approval seekers, workaholic, or binge workers (working at the last minute to meet deadlines). The typical pathological gambler is affable, self-centred, and often likeable. Most are male and many have committed illegal acts to support their habits. The signs associated with a person with a gambling addiction are as follows:

- Preoccupation with gambling
- Necessity to gamble with increasing amounts of money to experience the original thrill
- Failed attempts to cut back
- Restless when not gambling
- Lies to all concerned about the gambling
- Loss of a relationship, job, and/or money
- Reliance on others to get out of trouble

Individual cures are extremely difficult to come by. Gamblers Anonymous (GA), patterned after Alcoholics Anonymous, offers some hope, and Gam-Anon offers support for families of pathological gamblers. Few who only enter GA actually quit gambling, but if they enter GA and go to an inpatient treatment facility, recovery rates approach 50 per cent for those who complete the program. Families of pathological gamblers may have a better chance of adapting to the problems than the gambler has of stopping the creation of the problems.

Section 33.3

Intermittent Explosive Disorder

From "Impulse Control Disorders," © 2003 Queensland Health (www.health.qld.gov.au). Reprinted with permission. Reviewed by David A. Cooke, M.D., January 23, 2009. Dr. Cooke is not affiliated with Queensland Health.

This aptly named disorder is diagnosed if an individual manifests several obviously excessive and unjustified outbursts of anger that result in significant property damage or injury to others. Care must be taken in diagnosis to ensure that the outbursts cannot be better accounted for by another diagnosis or be substance-induced or the result of a medical condition. Voluntary acts for gain also do not qualify. The disorder does not necessarily interfere with aspects of the individual's life, although it obviously interferes with the lives of others. Some investigators believe that this disorder is a version of bipolar disorder, and have had some success treating the disorder with medication. However, it is fair to say that relatively little is certain about treatment of people with IED. Left untreated, symptoms of the disorder are certainly likely to recur.

Section 33.4

Kleptomania (Stealing)

From "Impulse Control Disorders," © 2003 Queensland Health (www.health.qld.gov.au). Reprinted with permission. Reviewed by David A. Cooke, M.D., January 23, 2009. Dr. Cooke is not affiliated with Queensland Health.

This is when a person will shoplift or steal from others even though the goods may be of little value or are unneeded. They steal for the thrill of stealing and they don't want to get caught. It is also done to relieve tension. Items may be hoarded or taken back secretly. They may feel guilty and worried about being caught. To be diagnosed, a person must have the typical pattern that involves having recurrent tension leading to the behaviour, which leads to relief or pleasure after performing the behaviour. This disorder may be associated with depression and/or bulimia. It is rare overall but is more common in females than in males.

The stealing is not accounted for by hunger or poverty or vengeance, or accounted for better by another disorder of which stealing is a part, e.g., antisocial personality disorder or a manic episode. It is difficult to document the precise number of people with kleptomania. People with kleptomania often have another psychiatric disorder, often a mood disorder. Treatment is largely untested, and the disorder often persists despite many convictions of shoplifting. It may decrease as the individual ages, however.

Section 33.5

Pyromania (Firesetting)

From "Impulse Control Disorders," © 2003 Queensland Health (www.health.qld.gov.au). Reprinted with permission. Reviewed by David A. Cooke, M.D., January 23, 2009. Dr. Cooke is not affiliated with Queensland Health.

Pyromania involves more planning than most of the impulse control disorders, so it is actually more compulsive than impulsive. It requires that the person set more than one deliberate fire (not in a barbecue or fireplace) that is also a destructive fire. It follows the usual impulse disorder sequence, which consists of a strong arousal before and pleasure or tension reduction after the act. People usually have a fascination, obsession, or attraction to fire and objects, people, or situations around fire. The fire setting is not done for monetary gain or an expression of anger, vengeance, personal gain, or psychosis, unless they meet the criteria above and the fire setting must not be accounted for by another diagnosis.

Section 33.6

Trichotillomania (Hair Pulling)

From "Impulse Control Disorders," © 2003 Queensland Health (www.health.qld.gov.au). Reprinted with permission. Reviewed by David A. Cooke, M.D., January 23, 2009. Dr. Cooke is not affiliated with Queensland Health.

Trichotillomania (T) has the usual features of impulse control disorders—that is relief after the behaviour, and usually a build up of tension before, at least when the individual is attempting to control the behaviour. T was thought to be rare, but earlier estimates may have been too low because victims are usually secretive about the behaviour.

Frequently, a stressful event can be associated with the onset, such as a change of schools, abuse, family conflict, or the death of a parent. The symptoms also may be triggered by pubertal hormonal changes. Most cases of hair pulling don't qualify as T, and many cases remit over time. Others continue indefinitely. In behavioural therapy, people learn a structured method of keeping track of the symptoms and associated behaviours, increasing awareness of pulling, substituting incompatible behaviours, and several other techniques aimed at reversing the "habit" of pulling. However, different treatments work for different people.

Chapter 34

Understanding Compulsive Sexual Behaviors

Introduction

Sexuality in the United States has never been more socially acceptable. Sex has become part of mainstream culture as reflected through the explicit coverage of sexual behaviors in the media, movies, newspapers, and magazines. In many ways, sexual expression has become a form of accepted entertainment similar to gambling, attending sporting events, or watching movies. Internet pornography has become a billion-dollar industry, stretching the limits of the imagination. Digital media offers portability, access, and visually explicit depictions of sexual acts in high-definition that leave nothing to the imagination. Sales and rental of adult movies through DVDs and pay-per-view services allow access to sex anywhere and at any time. The adult entertainment industry generates close to $4 billion per year and its acceptability in society is reflected in the mainstreaming of its products into traditional retail stores and the portrayal of its actors and actresses as role models and celebrities. Strip clubs have evolved from backroom cabarets into large multimillion dollar nightclubs and are present in virtually every state in the United States. Inside them, the degree of physical contact has also increased, as compared to a generation ago,

---

to the point where the boundaries of what constitutes sexual intercourse are blurred. Escort services, massage parlors, and street prostitution continue to be available in every major city in the United States. Strengthening their presence and availability is the Internet, which has created an information portal for these services through online dating services, classified ads, and discussion boards for those in pursuit of sexual gratification.

Together, these cultural changes have increased the acceptability and availability of sexual rewards. For some, though, this increase in availability has uncovered an inability to control sexual impulses resulting in continued engagement in these behaviors despite the creation of negative consequences—otherwise known as sexual addiction. This term has been used synonymously with others, such as compulsive sexual behaviors, hypersexuality, and excessive sexual desire disorder. It can take many forms, and although it may seem obvious to diagnose, standardized criteria have yet to be developed. Furthermore, debate is ongoing about where this behavioral pattern fits into the American Psychiatric Association's *Diagnostic and Statistical Manual* (*DSM-IV*), and how it should be classified and conceptualized. Is it an addictive disorder, an impulse-control disorder, or a variant of obsessive-compulsive disorders? Does it merit enough empirical evidence to stand alone as a separate disorder? Finally, what are the boundaries and limits that distinguish disease patterns, at-risk behaviors, and socially appropriate expression?

Compulsive sexual behavior has not yet received extensive attention from researchers and clinicians. To date, there have been very few formalized studies of compulsive sexual behaviors. As an example, a keyword search on PubMed, as of October, 2006, for "sexual addiction" yielded 518 articles, while "compulsive sexual behavior" yielded 264 (in comparison, "substance abuse" yields 164,104). Funding agencies, such as the National Institutes of Health (NIH), and pharmaceutical companies have not supported research into the etiology and mechanisms of compulsive sexual behavior and, as a result, evidenced-based treatments are limited. Despite the paucity of research, a significant number of patients with sexual addictions do present for treatment. This is evidenced by the number of treatment centers dedicated to the treatment of sexual addictions in both residential and intensive outpatient settings. Mental health professionals in any setting are likely to encounter patients with this hidden addiction and require better tools to diagnose and manage them. This article will review the terminology, the epidemiology, and the existing treatments that are currently available for compulsive sexual behaviors.

Defining Compulsive Sexual Behaviors

The *DSM-IV* currently does not list compulsive sexual behavior as a separate disorder with formal criteria. There are 12 listed sexual disorders and they are divided into disorders of sexual dysfunction, paraphilias, and gender identity disorder. Among these disorders, there is no mention of repetitive, continued sexual behaviors that cause clinical distress and impairment. In fact, the only place where compulsive sexual behaviors might be included is within the context of sexual disorder, not otherwise specified (NOS) or as part of a manic episode. In other words, hypersexuality, sexual addiction, or compulsive sexual behaviors are terms that are not found within the *DSM-IV*.

Some of the reasons for why there is a lack of formalized criteria include the lack of research as well as an agreed-upon terminology. This is due, in part, to the heterogeneous presentation of compulsive sexual behaviors. For instance, some patients present with clinical features that resemble an addictive disorder—i.e., continued engagement in the behavior despite physical or psychological consequences, a loss of control, and a preoccupation with the behavior. Others will demonstrate elements of an impulse control disorder, namely reporting irresistible urges and impulses, both physically and mentally, to act out sexually without regard to the consequences. Finally, there are patients who demonstrate sexual obsessions and compulsions to act out sexually in a way that resembles obsessive-compulsive disorders. They do so to quell anxiety and to minimize fears of harm. For these patients, the thoughts and urges to act out sexually are ego-dystonic, whereas other types of patients describe ego-syntonic feelings about their sexual behaviors.

One important feature to note is that hypersexuality is not necessarily symbolic or diagnostic of compulsive sexual behaviors. Libido and sexual drive can be seen as similar to other biological drives, such as sleep and appetite. States of hypersexuality induced by substances of abuse, mania, medications (e.g., dopamine agonists), or even other medical conditions (e.g., frontal-lobe tumors) can induce episodes of impulsive and excessive sexual behaviors. However, once those primary conditions are treated, the sexual behaviors return to normalcy in terms of frequency and intensity.

Clinical Features

Compulsive sexual behaviors can present in a variety of forms and degrees of severity, much like that of substance use disorders, mood disorders, or impulse-control disorders. Often, it may not be the primary reason for seeking treatment and the symptoms are not revealed unless inquired about. Despite the lack of formalized criteria, there are common clinical features that are typically seen in compulsive sexual behaviors.

One of the fundamental hallmarks of compulsive sexual behavior is continued engagement in sexual activities despite the negative consequences created by these activities. This is the same phenomenon seen in substance use and impulse control disorders. Psychologically, sexual behaviors serve to escape emotional or physical pain or are a way of dealing with life stressors. The irony is that the sexual behaviors becomes the primary way of coping and handling problems that, in turn, creates a cycle of more problems and increasing desperation, shame, and preoccupation.

Compulsive sexual behavior can be divided into paraphilic and non-paraphilic subtypes. Paraphilic behaviors refer to behaviors that are considered to be outside of the conventional range of sexual behaviors. These include the eight paraphilias recognized in the *DSM-IV*: Exhibitionism, voyeurism, pedophilia, sexual masochism, sexual sadism, transvestic fetishism, fetishism, and frotteurism. There are many other forms of paraphilias that are not listed in *DSM-IV* (e.g., gerontophilia, necrophilia, zoophilia) that exist but have not been yet recognized as clinical disorders. A key clinical feature in diagnosing a paraphilic sexual behavior is that it must be distressing and cause significant impairment in one's life, with the exception of pedophilia and fetishism. In other words, with the noted exceptions, engagement in these behaviors leads to sexual gratification but does not cause distress or impairment and do not represent clinical disorders. Thus, frequency, amount of time spent, and amount of money spent are not necessarily reliable indicators of the presence of a compulsive sexual disorder. Paraphilias begin in late adolescence and peak in the mid-20s. Commonly, paraphilias do not occur in isolation; as the expected course is characterized by multiple paraphilic and non-paraphilic behaviors.

Non-paraphilic behaviors represent engagement in commonly available sexual practices, such as attending strip clubs, compulsive masturbation, paying for sex through prostitution, excessive use of pornography, and repeated engagement in extramarital affairs. The onset, clinical course, and male predominance are fairly similar to paraphilic disorders. Various epidemiological studies estimate that close to six percent of the general population meet criteria but there are no national or large datasets to confirm this. Because of the variety of activities possible, non-paraphilic compulsive sexual behavior can present in a number of ways. This has the potential to confuse and cloud clinicians. In addition, a clinician that screens only for some but not all of the potentially problematic sexual behaviors is likely to miss important clinical information. Thus, asking about both paraphilic and non-paraphilic behaviors is critical in screening. In addition, it is important to assess the consequences as well as the nature of the behavior. A person who spends $1000 per week on strip clubs may at first glance appear to meet criteria, but if there are no notable adverse consequences in his or her life, then the disorder may not be present.

Identifying a compulsive sexual disorder is a challenge because of its sensitive and personal nature. Unless patients present specifically for treatment of this disorder, they are not likely to discuss it. Much like other impulse control disorders, the physical and psychological signs of compulsive sexual behaviors are often subtle or hidden. Even signs of excessive sexual behaviors (such as physical injury to the genital area) or the presence of sexually transmitted diseases does not necessarily indicate compulsive sexual activity. Their presence does signal the need to screen for those behaviors but one cannot assume a compulsive sexual disorder exists based on physical examination alone.

Consequences of compulsive sexual behaviors can vary with some being similar to that seen in other addictive disorders while others are unique. Medically, patients are at a higher risk for sexually transmitted diseases (STDs) and for physical injuries due to repetitive sexual practices. Human immunodeficiency virus (HIV), Hepatitis B and C, syphilis, and gonorrhea are particularly concerning consequences. Virtually unknown is the percentage of those individuals with STDs who meet criteria for compulsive sexual disorders.

Another significant consequence is the loss of time and productivity. It is not uncommon for patients to spend large amounts of time viewing pornography or cruising (also called mongering) for sexual gratification. Financial losses can mount quickly, and patients can accumulate several thousands of dollars of debt in a short amount of time. In addition, there is a long list of legal consequences, including arrest for solicitation and engaging in paraphilic acts that are illegal. One look at recent news headlines will likely reveal several stories focusing on illegal sexual activities or behaviors that jeopardize someone's livelihood or well-being.

The psychological consequences are numerous. Effects on the family and interpersonal relationships can be profound. Compulsive sexual behaviors can establish unhealthy and unrealistic expectations of what a satisfying sexual relationship should be. At the same time, the deception, secrecy, and violations of trust that occur with compulsive sexual behaviors may shatter intimacy and personal connections. The result is a warped view of intimacy that often leads to separation and divorce and, in turn, puts any future healthy relationship in doubt.

Finally, the shame and guilt that those with compulsive sexual behaviors experience is different from those with other addictive disorders. There are no substances of abuse to explain seemingly irrational behaviors. The stigma of not being able to control sexual impulses carries with it a connotation of depravity and moral selfishness. Stigmatization in the media and criminalization of "sexual offenders" creates an atmosphere that does not promote treatment and prevention. As a result, access to care and seeking care, even when one recognizes that sexual behaviors are out of control, is a decision faced with barriers and limitations.

Epidemiology

There have been no national studies documenting the past-year or lifetime prevalence of compulsive sexual behaviors in the general population. Regional and local surveys suggest that approximately five percent of the general population may meet criteria for a compulsive sexual disorder (using criteria that are similar to substance use disorders). Further replication of these data is needed but if true, these rates represent a significant percentage of the general population and would be higher than the rates for schizophrenia, bipolar disorder, and pathological gambling. One of the reasons why reliable epidemiological data are lacking is the inconsistency in defining criteria for compulsive sexual behaviors, lack of funding, and the lack of researchers committed to documenting the extent of this problem. Most of what is known about the epidemiological nature of this disorder comes from clinical treatment programs that focus on sexual addictions. Men appear to outnumber women with compulsive sexual behaviors. Comorbidities include substance use disorders and co-occurring impulse control disorders, and there is an association with histories of sexual abuse. Other significant epidemiological data is simply not known, such as the rate of compulsive sexual behaviors among prosecuted sex offenders or the rate among those who work within the adult entertainment industry.

Etiology

As with impulse control and substance use disorders, no single biological cause has yet been identified to explain the origins and maintenance of compulsive sexual behaviors. Neuroscience research, which would be an excellent approach to understand basic brain differences between those with and without compulsive sexual behaviors, has rarely been applied to this population. In particular, neuroimaging studies in patients with compulsive sexual behaviors would be interesting to compare with those involved in substance abuse and other behavioral addictions. To date though, most of the neuroimaging work has been done with nonclinical populations and has examined the biology of sexual arousal in healthy subjects.

Hypersexual behaviors have been reported in patients with frontal lobe lesion, tumors, and in those with neurological conditions that involve temporal lobes and midbrain areas such as seizure disorders, Huntington's disease, and dementia. Frontal lobe damage may trigger the expression of disinhibited behaviors, which could partially explain the increased sexual activity along with decreased control. Still, more investigation is needed to understand the specifics aberrances because there are certainly those individuals with frontal lobe injuries that do not experience the emergence of compulsive sexual behaviors.

Neurotransmitter studies in compulsive sexual behaviors have focused on the monoamines, namely serotonin, dopamine, and norepinephrine. Again, research in clinical populations is scant. Normal sexual functioning involves all of these monoamines as evidenced by selective serotonin reuptake inhibitor (SSRI)-induced sexual dysfunction and the increased sexuality observed among those on stimulants. Cases of hypersexual behavior have also been shown to be induced by medications for Parkinson's disease, implicating dopamine systems in compulsive sexual behaviors. What remains unclear is understanding how these perturbations in neurochemical functions differentiate compulsive sexual behaviors from those with hypersexuality alone without a negative life impact.

In addition to neurotransmitters, the sex hormones are obviously a critical component to sexual functioning. Testosterone levels have been correlated to sexual functioning but curiously, levels do not necessarily correlate to libido and sexual desires. The implication of these hormones in compulsive sexual behaviors is critical to understand. It may be that regions of reward and pleasure are modulated by these hormones through facilitating or enhancing the response to sex and the desire for sex.

Clinical Assessment Measures

There are existing screening instruments, which are only as valid as the responder's honesty and integrity. Although this is true of all psychiatric screening instruments, revealing sexual practices is probably the most humbling because of its private nature. Questions about time spent on sexual activities and impact of functioning are important clinically, but also rely on self-report. Patrick Carnes, one of the pioneers in the field of compulsive sexual behavior research, developed the Sexual Addiction Screening Test, which is a 25-item, self-report symptom checklist that can be used to identify those at risk to develop compulsive sexual behaviors. The Sexual Addiction Screening Test has also been modified for women and for internet sexual behaviors. Kafka has suggested a behavioral screening test (i.e., Total Sexual Outlet) in which a total of seven sexual orgasms per week, regardless of how they are achieved, could represent at-risk behavior and requires further clinical exploration.

Treatment: Psychosocial

Various types of psychosocial treatments are available for individuals suffering from compulsive sexual behaviors. The most widely available and accessible are Sexual Addicts Anonymous, Sex and Love Addicts Anonymous, and Sexaholics Anonymous. All three are modeled after 12-step theory and practice, and are available throughout the United States. There is almost no data evaluating their efficacy or effectiveness. Nevertheless, participation in these groups is usually recommended because they provide a place for fellowship, support, structure, and accountability, and they are free of charge.

Inpatient and intensive outpatient treatment programs for compulsive sexual behaviors usually focus on helping to identify core triggers and beliefs about sexual addiction and to develop healthier choices and coping skills to minimize urges and deal with the preoccupation of sexual addiction.

Individual psychotherapy for compulsive sexual behaviors is varied but the two most common approaches are cognitive behavioral therapy (CBT) and psychodynamic psychotherapy. CBT in compulsive sexual behaviors borrows greatly from treatment with substance use disorders, focuses on identifying triggers to sexual behaviors and reshaping cognitive distortions about sexual behaviors (e.g., “I’m not really cheating on my spouse if I go to a massage parlor”), and emphasizes relapse prevention. Psychodynamic psychotherapy in compulsive sexual behaviors explores the core conflicts that drive dysfunctional sexual expression. Themes of shame, avoidance, anger, and impaired self-esteem and efficacy are common. Note that these types of therapy are not sex therapy, but individual therapy that focuses on reducing or controlling compulsive sexual behaviors.

Other forms of therapy may helpful, as well. For example, family therapy and couples therapy may restore trust, minimize shame/guilt, and establish a healthy sexual relationship between partners.

As for the assessment of treatment outcome, one of the unique difficulties in compulsive sexual behavior is determining when a patient has relapsed. Since there are no biological tests to indicate relapse, collateral history and functioning within the patient's significant relationship tends to be the most reliable markers. Despite the availability of psychosocial treatments, there are little data documenting treatment outcomes, success rates, predictors of treatment outcome.

Treatment: Pharmacotherapy

There are no U.S. Food and Drug Administration (FDA)-approved medications for compulsive sexual behaviors. While preliminary case reports and open-label trials that have been conducted, no known randomized, double-blind placebo-controlled trials have been published. Various classes of medications have been tried, including antidepressants, mood stabilizers, antipsychotics, and antiandrogens. The rationales for these drugs are based on clinical phenomenology and symptoms seen in other disorders, such as substance use or obsessive-compulsive disorders.

SSRIs have been tried for both paraphilic and non-paraphilic compulsive sexual behaviors through both case series and open-label studies. No one SSRI has demonstrated superior efficacy to another. Theoretically, SSRIs may decrease the urges/craving and preoccupation associated with sexual addiction. Attempting to use SSRIs to create sexual dysfunction through their side effect profile and thus to reduce compulsive sexual behaviors does not appear to be effective. Clinical experience suggests that patients who respond best to SSRIs have co-occurring psychiatric disorders, such as depression, anxiety, or obsessive-compulsive disorders. Those who do not have sexual dysfunction from SSRIs have the best treatment response.

In addition to SSRIs, naltrexone, an opiate antagonist, has been evaluated in the treatment of compulsive sexual behaviors. Grant describes a case report of co-occurring kleptomania and compulsive sexual behaviors treated successfully with naltrexone after treatment failure with SSRIs and psychotherapy. The rationale for using this medication is based on previous work in substance abuse populations and pathological gamblers, where the intent is to reduce the cravings and urges by blocking the euphoria associated with the behavior. In an open-label trial of naltrexone with adolescent sexual offenders, 15 out of 21 patients noted reductions in sexual impulses and arousal. There have also been studies examining the efficacy of intramuscular naltrexone in this clinical population.

Mood stabilizers, such as valproic acid and lithium, appear promising in the treatment of patients with bipolar disorder and compulsive sexual behaviors. Whether this class of medications has an independent effect on reducing compulsive sexual behaviors in patients without comorbid bipolar disorder remains to be seen. Other medications, such as topiramate and nefazodone, have also been tried, but further replication is needed to determine their effectiveness.

In the treatment of paraphilic compulsive sexual behaviors, some pharmacotherapy strategies have focused on altering or attenuating sexual hormone function. Anti-androgens, such as medroxyprogesterone acetate (300-500 mg per week, intramuscularly) or cyproterone acetate (300-600 mg per week, intramuscularly), lower serum testosterone levels and diminish sexual drive and desire. On a more drastic level, surgical intervention (castration) has been shown to reduce recidivism in sexual offenders by theoretically lowering testosterone levels to reduce urges and cravings. There are no known double-blind, randomized studies of anti-androgenic agents in the treatment of non-paraphilic compulsive sexual behaviors. However, case reports and open label studies suggest these may be effective treatments. Of importance to note, this treatment approach is temporary. Once the medications are stopped, testosterone levels will return to normal levels. This treatment approach has not been utilized in the non-paraphilic sexual behaviors.

Conclusions and Future Directions

We have much to learn about compulsive sexual behaviors, particularly their neurobiological roots, psychological risk factors, and the impact of societal values on their emergence. For now, compulsive sexual behaviors are the extreme end of a wide range of sexual experience. These behaviors can present in a variety of manners and undoubtedly have many different subtypes, severities, and clinical courses. Clinicians can enhance the identification and treatment of these disorders by implementing formal screening practices, becoming familiar with the warning signs, and knowing which types of patients are vulnerable. In time, research will begin to uncover the different subtypes of compulsive sexual behaviors as well as determine which treatment and prevention practices work the best. Currently, since there are no guidelines from which clinicians can work, we are left to review the work of those who specialize in the treatment of compulsive sexual behaviors.

Chapter 35

Self-Harm

Hurting yourself, sometimes called self-injury, is when a person deliberately hurts his or her own body. Some self-injuries can leave scars that won't go away, while others leave marks or bruises that eventually will go away. These are some forms of self-injury:

- cutting yourself (such as using a razor blade, knife or other sharp object to cut the skin);
- punching yourself or other objects;
- burning yourself with cigarettes, matches, or candles;
- pulling out your hair;
- poking objects through body openings;
- breaking your bones or bruising yourself; and
- plucking hair for hours.

Why do some people want to hurt themselves?

Many people cut themselves because it gives them a sense of relief. Some people use cutting as a means to cope with any problem.

From "Cutting and Hurting Yourself," by the Office of Women's Health (www.girlshealth.gov), part of the U.S. Department of Health and Human Services, March 12, 2008.

Some people say that when they hurt themselves, they are trying to stop feeling lonely, angry, or hopeless. Some people who hurt themselves have low self-esteem, they may feel unloved by their family and friends, and they may have an eating disorder, an alcohol or drug problem, or may have been victims of abuse.

People who hurt themselves often keep their feelings "bottled up" inside and have a hard time letting their feelings show. Some people who hurt themselves say that feeling the pain provides a sense of relief from intense feelings. Cutting can relieve the tension from bottled up sadness or anxiety. Others hurt themselves in order to "feel." Often people who hold back strong emotions can begin feeling numb, and cutting can be a way to cope with this because it causes them to feel something. Some people also may hurt themselves because they want to fit in with others who do it.

If you are hurting yourself, please get help. It is possible to overcome the urge to cut. There are other ways to find relief and cope with your emotions. Please talk to your parents, your doctor, or an adult you trust, like a teacher or religious leader.

Who are the people who hurt themselves?

People who hurt themselves come from all walks of life, no matter their age, gender, race, or ethnicity. About one in 100 people hurts himself or herself on purpose. More females hurt themselves than males. Teens usually hurt themselves by cutting with sharp objects.

What are the signs of self-injury?

These are some signs of self-injury:

- cuts or scars on the arms or legs;
- hiding cuts or scars by wearing long sleeved shirts or pants, even in hot weather; and
- making poor excuses about how the injuries happened.

Self-injury can be dangerous—cutting can lead to infections, scars, numbness, and even hospitalization and death. People who share tools to cut themselves are at risk of getting and spreading diseases like HIV [human immunodeficiency virus]and hepatitis. Teens who continue to hurt themselves are less likely to learn how to cope with negative feelings.

Are you or a friend depressed, angry, or having a hard time coping with life?

If you are thinking about hurting yourself, please ask for help! Talk with an adult you trust, like a teacher or minister or doctor. There is nothing wrong with asking for help—everyone needs help sometimes. You have a right to be strong, safe, and happy!

Do you have a friend who hurts herself or himself?

Please try to get your friend to talk to a trusted adult. Your friend may need professional counseling and treatment. Help is available—counselors can teach positive ways to cope with problems without turning to self-injury.

Have you been pressured to cut yourself by others who do it?

If so, think about how much you value that friendship or relationship. Do you really want a friend who wants you to hurt yourself, cause you pain, and put you in danger? Try to hang out with other friends who don't pressure you in this way.

Chapter 36

Alcohol Addiction

Alcoholism, also known as "alcohol dependence," is a disease that includes four symptoms:

- **Craving:** A strong need, or compulsion, to drink.
- **Loss of control:** The inability to limit one's drinking on any given occasion.
- **Physical dependence:** Withdrawal symptoms, such as nausea, sweating, shakiness, and anxiety, occur when alcohol use is stopped after a period of heavy drinking.
- **Tolerance:** The need to drink greater amounts of alcohol in order to "get high."

People who are not alcoholic sometimes do not understand why an alcoholic can't just "use a little willpower" to stop drinking. However, alcoholism has little to do with willpower. Alcoholics are in the grip of a powerful "craving," or uncontrollable need, for alcohol that overrides their ability to stop drinking. This need can be as strong as the need for food or water.

Although some people are able to recover from alcoholism without help, the majority of alcoholics need assistance. With treatment

From "Health Risks and Benefits of Alcohol Consumption," by the National Institute on Alcohol Abuse and Alcoholism (NIAAA, www.niaaa.nih.gov), part of the National Institutes of Health, *Alcohol Research and Health,* Vol. 24, No. 1, 2000. Reviewed by David A. Cooke, M.D., January 10, 2009.

and support, many individuals are able to stop drinking and rebuild their lives.

Many people wonder why some individuals can use alcohol without problems but others cannot. One important reason has to do with genetics. Scientists have found that having an alcoholic family member makes it more likely that if you choose to drink you too may develop alcoholism. Genes, however, are not the whole story. In fact, scientists now believe that certain factors in a person's environment influence whether a person with a genetic risk for alcoholism ever develops the disease. A person's risk for developing alcoholism can increase based on the person's environment, including where and how he or she lives; family, friends, and culture; peer pressure; and even how easy it is to get alcohol.

Statistics

Almost half of Americans aged 12 or older reported being current drinkers of alcohol in the 2001 survey (48.3 percent). This translates to an estimated 109 million people. Both the rate of alcohol use and the number of drinkers increased from 2000, when 104 million, or 46.6 percent, of people aged 12 or older reported drinking in the past 30 days.

Approximately one fifth (20.5 percent) of persons aged 12 or older participated in binge drinking at least once in the 30 days prior to the survey. Although the number of current drinkers increased between 2000 and 2001, the number of those reporting binge drinking did not change significantly.

Heavy drinking was reported by 5.7 percent of the population aged 12 or older, or 12.9 million people. These 2001 estimates are similar to the 2000 estimates.

The prevalence of current alcohol use in 2001 increased with increasing age for youths, from 2.6 percent at age 12 to a peak of 67.5 percent for persons 21 years old. Unlike prevalence patterns observed for cigarettes and illicit drugs, current alcohol use remained steady among older age groups. For people aged 21 to 25 and those aged 26 to 34, the rates of current alcohol use in 2001 were 64.3 and 59.9 percent, respectively. The prevalence of alcohol use was slightly lower for persons in their 40s. Past month drinking was reported by 45.6 percent of respondents aged 60 to 64, and 33.0 percent of persons 65 or older.

The highest prevalence of both binge and heavy drinking in 2001 was for young adults aged 18 to 25, with the peak rate occurring at age 21. The rate of binge drinking was 38.7 percent for young adults and 48.2 percent at age 21. Heavy alcohol use was reported by 13.6

percent of persons aged 18 to 25, and by 17.8 percent of persons aged 21. Binge and heavy alcohol use rates decreased faster with increasing age than did rates of past month alcohol use. While 55.2 percent of the population aged 45 to 49 in 2001 were current drinkers, 19.1 percent of persons within this age range binge drank and 5.4 percent drank heavily. Binge and heavy drinking were relatively rare among people aged 65 or older, with reported rates of 5.8 and 1.4 percent, respectively.

Among youths aged 12 to 17, an estimated 17.3 percent used alcohol in the month prior to the survey interview. This rate was higher than the rate of youth alcohol use reported in 2000 (16.4 percent). Of all youths, 10.6 percent were binge drinkers, and 2.5 percent were heavy drinkers. These are roughly the same percentages as those reported in 2000 (10.4 and 2.6 percent, respectively).

Forty-four percent of the adult U.S. population (aged 18 and over) are current drinkers who have consumed at least 12 drinks in the preceding year. Although most people who drink do so safely, the minority who consume alcohol heavily produce an impact that ripples outward to encompass their families, friends, and communities. The following statistics give a glimpse of the magnitude of problem drinking:

- Approximately 14 million Americans—7.4 percent of the population—meet the diagnostic criteria for alcohol abuse or alcoholism.
- More than one-half of American adults have a close family member who has or has had alcoholism.
- Approximately one in four children younger than 18 years old in the United States is exposed to alcohol abuse or alcohol dependence in the family.

Alcohol consumption has consequences for the health and well-being of those who drink and, by extension, the lives of those around them.

Short-Term Effects

Short-term effects of alcohol use include:

- distorted vision, hearing, and coordination
- altered perceptions and emotions
- impaired judgment
- bad breath; hangovers

Alcohol abuse is a pattern of problem drinking that results in health consequences, social, problems, or both. However, alcohol dependence, or alcoholism, refers to a disease that is characterized by abnormal alcohol-seeking behavior that leads to impaired control over drinking.

Long-Term Effects

Some problems, like those mentioned earlier, can occur after drinking over a relatively short period of time. But other problems—such as liver disease, heart disease, certain forms of cancer, and pancreatitis—often develop more gradually and may become evident only after long-term heavy drinking. Women may develop alcohol-related health problems after consuming less alcohol than men do over a shorter period of time. Because alcohol affects many organs in the body, long-term heavy drinking puts you at risk for developing serious health problems, some of which are described in the following text.

Alcohol-related liver disease: More than 2 million Americans suffer from alcohol-related liver disease. Some drinkers develop alcoholic hepatitis, or inflammation of the liver, as a result of long-term heavy drinking. Its symptoms include fever, jaundice (abnormal yellowing of the skin, eyeballs, and urine), and abdominal pain. Alcoholic hepatitis can cause death if drinking continues. If drinking stops, this condition often is reversible. About 10 to 20 percent of heavy drinkers develop alcoholic cirrhosis, or scarring of the liver. Alcoholic cirrhosis can cause death if drinking continues. Although cirrhosis is not reversible, if drinking stops, one's chances of survival improve considerably. Those with cirrhosis often feel better, and the functioning of their liver may improve, if they stop drinking. Although liver transplantation may be needed as a last resort, many people with cirrhosis who abstain from alcohol may never need liver transplantation. In addition, treatment for the complications of cirrhosis is available.

Heart disease: Moderate drinking can have beneficial effects on the heart, especially among those at greatest risk for heart attacks, such as men over the age of 45 and women after menopause. But long-term heavy drinking increases the risk for high blood pressure, heart disease, and some kinds of stroke.

Cancer: Long-term heavy drinking increases the risk of developing certain forms of cancer, especially cancer of the esophagus, mouth, throat, and voice box. Women are at slightly increased risk of developing breast cancer if they drink two or more drinks per day. Drinking may also increase the risk for developing cancer of the colon and rectum.

Pancreatitis: The pancreas helps to regulate the body's blood sugar levels by producing insulin. The pancreas also has a role in digesting the food we eat. Long-term heavy drinking can lead to pancreatitis, or inflammation of the pancreas. This condition is associated with severe abdominal pain and weight loss and can be fatal.

Chapter 37

Drug Addiction

Many people do not understand why individuals become addicted to drugs or how drugs change the brain to foster compulsive drug abuse. They mistakenly view drug abuse and addiction as strictly a social problem and may characterize those who take drugs as morally weak. One very common belief is that drug abusers should be able to just stop taking drugs if they are only willing to change their behavior. What people often underestimate is the complexity of drug addiction—that it is a disease that impacts the brain and because of that, stopping drug abuse is not simply a matter of willpower. Through scientific advances we now know much more about how exactly drugs work in the brain, and we also know that drug addiction can be successfully treated to help people stop abusing drugs and resume their productive lives.

Drug abuse and addiction are a major burden to society. Estimates of the total overall costs of substance abuse in the United States—including health- and crime-related costs as well as losses in productivity—exceed half a trillion dollars annually. This includes approximately $181 billion for illicit drugs, $168 billion for tobacco, and $185 billion for alcohol. Staggering as these numbers are, however, they do not fully describe the breadth of deleterious public health—and safety—implications, which include family disintegration, loss of

---

From "Understanding Drug Abuse and Addiction," by the National Institute on Drug Abuse (NIDA, www.nida.nih.gov), part of the National Institutes of Health, June 2008.

employment, failure in school, domestic violence, child abuse, and other crimes.

What Is Drug Addiction?

Addiction is a chronic, often relapsing brain disease that causes compulsive drug seeking and use despite harmful consequences to the individual who is addicted and to those around them. Drug addiction is a brain disease because the abuse of drugs leads to changes in the structure and function of the brain. Although it is true that for most people the initial decision to take drugs is voluntary, over time the changes in the brain caused by repeated drug abuse can affect a person's self-control and ability to make sound decisions, and at the same time send intense impulses to take drugs.

It is because of these changes in the brain that it is so challenging for a person who is addicted to stop abusing drugs. Fortunately, there are treatments that help people to counteract addiction's powerful disruptive effects and regain control. Research shows that combining addiction treatment medications, if available, with behavioral therapy is the best way to ensure success for most patients. Treatment approaches that are tailored to each patient's drug abuse patterns and any co-occurring medical, psychiatric, and social problems can lead to sustained recovery and a life without drug abuse.

Similar to other chronic, relapsing diseases, such as diabetes, asthma, or heart disease, drug addiction can be managed successfully. And, as with other chronic diseases, it is not uncommon for a person to relapse and begin abusing drugs again. Relapse, however, does not signal failure—rather, it indicates that treatment should be reinstated, adjusted, or that alternate treatment is needed to help the individual regain control and recover.

What Happens to Your Brain When You Take Drugs?

Drugs are chemicals that tap into the brain's communication system and disrupt the way nerve cells normally send, receive, and process information. There are at least two ways that drugs are able to do this: (1) by imitating the brain's natural chemical messengers, and/or (2) by overstimulating the "reward circuit" of the brain. Some drugs, such as marijuana and heroin, have a similar structure to chemical messengers, called neurotransmitters, which are naturally produced by the brain. Because of this similarity, these drugs are able to "fool" the brain's receptors and activate nerve cells to send abnormal messages.

Other drugs, such as cocaine or methamphetamine, can cause the nerve cells to release abnormally large amounts of natural neurotransmitters, or prevent the normal recycling of these brain chemicals, which is needed to shut off the signal between neurons. This disruption produces a greatly amplified message that ultimately disrupts normal communication patterns.

Nearly all drugs, directly or indirectly, target the brain's reward system by flooding the circuit with dopamine. Dopamine is a neurotransmitter present in regions of the brain that control movement, emotion, motivation, and feelings of pleasure. The overstimulation of this system, which normally responds to natural behaviors that are linked to survival (eating, spending time with loved ones, etc.), produces euphoric effects in response to the drugs. This reaction sets in motion a pattern that "teaches" people to repeat the behavior of abusing drugs.

As a person continues to abuse drugs, the brain adapts to the overwhelming surges in dopamine by producing less dopamine or by reducing the number of dopamine receptors in the reward circuit. As a result, dopamine's impact on the reward circuit is lessened, reducing the abuser's ability to enjoy the drugs and the things that previously brought pleasure. This decrease compels those addicted to drugs to keep abusing drugs in order to attempt to bring their dopamine function back to normal. And, they may now require larger amounts of the drug than they first did to achieve the dopamine high—an effect known as tolerance.

Long-term abuse causes changes in other brain chemical systems and circuits as well. Glutamate is a neurotransmitter that influences the reward circuit and the ability to learn. When the optimal concentration of glutamate is altered by drug abuse, the brain attempts to compensate, which can impair cognitive function. Drugs of abuse facilitate nonconscious (conditioned) learning, which leads the user to experience uncontrollable cravings when they see a place or person they associate with the drug experience, even when the drug itself is not available. Brain imaging studies of drug-addicted individuals show changes in areas of the brain that are critical to judgment, decision-making, learning and memory, and behavior control. Together, these changes can drive an abuser to seek out and take drugs compulsively despite adverse consequences—in other words, to become addicted to drugs.

Why Do Some People Become Addicted and Others Do Not?

No single factor can predict whether or not a person will become addicted to drugs. Risk for addiction is influenced by a person's biology, social environment, and age or stage of development. The more risk factors an individual has, the greater the chance that taking drugs can lead to addiction. For example:

- **Biology:** The genes that people are born with—in combination with environmental influences—account for about half of their addiction vulnerability. Additionally, gender, ethnicity, and the presence of other mental disorders may influence risk for drug abuse and addiction.
- **Environment:** A person's environment includes many different influences—from family and friends to socioeconomic status and quality of life in general. Factors such as peer pressure, physical and sexual abuse, stress, and parental involvement can greatly influence the course of drug abuse and addiction in a person's life.
- **Development:** Genetic and environmental factors interact with critical developmental stages in a person's life to affect addiction vulnerability, and adolescents experience a double challenge. Although taking drugs at any age can lead to addiction, the earlier that drug use begins, the more likely it is to progress to more serious abuse. And because adolescents' brains are still developing in the areas that govern decision-making, judgment, and self-control, they are especially prone to risk-taking behaviors, including trying drugs of abuse.

Prevention Is the Key

Drug addiction is a preventable disease. Results from NIDA-funded research have shown that prevention programs that involve families, schools, communities, and the media are effective in reducing drug abuse. Although many events and cultural factors affect drug abuse trends, when youths perceive drug abuse as harmful, they reduce their drug taking. It is necessary, therefore, to help youth and the general public to understand the risks of drug abuse, and for teachers, parents, and healthcare professionals to keep sending the message that drug addiction can be prevented if a person never abuses drugs.

Chapter 38

Dual Diagnosis: Substance Abuse Problems and Mental Health Disorders

Chapter Contents

Section 38.1

What Is Dual Diagnosis?

"Dual Diagnosis and Integrated Treatment of Mental Illness and Substance Abuse Disorder," © 2003 NAMI: The Nation's Voice on Mental Illness (www.nami.org). Reprinted with permission. Reviewed by Robert Drake, M.D., September 2003. Reviewed by David A. Cooke, M.D., January 2, 2009. Dr. Cooke is not affiliated with NAMI.

What are dual diagnosis services?

Dual diagnosis services are treatments for people who suffer from co-occurring disorders—mental illness and substance abuse. Research has strongly indicated that to recover fully, a consumer with co-occurring disorder needs treatment for both problems—focusing on one does not ensure the other will go away. Dual diagnosis services integrate assistance for each condition, helping people recover from both in one setting, at the same time.

Dual diagnosis services include different types of assistance that go beyond standard therapy or medication: assertive outreach, job and housing assistance, family counseling, even money and relationship management. The personalized treatment is viewed as long-term and can be begun at whatever stage of recovery the consumer is in. Positivity, hope, and optimism are at the foundation of integrated treatment.

How often do people with severe mental illnesses also experience a co-occurring substance abuse problem?

There is a lack of information on the numbers of people with co-occurring disorders, but research has shown the disorders are very common. According to reports published in the *Journal of the American Medical Association* (*JAMA*):

- Roughly 50 percent of individuals with severe mental disorders are affected by substance abuse.
- Thirty-seven percent of alcohol abusers and 53 percent of drug abusers also have at least one serious mental illness.

- Of all people diagnosed as mentally ill, 29 percent abuse either alcohol or drugs.

The best data available on the prevalence of co-occurring disorders are derived from two major surveys: the Epidemiologic Catchment Area (ECA) Survey (administered 1980-1984), and the National Comorbidity Survey (NCS), administered between 1990 and 1992.

Results of the NCS and the ECA Survey indicate high prevalence rates for co-occurring substance abuse disorders and mental disorders, as well as the increased risk for people with either a substance abuse disorder or mental disorder for developing a co-occurring disorder. For example, the NCS found that:

- 42.7 percent of individuals with a 12-month addictive disorder had at least one 12-month mental disorder.
- 14.7 percent of individuals with a 12-month mental disorder had at least one 12-month addictive disorder.

The ECA Survey found that individuals with severe mental disorders were at significant risk for developing a substance use disorder during their lifetime. Specifically:

- 47 percent of individuals with schizophrenia also had a substance abuse disorder (more than four times as likely as the general population).
- 61 percent of individuals with bipolar disorder also had a substance abuse disorder (more than five times as likely as the general population).

Continuing studies support these findings, that these disorders do appear to occur much more frequently then previously realized, and that appropriate integrated treatments must be developed.

What are the consequences of co-occurring severe mental illness and substance abuse?

For the consumer, the consequences are numerous and harsh. Persons with a co-occurring disorder have a statistically greater propensity for violence, medication noncompliance, and failure to respond to treatment than consumers with just substance abuse or a mental illness. These problems also extend out to these consumers' families, friends, and co-workers.

Purely healthwise, having a simultaneous mental illness and a substance abuse disorder frequently leads to overall poorer functioning and a greater chance of relapse. These consumers are in and out of hospitals and treatment programs without lasting success. People with dual diagnoses also tend to have tardive dyskinesia (TD) and physical illnesses more often than those with a single disorder, and they experience more episodes of psychosis. In addition, physicians often don't recognize the presence of substance abuse disorders and mental disorders, especially in older adults.

Socially, people with mental illnesses often are susceptible to co-occurring disorders due to "downward drift." In other words, as a consequence of their mental illness they may find themselves living in marginal neighborhoods where drug use prevails. Having great difficulty developing social relationships, some people find themselves more easily accepted by groups whose social activity is based on drug use. Some may believe that an identity based on drug addiction is more acceptable than one based on mental illness.

Consumers with co-occurring disorders are also much more likely to be homeless or jailed. An estimated 50 percent of homeless adults with serious mental illnesses have a co-occurring substance abuse disorder. Meanwhile, 16 percent of jail and prison inmates are estimated to have severe mental and substance abuse disorders. Among detainees with mental disorders, 72 percent also have a co-occurring substance abuse disorder.

Consequences for society directly stem from the above. Just the back-and-forth treatment alone currently given to non-violent persons with dual diagnosis is costly. Moreover, violent or criminal consumers, no matter how unfairly afflicted, are dangerous and also costly. Those with co-occurring disorders are at high risk to contract AIDS [acquired immunodeficiency syndrome], a disease that can affect society at large. Costs rise even higher when these persons, as those with co-occurring disorders have been shown to do, recycle through healthcare and criminal justice systems again and again. Without the establishment of more integrated treatment programs, the cycle will continue.

Why is an integrated approach to treating severe mental illnesses and substance abuse problems so important?

Despite much research that supports its success, integrated treatment is still not made widely available to consumers. Those who struggle both with serious mental illness and substance abuse face problems of enormous proportions. Mental health services tend not to be well prepared to deal with patients having both afflictions. Often only one of the two problems is identified. If both are recognized, the individual may bounce back and forth between services for mental illness and those for substance abuse, or they may be refused treatment by each of them. Fragmented and uncoordinated services create a service gap for persons with co-occurring disorders.

Providing appropriate, integrated services for these consumers will not only allow for their recovery and improved overall health, but can ameliorate the effects their disorders have on their family, friends, and society at large. By helping these consumers stay in treatment, find housing and jobs, and develop better social skills and judgment, we can potentially begin to substantially diminish some of the most sinister and costly societal problems: crime, HIV [human immunodeficiency virus]/AIDS, domestic violence, and more.

There is much evidence that integrated treatment can be effective. For example:

- Individuals with a substance abuse disorder are more likely to receive treatment if they have a co-occurring mental disorder.
- Research shows that when consumers with dual diagnosis successfully overcome alcohol abuse, their response to treatment improves remarkably.

With continued education on co-occurring disorders, hopefully, more treatments and better understanding are on the way.

What does effective integrated treatment entail?

Effective integrated treatment consists of the same health professionals, working in one setting, providing appropriate treatment for both mental health and substance abuse in a coordinated fashion. The caregivers see to it that interventions are bundled together; the consumers, therefore, receive consistent treatment, with no division between mental health or substance abuse assistance. The approach, philosophy, and recommendations are seamless, and the need to consult with separate teams and programs is eliminated.

Integrated treatment also requires the recognition that substance abuse counseling and traditional mental health counseling are different approaches that must be reconciled to treat co-occurring disorders. It is not enough merely to teach relationship skills to a person with bipolar disorder. They must also learn to explore how to avoid the relationships that are intertwined with their substance abuse.

Providers should recognize that denial is an inherent part of the problem. Patients often do not have insight as to the seriousness and scope of the problem. Abstinence may be a goal of the program but should not be a precondition for entering treatment. If dually diagnosed clients do not fit into local Alcoholics Anonymous (AA) and Narcotics Anonymous (NA) groups, special peer groups based on AA principles might be developed.

Clients with a dual diagnosis have to proceed at their own pace in treatment. An illness model of the problem should be used rather than a moralistic one. Providers need to convey understanding of how hard it is to end an addiction problem and give credit for any accomplishments. Attention should be given to social networks that can serve as important reinforcers. Clients should be given opportunities to socialize, have access to recreational activities, and develop peer relationships. Their families should be offered support and education, while learning not to react with guilt or blame but to learn to cope with two interacting illnesses.

What are the key factors in effective integrated treatment?

There are a number of key factors in an integrated treatment program.

Treatment must be approached in stages. First, a trust is established between the consumer and the caregiver. This helps motivate the consumer to learn the skills for actively controlling their illnesses and focus on goals. This helps keep the consumer on track, preventing relapse. Treatment can begin at any one of these stages; the program is tailored to the individual.

Assertive outreach has been shown to engage and retain clients at a high rate, while those that fail to include outreach lose clients. Therefore, effective programs, through intensive case management, meeting at the consumer's residence, and other methods of developing a dependable relationship with the client, ensure that more consumers are consistently monitored and counseled.

Effective treatment includes motivational interventions, which, through education, support, and counseling, help empower deeply demoralized clients to recognize the importance of their goals and illness self-management.

Of course, counseling is a fundamental component of dual diagnosis services. Counseling helps develop positive coping patterns, as well as promotes cognitive and behavioral skills. Counseling can be in the form of individual, group, or family therapy or a combination of these.

A consumer's social support is critical. Their immediate environment has a direct impact on their choices and moods; therefore consumers need help strengthening positive relationships and jettisoning those that encourage negative behavior.

Effective integrated treatment programs view recovery as a long-term, community-based process, one that can take months or, more likely, years to undergo. Improvement is slow even with a consistent treatment program. However, such an approach prevents relapses and enhances a consumer's gains.

To be effective, a dual diagnosis program must be comprehensive, taking into account a number of life's aspects: stress management, social networks, jobs, housing, and activities. These programs view substance abuse as intertwined with mental illness, not a separate issue, and therefore provide solutions to both illnesses together at the same time.

Finally, effective integrated treatment programs must contain elements of cultural sensitivity and competence to even lure consumers, much less retain them. Various groups such as African-Americans, homeless, women with children, Hispanics, and others can benefit from services tailored to their particular racial and cultural needs.

Section 38.2

Mood Disorders Predict Later Substance Abuse Problems

From "Mood Disorders Predict Later Substance Abuse Problems," from the National Institute of Mental Health (NIMH, www.nimh.nih.gov), part of the National Institutes of Health, January 9, 2008.

People with manic symptoms and bipolar disorder type II are at significant risk of later developing an alcohol abuse or dependence problem, a long-term study conducted in Switzerland confirms. The study was published in the January 2008 issue of the *Archives of General Psychiatry.*

Extensive research using retrospective reports has demonstrated a clear association between mood disorders and substance abuse. But few prospective long-term studies have been able to show evidence of this.

Kathleen Merikangas, Ph.D., of the NIMH Mood and Anxiety Disorders Program, collaborated with colleagues to follow 591 people (292 men and 299 women) over two decades, beginning in 1978 when the participants were 19 or 20 years old. The participants were interviewed six times between 1979 and 1999.

By 1993, almost 10 percent met criteria for major depression. Although bipolar disorder type I was very rare, 4 percent met criteria for bipolar disorder II—a milder form of the disorder. In addition, 24 percent had symptoms of mania but did not meet specific criteria for bipolar disorder.

By 1999, when participants were about 40 years old, 18 percent met criteria for alcohol abuse or dependence problems, while 8 percent met criteria for cannabis (marijuana) abuse and 3 percent met criteria for benzodiazepine abuse.

Merikangas and colleagues found that people who showed symptoms of mania, but who did not meet criteria for bipolar disorder, were at significantly greater risk for later developing an alcohol abuse or dependence problem. Those with bipolar disorder II were even more at risk of developing an alcohol problem or benzodiazepine abuse problem. Major depression was associated only with developing a benzodiazepine abuse problem among this population.

"The findings confirm the link between mood disorders and substance abuse or dependence problems," said Dr. Merikangas. "They also suggest that earlier detection of bipolar symptoms could help to prevent consequent substance abuse problems."

The study was known as the Zurich Cohort Study.

Reference

Merikangas, KR, Herrell R, Swendsen J, Rossler W, Ajdacic-Gross V, Angst J. Specificity of bipolar spectrum conditions in the comorbidity of mood and substance abuse disorders. *Archives of General Psychiatry.* 2008;65(1): 47–52.

Part Five

Personality and Schizophrenic Disorders

Chapter 39

What Are Personality Disorders?

Mental health professionals use the term "personality disorders" to refer to personality traits that are extreme or that create so much difficulty in life as to be considered disabling. Personality disorders are more severe than the negative personality traits that we all show at various times throughout our lives, or the "problem" people that we sometimes have to deal with at work. Personality disorders are medically defined as long-term, pervasive, inflexible patterns of thoughts and behaviors that are not well adapted or do not fit within the range of behavior considered normal. These patterns lead to significant difficulties in the ability to reason or interact with others or to behave appropriately.

Personality disorders can surface at any time, including old age. As many as 10% of older adults living at home may have a personality disorder. This figure is even higher among older adults living in nursing homes.

People with personality disorders are often involved in repeated episodes of disruptive or difficult behavior. Others often consider these people overbearing, dramatic, or even obnoxious. Personality disorders are categorized according to the types of behaviors that are seen:

"Personality Disorders," http://www.healthinaging.org/agingintheknow/chapters_ch_trial.asp?ch=35, Chapter 35 from *Aging in the Know*, http://www.healthinaging.org/agingintheknow/, from the American Geriatrics Society Foundation for Health in Aging (www.healthinaging.org), © 2005. Reprinted with permission. For more information visit the American Geriatrics Society at www.americangeriatrics.org.

- Paranoid
- Narcissistic
- Schizoid
- Avoidant
- Schizotypal
- Dependent
- Antisocial
- Obsessive-compulsive
- Borderline
- Passive-aggressive
- Histrionic
- Depressive

People who show paranoid behavior are always suspicious of others, and often become irritable and hostile. Older adults may have paranoid delusions, become very agitated, or even assault someone. People who show schizoid behavior are not usually interested in social relationships and may behave oddly or in ways that tend to keep them isolated and separate from others. Older adults with schizoid behavior may have poor, strained, or sometimes no relationships with caregivers. In schizotypal behavior, people may have strange, unusual, or inappropriate behaviors or beliefs that may lead to having conflicts with other people, including caregivers.

Behavior that is antisocial shows little regard or respect for standard rules and laws of society. In addition, antisocial people often do not seem to have a conscience or care about others. People who show borderline behavior have unstable emotions, which lead to unstable relationships. They may have emotional outbursts or injure themselves. People who show histrionic behavior are over emotional and want to be the center of attention. They are often disorganized and lack inhibitions. People who are narcissistic think that they should have and, in fact, are entitled to whatever they want. They often act superior, self-important, and arrogant. They do not seem to care about others. Older adults who are narcissistic may appear hostile, extremely angry, paranoid, or depressed.

People who show avoidant behavior are shy, inhibited, and very sensitive to rejection and how others look at them. In older adults, this often leads to having not many social relationships and little support. People who show dependent behavior rely completely or almost completely on others to make decisions and for support. Older adults may be demanding or clinging, as well as depressed. People who are obsessive-compulsive are constantly worried about cleanliness and keeping everything in order. They are perfectionists and do not want to compromise, especially under stress. Older adults may show obsessive-compulsive behavior in response to an illness or moving to a nursing home or other new environment.

In passive-aggressive behavior, people tend to resist authority or any demands placed on them by not taking any action, i.e., procrastinating. These people often criticize and resent others. People who show depressive behavior view life as always gloomy and miserable, with no hope of change in the future. These people often have low self-esteem and feel guilty. They often have major or clinical depression in later life.

Personality disorders are sometimes grouped into clusters:

- Cluster A includes the paranoid, schizoid, and schizotypal personality disorders. Individuals with these conditions often appear odd or eccentric.
- Cluster B includes the antisocial, borderline, histrionic and narcissistic personality disorders. Individuals with these disorders often appear dramatic, emotional, or erratic.
- Cluster C includes the avoidant, dependent, and obsessive-compulsive personality disorders. Individuals with these disorders often appear anxious or fearful.

Causes of Personality Disorders

The roots of personality disorder lie in both early life experiences and genetic (i.e., inherited) factors. However, severe changes in personality may develop during later life because of the unique stresses experienced by older adults. Many older adults become overwhelmed by losses (e.g., deaths among friends and loved ones), medical problems, and stresses that build up over time. This is especially true for people who are not able to cope well or do not have the personal, social, or financial resources to act as a cushion or buffer against these stresses. Being admitted to a hospital or nursing home can be a particularly stressful event, because of the loss of familiar environment, personal items, privacy, and the control over one's schedule.

In institutional settings, personality disorders can show up when an older adult tries to cope with the stresses in their new environment by exaggerating strong personality traits. For example, a person with obsessive-compulsive tendencies might try to keep a sense of control by demanding that schedules and rules of hygiene are followed exactly. People who have dependent personalities may feel helpless and panicked if they don't receive enough attention, and respond by clinging or by constantly asking questions or asking for help. People who have paranoid, antisocial, or borderline personalities may refuse to cooperate with treatment plans or institutional rules.

Diagnosis of Personality Disorders

Personality disorders can typically be diagnosed only by a mental health professional such as a psychiatrist. Even then, the diagnosis can be very difficult in older adults. It requires a detailed lifetime history, which is often beyond the ability of the affected person, or the knowledge of their family and caregivers to provide. In addition, this history often becomes less accurate and distorted because of memory problems or the tendency that we all have to put the "best face" on past behaviors. People with some types of personality disorders (e.g., paranoid) may also be reluctant to speak openly with a mental health professional, aggravating the problem. This means that mental health professionals often need to observe someone for a fairly long time under various circumstances before being able to make a diagnosis.

Separating personality disorders from underlying medical or psychological problems is also difficult. For example, major or clinical depression, psychosis, or other psychiatric problems can distort personality features considerably. Alzheimer's disease and other dementias are often associated with personality changes, including loss of interest, increased self-image, or impulsive behaviors. Similarly, physical pain and disability can lead to dependency or withdrawal, which can resemble symptoms seen in personality disorders. Brain damage or tumors can also lead to dramatic changes in personality.

Remember that in true personality disorder, extreme, inflexible, and difficult personality traits become a lasting part of someone's overall personality. Many older adults who appear to have troubling personality problems do not have a personality disorder. Some people just have trouble adapting to changes, which is a condition called "adjustment disorder." An adjustment disorder develops when a previously healthy and well-adjusted person suddenly shows personality changes as a result of severe stress.

Treatment of Personality Disorders

Personality disorders may continue unchanged over time, or they may seem to get a little better, then a little worse, then a little better, etc. The treatment of personality disorders in later life is complicated and, sometimes, success is limited. In addition, underlying mental disorders such as clinical depression or dementia further complicate treatment for personality disorders, and vice versa.

Treatment in older adults usually focuses on short-term goals meant to decrease stress and the frequency and intensity of difficult behaviors, rather than to cure the disorder. The first step should always be to confirm the diagnosis and then to identify recent stresses that may account for the current behavior problem(s). Treatment for personality disorders includes many forms of psychotherapy, depending on the situation. A variety of possible drug treatments are also available, including medications for depression, anxiety, and psychoses. However, medications are used cautiously, because of the potential for side effects or drug interactions, as well as the possibility of affecting other medical problems. The best treatment approach often involves a combination of psychotherapy and drug treatment.

Family members and other caregivers (e.g., visiting nurses or social workers) need to communicate closely with healthcare providers during the treatment of personality disorders. However, if the affected older adult has a conflict with certain family members or caregivers, this can complicate treatment. Treatment is often most effective in long-term care settings such as nursing homes because of the constant supervision and professional communication among staff members. In these settings, difficult or disruptive behaviors can sometimes be traced to particular activities or staff interactions, which can then be changed as part of the treatment strategy.

Chapter 40

Types of Personality Disorders

Chapter Contents

Section 40.1

Antisocial Personality Disorder

Alternative Names

Psychopathic personality; Sociopathic personality; Personality disorder—antisocial

Definition

Antisocial personality disorder is a psychiatric condition characterized by chronic behavior that manipulates, exploits, or violates the rights of others. This behavior is often criminal.

Causes

Personality disorders are chronic behavioral and relationship patterns that interfere with a person's life over many years. To receive a diagnosis of antisocial personality disorder, a person must have exhibited behavior that qualifies for a diagnosis of conduct disorder during childhood.

The cause of antisocial personality disorder is unknown, but genetic factors and child abuse are believed to contribute to the development of this condition.

People with an antisocial or alcoholic parent are at increased risk. Far more men than women are affected, and unsurprisingly, the condition is common in prison populations. Fire-setting and cruelty to animals during childhood are linked to the development of antisocial personality.

Symptoms

A person with antisocial personality disorder:

- Breaks the law repeatedly
- Lies, steals, and fights often

- Disregards the safety of self and others
- Demonstrates a lack of guilt
- Had a childhood diagnosis (or symptoms consistent with) conduct disorder

Exams and Tests

Individuals with antisocial personality disorder are often angry and arrogant, but may be capable of superficial wit and charm. They may be adept at flattery and manipulating the emotions of others. People with antisocial personality disorder often have extensive substance abuse and legal problems.

Treatment

Antisocial personality disorder is one of the most difficult personality disorders to treat. Individuals rarely seek treatment on their own and may only initiate therapy when mandated by a court. The efficacy of treatment for antisocial personality disorder is largely unknown.

Outlook (Prognosis)

Symptoms tend to peak during the late teenage years and early 20s and may improve on their own by a person's 40s.

Possible Complications

Complications can include incarceration and drug abuse.

When to Contact a Medical Professional

Call for an appointment with a mental health professional if you have symptoms suggestive of antisocial personality disorder, or if your child exhibits behaviors that indicate a risk for developing this disorder.

Section 40.2

Borderline Personality Disorder (BPD)

From the National Institute of Mental Health (NIMH, www.nimh.nih.gov), part of the National Institutes of Health, June 26, 2008.

Raising Questions, Finding Answers

Borderline personality disorder (BPD) is a serious mental illness characterized by pervasive instability in moods, interpersonal relationships, self-image, and behavior. This instability often disrupts family and work life, long-term planning, and the individual's sense of self-identity. Originally thought to be at the "borderline" of psychosis, people with BPD suffer from a disorder of emotion regulation. While less well known than schizophrenia or bipolar disorder (manic-depressive illness), BPD is more common, affecting 2 percent of adults, mostly young women. There is a high rate of self-injury without suicide intent, as well as a significant rate of suicide attempts and completed suicide in severe cases. Patients often need extensive mental health services, and account for 20 percent of psychiatric hospitalizations. Yet, with help, many improve over time and are eventually able to lead productive lives.

Symptoms

While a person with depression or bipolar disorder typically endures the same mood for weeks, a person with BPD may experience intense bouts of anger, depression, and anxiety that may last only hours, or at most a day. These may be associated with episodes of impulsive aggression, self-injury, and drug or alcohol abuse. Distortions in cognition and sense of self can lead to frequent changes in long-term goals, career plans, jobs, friendships, gender identity, and values. Sometimes people with BPD view themselves as fundamentally bad, or unworthy. They may feel unfairly misunderstood or mistreated, bored, empty, and have little idea who they are. Such symptoms are most acute when people with BPD feel isolated and lacking in social support, and may result in frantic efforts to avoid being alone.

People with BPD often have highly unstable patterns of social relationships. While they can develop intense but stormy attachments, their attitudes towards family, friends, and loved ones may suddenly shift from idealization (great admiration and love) to devaluation (intense anger and dislike). Thus, they may form an immediate attachment and idealize the other person, but when a slight separation or conflict occurs, they switch unexpectedly to the other extreme and angrily accuse the other person of not caring for them at all. Even with family members, individuals with BPD are highly sensitive to rejection, reacting with anger and distress to such mild separations as a vacation, a business trip, or a sudden change in plans. These fears of abandonment seem to be related to difficulties feeling emotionally connected to important persons when they are physically absent, leaving the individual with BPD feeling lost and perhaps worthless. Suicide threats and attempts may occur along with anger at perceived abandonment and disappointments.

People with BPD exhibit other impulsive behaviors, such as excessive spending, binge eating, and risky sex. BPD often occurs together with other psychiatric problems, particularly bipolar disorder, depression, anxiety disorders, substance abuse, and other personality disorders.

Treatment

Treatments for BPD have improved in recent years. Group and individual psychotherapy are at least partially effective for many patients. Within the past 15 years, a new psychosocial treatment termed dialectical behavior therapy (DBT) was developed specifically to treat BPD, and this technique has looked promising in treatment studies. Pharmacological treatments are often prescribed based on specific target symptoms shown by the individual patient. Antidepressant drugs and mood stabilizers may be helpful for depressed and/or labile mood. Antipsychotic drugs may also be used when there are distortions in thinking.

Recent Research Findings

Although the cause of BPD is unknown, both environmental and genetic factors are thought to play a role in predisposing patients to BPD symptoms and traits. Studies show that many, but not all individuals with BPD report a history of abuse, neglect, or separation as young children. Forty to 71 percent of BPD patients report having been sexually abused, usually by a non-caregiver. Researchers believe that BPD results from a combination of individual vulnerability to environmental stress, neglect, or abuse as young children, and a series of events that trigger the onset of the disorder as young adults. Adults with BPD are also considerably more likely to be the victim of violence, including rape and other crimes. This may result from both harmful environments as well as impulsivity and poor judgment in choosing partners and lifestyles.

NIMH-funded neuroscience research is revealing brain mechanisms underlying the impulsivity, mood instability, aggression, anger, and negative emotion seen in BPD. Studies suggest that people predisposed to impulsive aggression have impaired regulation of the neural circuits that modulate emotion. The amygdala, a small almond-shaped structure deep inside the brain, is an important component of the circuit that regulates negative emotion. In response to signals from other brain centers indicating a perceived threat, it marshals fear and arousal. This might be more pronounced under the influence of drugs like alcohol or stress. Areas in the front of the brain (prefrontal area) act to dampen the activity of this circuit. Recent brain imaging studies show that individual differences in the ability to activate regions of the prefrontal cerebral cortex thought to be involved in inhibitory activity predict the ability to suppress negative emotion.

Serotonin, norepinephrine, and acetylcholine are among the chemical messengers in these circuits that play a role in the regulation of emotions, including sadness, anger, anxiety, and irritability. Drugs that enhance brain serotonin function may improve emotional symptoms in BPD. Likewise, mood-stabilizing drugs that are known to enhance the activity of GABA [gamma aminobutyric acid], the brain's major inhibitory neurotransmitter, may help people who experience BPD-like mood swings. Such brain-based vulnerabilities can be managed with help from behavioral interventions and medications, much like people manage susceptibility to diabetes or high blood pressure.

Future Progress

Studies that translate basic findings about the neural basis of temperament, mood regulation, and cognition into clinically relevant insights which bear directly on BPD represent a growing area of NIMH-supported research. Research is also underway to test the efficacy of combining medications with behavioral treatments like DBT, and gauging the effect of childhood abuse and other stress in BPD on brain hormones. Data from the first prospective, longitudinal study of BPD, which began in the early 1990s, is expected to reveal how treatment affects the course of the illness. It will also pinpoint specific environmental factors and personality traits that predict a more favorable outcome. The Institute is also collaborating with a private foundation to help attract new researchers to develop a better understanding and better treatment for BPD.

Section 40.3

Paranoid Personality Disorder

Alternative Names

Personality disorder—paranoid

Definition

Paranoid personality disorder is a psychiatric condition characterized by extreme distrust and suspicion of others.

Causes

Personality disorders are chronic patterns of behavior that cause lasting problems with work and relationships. The cause of paranoid personality disorder is unknown, but it appears to be more common in families with psychotic disorders like schizophrenia and delusional disorder, which suggests a genetic influence.

Symptoms

People with paranoid personality disorder are highly suspicious of other people. They are usually unable to acknowledge their own negative feelings towards other people.

Other common symptoms include:

- Concern that other people have hidden motives
- Expectation to be exploited by others
- Inability to collaborate
- Poor self-image
- Social isolation
- Detachment
- Hostility

Exams and Tests

Personality disorders are diagnosed based on psychological evaluation and the history and severity of the symptoms.

Treatment

Treatment is difficult because people with this condition are often extremely suspicious of doctors. If accepted, medications and talk therapy can both be effective.

Outlook (Prognosis)

Therapy can limit the impact of the paranoia on the person's daily functioning.

Possible Complications

- Extreme social isolation
- Potential for violence

When to Contact a Medical Professional

If suspicions are interfering with relationships or work, a health care provider or mental health professional should be consulted.

Chapter 41

Dissociation and Dissociative Disorders

What is dissociation?

Dissociation is a word that is used to describe the disconnection or lack of connection between things usually associated with each other. Dissociated experiences are not integrated into the usual sense of self, resulting in discontinuities in conscious awareness. In severe forms of dissociation, disconnection occurs in the usually integrated functions of consciousness, memory, identity, or perception. For example, someone may think about an event that was tremendously upsetting yet have no feelings about it. Clinically, this is termed emotional numbing, one of the hallmarks of post-traumatic stress disorder. Dissociation is a psychological process commonly found in persons seeking mental health treatment.

Dissociation may affect a person subjectively in the form of "made" thoughts, feelings, and actions. These are thoughts or emotions seemingly coming out of nowhere, or finding oneself carrying out an action as if it were controlled by a force other than oneself. Typically, a person feels "taken over" by an emotion that does not seem to make

"FAQ: Dissociation and Dissociative Disorders," http://www.isst-d.org/education/faq-dissociation.htm, is reprinted with permission from the International Society for the Study of Trauma and Dissociation. © 2004. For more information, contact ISSTD Headquarters, 8400 Westpark Drive, Second Floor, McLean, Virginia 22102; ph: 703-610-0250; fax: 703-610-0234, or visit their website at www.isst-d.org. Reviewed by David A. Cooke, M.D., January 23, 2009. Dr. Cooke is not affiliated with the International Society for the Study of Trauma and Dissociation.

sense at the time. Feeling suddenly, unbearably sad, without an apparent reason, and then having the sadness leave in much the same manner as it came, is an example. Or someone may find himself or herself doing something that they would not normally do but unable to stop themselves, almost as if they are being compelled to do it. This is sometimes described as the experience of being a "passenger" in one's body, rather than the driver.

There are five main ways in which the dissociation of psychological processes changes the way a person experiences living: depersonalization, derealization, amnesia, identity confusion, and identity alteration. These are the main areas of investigation in the Structured Clinical Interview for Dissociative Disorders (SCID-D). A dissociative disorder is suggested by the robust presence of any of the five features.

What is depersonalization?

Depersonalization is the sense of being detached from, or "not in" one's body. This is what is often referred to as an "out-of-body" experience. However, some people report rather profound alienation from their bodies, a sense that they do not recognize themselves in the mirror, recognize their face, or simply feel not "connected" to their bodies in ways which are challenging to articulate.

What is derealization?

Derealization is the sense of the world not being real. Some people say the world looks phony, foggy, far away, or as if seen through a veil. Some people describe seeing the world as if they are detached, or as if they were watching a movie.

What is dissociative amnesia?

Amnesia refers to the inability to recall important personal information that is so extensive that it is not due to ordinary forgetfulness. Most of the amnesias typical of dissociative disorders are not of the classic fugue variety, where people travel long distances, and suddenly become alert, disoriented as to where they are and how they got there. Rather, the amnesias are often an important event that is forgotten, such as a wedding, or birthday party that was attended, or a block of time, from minutes to years. More typically, there are microamnesias where the discussion engaged in is not remembered, or the content of a conversation is forgotten from one moment to the next.

Some people report that these kinds of experiences often leave them scrambling to figure out what was being discussed. Meanwhile, they try not to let the person with whom they are talking realize they haven't a clue as to what was just said.

What are identity confusion and identity alteration?

Identity confusion is a sense of confusion about who a person is. An example of identity confusion is when a person sometimes feels a thrill while engaged in an activity (e.g., reckless driving, drug use) which at other times would be repugnant. Identity alteration is the sense of being markedly different from another part of oneself. This can be unnerving to clinicians. A person may shift into an alternate personality, become confused, and demand of the clinician, "Who the dickens are you, and what am I doing here?" In addition to these observable changes, the person may experience distortions in time, place, and situation. For example, in the course of an initial discovery of the experience of identity alteration, a person might incorrectly believe they were 5 years old, in their childhood home and not the therapist's office, and expecting a deceased person whom they fear to appear at any moment.

More frequently, subtler forms of identity alteration can be observed when a person uses different voice tones, range of language, or facial expressions. These may be associated with a change in the patient's world view. For example, during a discussion about fear, a client may initially feel young, vulnerable, and frightened, followed by a sudden shift to feeling hostile and callous. The person may express confusion about their feelings and perceptions, or may have difficulty remembering what they have just said, even though they do not claim to be a different person or have a different name. The patient may be able to confirm the experience of identity alteration, but often the part of the self that presents for therapy is not aware of the existence of dissociated self-states. If identity alteration is suspected, it may be confirmed by observation of amnesia for behavior and distinct changes in affect, speech patterns, demeanor and body language, and relationship to the therapist. The therapist can gently help the patient become aware of these changes.

What is the cause of dissociation and dissociative disorders?

Research tends to show that dissociation stems from a combination of environmental and biological factors. The likelihood that a tendency to dissociate is inherited genetically is estimated to be zero.

Most commonly, repetitive childhood physical and/or sexual abuse and other forms of trauma are associated with the development of dissociative disorders. In the context of chronic, severe childhood trauma, dissociation can be considered adaptive because it reduces the overwhelming distress created by trauma. However, if dissociation continues to be used in adulthood, when the original danger no longer exists, it can be maladaptive. The dissociative adult may automatically disconnect from situations that are perceived as dangerous or threatening, without taking time to determine whether there is any real danger. This leaves the person "spaced out" in many situations in ordinary life, and unable to protect themselves in conditions of real danger.

Dissociation may also occur when there has been severe neglect or emotional abuse, even when there has been no overt physical or sexual abuse. Children may also become dissociative in families in which the parents are frightening, unpredictable, are dissociative themselves, or make highly contradictory communications.

The development of dissociative disorders in adulthood appears to be related to the intensity of dissociation during the actual traumatic event(s); severe dissociation during the traumatic experience increases the likelihood of generalization of such mechanisms following the event(s). The experience of ongoing trauma in childhood significantly increases the likelihood of developing dissociative disorders in adulthood.

How does affect dysregulation influence dissociation?

One of the core problems for the person with a dissociative disorder is affect dysregulation, or difficulty tolerating and regulating intense emotional experiences. This problem results in part from having had little opportunity to learn to soothe oneself or modulate feelings, due to growing up in an abusive or neglectful family, where parents did not teach these skills. Problems in affect regulation are compounded by the sudden intrusion of traumatic memories and the overwhelming emotions accompanying them.

The inability to manage intense feelings may trigger a change in self-state from one prevailing mood to another. Depersonalization, derealization, amnesia, and identity confusion can all be thought of as efforts at self-regulation when affect regulation fails. Each psychological adaptation changes the ability of the person to tolerate a particular emotion, such as feeling threatened. As a last alternative for an overwhelmed mind to escape from fear when there is no escape, a person may unconsciously adapt by believing, incorrectly, that they are somebody else. Becoming aware of this kind of fear is terrifying. Therein lies one of the central problems in treatment for a person with a dissociative disorder: "How do I learn to approach things I fear when to understand that I am afraid is itself frightening?" Skillful clinical approaches are required to help build confidence in a person's ability to tolerate their feelings, learn, and grow as a person.

How is dissociation different from hypnosis?

Dissociative experiences are often confused with those of hypnosis. While the two experiences may exist together, they are not the same. For example, hypnotic absorption may be present in someone who is experiencing identity alteration, but it is not equivalent. To be hypnotically absorbed is to lose track of the background events and be completely absorbed by the foreground (e.g., highway hypnosis, where a person drives by the exit they had taken many times, only to discover they had missed the exit and are further down the road). A person capable of hypnotic absorption may be absorbed in their thoughts while maintaining control of their body (and their driving), but what they are doing is not in their awareness. Thus there is a disconnection between mind (conscious awareness) and body. This disconnection in hypnotic absorption is an example of a dissociative process, but the absorption itself is not indicative of a dissociative disorder. Rather, absorption is an example of everyday hypnotic experience and is part of the continuum of the dissociation of psychological functions that can be seen during hypnosis.

What are the different types of dissociative disorders?

There are four main categories of dissociative disorders as defined in the standard catalogue of psychological diagnoses used by mental health professionals in North America, the *Diagnostic and Statistical Manual of Mental Disorders, Fourth Edition, Text Revision* (*DSM-IV-TR*). The four dissociative disorders are: dissociative amnesia, dissociative fugue, dissociative identity disorder, and depersonalization disorder.

Dissociative amnesia (psychogenic amnesia) is characterized by an inability to recall important personal information, usually of a traumatic or stressful nature, that is too extensive to be explained by ordinary forgetfulness. The amnesia must be too extensive to be characterized as typical forgetfulness and cannot be due to an organic disorder or DID [dissociative identity disorder]. It is the most common of all dissociative disorders, frequently seen in hospital emergency rooms. In addition, dissociative amnesia is often embedded within other psychological disorders (e.g., anxiety disorders, other dissociative disorders). Individuals suffering from dissociative amnesia are generally aware of their memory loss. The memory loss is usually reversible because the memory difficulties are in the retrieval process, not the encoding process. Duration of disorder varies from a few days to a few years.

Dissociative fugue (psychogenic fugue) is characterized by a sudden, unexpected travel away from home or one's customary place of work, accompanied by an inability to recall one's past and confusion about personal identity or the assumption of a new identity. Individual's suffering from dissociative fugue appear "normal" to others. That is, their psychopathology is not obvious. They are generally unaware of their memory loss/amnesia.

Depersonalization disorder is characterized by a persistent or recurrent feeling of being detached from one's own mental processes or body. Individuals suffering from depersonalization disorder relate feeling as if they are watching their lives from outside of their bodies, similar to watching a movie. Individuals with depersonalization disorder often report problems with concentration, memory, and perception. The depersonalization must occur independently of DID, substance abuse disorders, and schizophrenia.

Dissociative identity disorder (previously known as multiple personality disorder) is the most severe and chronic manifestation of dissociation, characterized by the presence of two or more distinct identities or personality states that recurrently take control of the individual's behavior, accompanied by an inability to recall important personal information that is too extensive to be explained by ordinary forgetfulness. It is now recognized that these dissociated states are not fully-formed personalities, but rather represent a fragmented sense of identity. The amnesia typically associated with dissociative identity disorder is asymmetrical, with different identity states remembering different aspects of autobiographical information. There is usually a host personality who identifies with the client's real name. Typically, the host personality is not aware of the presence of other alters. The different personalities may serve distinct roles in coping with problem areas. An average of 2 to 4 personalities/alters are present at diagnosis, with an average of 13 to 15 personalities emerging over the course of treatment. Environmental events usually trigger a sudden shifting from one personality to another. Dissociative Disorder Not Otherwise Specified (DDNOS): DDNOS includes dissociative presentations that do not meet the full criteria for any other dissociative disorder. In clinical practice, this appears to be the most commonly presented dissociative disorder, and may often be better characterized by major dissociative disorder with partially dissociated self states.

What is the prevalence of dissociative disorders?

Some studies indicate that diagnosable dissociation occurs in approximately two to three percent of the general population. Other studies have estimated a prevalence rate of 10% for all dissociative disorders in the general population.

Dissociation may exist in either acute or chronic forms. Immediately following severe trauma, the incidence of dissociative phenomena is remarkably high. Approximately 73% of individuals exposed to a traumatic incident will experience dissociative states during the incident or in the hours, days, and weeks following. However, for most people these dissociative experiences will subside on their own within a few weeks after the traumatic incident subsides.

Some prevalence rates have been calculated individually for the four types of dissociative disorders:

- **Dissociative amnesia:** No exact prevalence rates have been empirically demonstrated for dissociative amnesia.
- **Dissociative fugue:** Prevalence rate of 0.2% in the general population. The prevalence is thought to be higher during periods of extreme stress.
- **Dissociative identity disorder:** Prevalence rates of .01 to 1% in the general population. Studies have indicated a prevalence rate of .5 to 1.0% in psychiatric settings.
- **Depersonalization disorder:** Exact prevalence is unknown. Some researchers have suggested that depersonalization disorder is the third most common psychological disorder following depression and anxiety.

What are treatments specific to the types of dissociative disorder?

For more general treatment guidelines please refer to the Treatment Guidelines of the International Society for the Study of Trauma and Dissociation.

Dissociative amnesia: No empirical studies have assessed the treatment of dissociative amnesia. Current information is based upon case studies and will be discussed briefly. Prior to beginning treatment, it is essential to determine that the amnesia is dissociative in origin. That is, neurological and/or medical causes must be ruled out. Clients with acute onset are typically treated more aggressively than clients presenting with chronic amnesia.

- **Acute amnesia:** In clients with acute presentation of amnesia it is first necessary to provide a safe therapeutic environment. In fact, researchers have demonstrated that sometimes simply removing threatening stimuli and providing an individual with a safe environment has enabled spontaneous retrieval of memory. Barbiturates can be used to pharmacologically facilitate the interviewing process. Most commonly used are sodium amobarbital and sodium pentobarbital. No studies have empirically investigated the effectiveness of hypnosis in treating dissociative amnesia. However, hypnosis has been used successfully in the recovery of dissociated and repressed memories. Once the amnesia has been reversed it is important to explore and identify events that triggered the dissociative amnesia. The therapist should reinforce the use of effective coping mechanisms and the clients' failure to use dissociation as their primary coping strategy.
- **Chronic amnesia:** Pharmacologically facilitated intervention is not recommended. Hypnosis may be beneficial in recovering and working through traumatic memories at a pace comfortable for the client. Reframing of the traumatic experiences can occur during the hypnotic process. The goal of therapy is the integration of dissociated material. Treatment of chronic dissociative amnesia is typically long-term.

Dissociative fugue: To date, there are no empirical studies that have addressed the treatment of dissociative fugue. All current information is derived from case studies and will be briefly discussed.

A safe therapeutic environment, strong therapeutic alliance, recovery of one's own identity, identification of triggers associated with fugue onset, reprocessing trauma and integrating trauma into one's current being are essential components in the treatment of dissociative fugue. Drug-facilitated interviews and hypnosis may be helpful. Treatment should begin as soon as possible following the fugue.

Dissociative identity disorder: Treatment of dissociative identity disorder typically includes the following components: a strong therapeutic relationship, a safe therapeutic environment, appropriate boundaries, development of no self- or other-harm contracts, an understanding of the personality structures, working through traumatic and dissociated material, the development of more mature psychological defenses, and the integration of states of self. Guidelines for treatment of adults and children are available from the International Society for the Study of Trauma and Dissociation, www.ISST-D.org. Integration of traumatic memories is an essential aspect of treatment. Hypnosis can aid in allowing the client to gain control over the dissociative episodes and in the integration of memories. Treatment of dissociative identity disorder is typically long and challenging. Spontaneous remission will not occur. Studies have shown that cognitive behavioral treatment of dissociative identity disorder can be beneficial. Electroconvulsive therapy (ECT) is not generally recommended. Eye-movement desensitization and reprocessing (EMDR) can be used in the treatment of DID although it needs to be implemented with great caution. EMDR is a newer psychological treatment designed to accelerate the processing of information and to facilitate integration of fragmented trauma memories.

Depersonalization disorder: As holds true for the other dissociative disorders, no controlled studies have addressed the treatment of depersonalization disorder. Treatments currently used include a variety of models including cognitive and behavioral approaches, psychoanalysis, and psychopharmacology. Clinical findings are inconsistent. The lack of empirical treatment studies on depersonalization adversely impacts the understanding and treatment of other dissociative disorders due to the fact that depersonalization is often a component of these disorders. Depersonalization disorder has been described as resistant to psychopharmacological and psychotherapeutic treatment interventions.

Chapter 42

Munchausen by Proxy Syndrome

By the time she was 8 years old, J.B. had been hospitalized 200 times and had undergone more than 40 operations, including the removal of most of her intestines.

K.C., a 2-year-old boy, was hospitalized more than 20 times due to complications from asthma, severe pneumonia, mysterious infections, and sudden fevers. His doctors were baffled and unable to determine the cause of these illnesses.

What do these seemingly unrelated cases have in common? They were the result of Munchausen by proxy syndrome (MBPS), or Factitious Disorder by Proxy, as it's listed in the American Psychiatric Association's *Diagnostic and Statistical Manual of Mental Disorders* (Fourth Edition, Text Revision, also known as DSM-IV-TR).

This relatively uncommon condition involves the exaggeration or fabrication of illnesses or symptoms by a primary caretaker. One of the most harmful forms of child abuse, Munchausen by proxy syndrome—also commonly called Munchausen syndrome by proxy (MSBP)—was named after Baron von Munchausen, an eighteenth-century German dignitary known for telling outlandish stories.

J.B.'s medical history was traced to her mother, who manufactured her daughter's illnesses. Similarly, when K.C. was thought to have AIDS [acquired immunodeficiency syndrome], he eventually complained to his mother's friend that his thigh was sore because "Mommy gave me shots" (indicating that the mother was giving her son something to cause his symptoms).

About MBPS

In MBPS, an individual—usually a mother—deliberately makes another person (most often his or her own preschool child) sick or convinces others that the person is sick. The parent or caregiver misleads others into thinking that the child has medical problems by lying and reporting fictitious episodes. He or she may exaggerate, fabricate, or induce symptoms. As a result, doctors usually order tests, try different types of medications, and may even hospitalize the child or perform surgery to determine the cause.

Typically, the perpetrator feels satisfied by gaining the attention and sympathy of doctors, nurses, and others who come into contact with him or her and the child. Some experts believe that it isn't just the attention that's gained from the "illness" of the child that drives this behavior, but also the satisfaction in being able to deceive individuals that they consider to be more important and powerful than themselves.

Because the parent or caregiver appears to be so caring and attentive, often no one suspects any wrongdoing. A perplexing aspect of the syndrome is the ability of the parent or caregiver to fool and manipulate doctors. Frequently, the perpetrator is familiar with the medical profession and is very good at fooling the doctors. Even the most experienced doctors can miss the meaning of the inconsistencies in the child's symptoms. It's not unusual for medical personnel to overlook the possibility of Munchausen by proxy syndrome because it goes against the belief that a parent or caregiver would never deliberately hurt his or her child.

Children who are subject to MBPS are typically preschool age, although there have been reported cases in children up to 16 years old. There are equal numbers of boys and girls; however, 98% of the perpetrators are female.

Diagnosis is very difficult, but would involve some of the following:

- a child who has multiple medical problems that don't respond to treatment or that follow a persistent and puzzling course

- physical or laboratory findings that are highly unusual, don't correspond with the child's medical history, or are physically or clinically impossible
- short-term symptoms that tend to stop when the perpetrator isn't around
- a parent or caregiver who isn't reassured by "good news" when test results find no medical problems, but continues to believe that the child is ill
- a parent or caregiver who appears to be medically knowledgeable or fascinated with medical details or appears to enjoy the hospital environment
- a parent or caregiver who's unusually calm in the face of serious difficulties with the child's health
- a parent or caregiver who's highly supportive and encouraging of the doctor, or one who is angry and demands further intervention, more procedures, second opinions, or transfers to more sophisticated facilities

Causes of MBPS

In some cases, the parents or caregivers themselves were abused, both physically and sexually, as children. They may have come from families in which being sick was a way to get love. The parent's or caregiver's own personal needs overcome his or her ability to see the child as a person with feelings and rights, possibly because the parent or caregiver may have grown up being treated like he or she wasn't a person with rights or feelings.

Other theories say that Munchausen by proxy syndrome is a cry for help on the part of the parent or caregiver, who may be experiencing anxiety or depression or have feelings of inadequacy as a parent or caregiver of a young child. Some may feel a sense of acknowledgement when the child's doctor confirms their caregiving skills. Or, the parent or caregiver may just enjoy the attention that the sick child—and, therefore, he or she—gets.

The suspected person may also have symptoms similar to the child's own medical problems or an illness history that's puzzling and unusual. He or she frequently has an emotionally distant relationship with a spouse, who often fails to visit the seriously ill child or have contact with doctors.

What Happens to the Child?

In the most severe instances, parents or caregivers with Munchausen by proxy syndrome may go to great lengths to make their children sick. When cameras were placed in some children's hospital rooms, some perpetrators were filmed switching medications, injecting kids with urine to cause an infection, or placing drops of blood in urine specimens.

Some perpetrators aggravate an existing problem, such as manipulating a wound so that it doesn't heal. One parent discovered that scrubbing the child's skin with oven cleaner would cause a baffling, long-lasting rash.

Whatever the course, the child's symptoms—whether created or faked—don't happen when the parent isn't present, and they usually go away during periods of separation from the parent. When confronted, the parent usually denies knowing how the illness occurred.

According to the DSM-IV-TR, some of the most common conditions and symptoms that are created or faked by parents or caregivers with Munchausen by proxy syndrome include: failure to thrive, allergies, asthma, vomiting, diarrhea, seizures, and infections.

The long-term prognosis for these children depends on the degree of damage created by the perpetrator and the amount of time it takes to recognize and diagnose MBPS. Some extreme cases have been reported in which children developed destructive skeletal changes, limps, mental retardation, brain damage, and blindness from symptoms caused by the parent or caregiver. Often, these children require multiple surgeries, each with the risk for future medical problems.

If the child lives to be old enough to comprehend what's happening, the psychological damage can be significant. The child may come to feel that he or she will only be loved when ill and may, therefore, help the parent try to deceive doctors, using self-abuse to avoid being abandoned. And so, some victims of Munchausen by proxy syndrome later become perpetrators themselves.

Getting Help for the Child

If Munchausen by proxy syndrome is suspected, health care providers are required by law to report their concerns. However, after a parent or caregiver is charged, the child's symptoms may increase as the person who is accused attempts to prove the presence of the illness. If the parent or caregiver repeatedly denies the charges, the child should be removed from the home and legal action should be taken on the child's behalf.

In some cases, the parent or caregiver may deny the charges and move to another location, only to continue the behavior. Even if the child is returned to the perpetrator's custody while protective services are still involved, the child may continue to be a victim of abuse. For these reasons, it's always advised that these cases be resolved quickly.

Getting Help for the Parent or Caregiver

Most often, abusive Munchausen by proxy syndrome cases are resolved in one of three ways:

1. the perpetrator is apprehended
2. the perpetrator moves on to a younger child when the original victim gets old enough to "tell"
3. the child dies

To get help, the parent or caregiver must admit to the abuse and seek psychological treatment. But if the perpetrator doesn't admit to the wrongdoing, psychological treatment has little chance of remedying the situation. Psychotherapy depends on truth, and MBPS perpetrators generally live in denial.

Chapter 43

Schizophrenic Disorders

Chapter Contents

Section 43.1

All about Schizophrenia

Excerpted from the booklet "Schizophrenia," by the National Institute of Mental Health (NIMH, www.nimh.nih.gov), part of the National Institutes of Health, 2006.

What is schizophrenia?

Schizophrenia is a chronic, severe, and disabling brain disorder that has been recognized throughout recorded history. It affects about 1 percent of Americans.

People with schizophrenia may hear voices other people don't hear or they may believe that others are reading their minds, controlling their thoughts, or plotting to harm them. These experiences are terrifying and can cause fearfulness, withdrawal, or extreme agitation. People with schizophrenia may not make sense when they talk, may sit for hours without moving or talking much, or may seem perfectly fine until they talk about what they are really thinking. Because many people with schizophrenia have difficulty holding a job or caring for themselves, the burden on their families and society is significant as well.

Available treatments can relieve many of the disorder's symptoms, but most people who have schizophrenia must cope with some residual symptoms as long as they live. Nevertheless, this is a time of hope for people with schizophrenia and their families. Many people with the disorder now lead rewarding and meaningful lives in their communities. Researchers are developing more effective medications and using new research tools to understand the causes of schizophrenia and to find ways to prevent and treat it.

This text presents information on the symptoms of schizophrenia, when the symptoms appear, how the disease develops, current treatments, support for patients and their loved ones, and new directions in research.

What are the symptoms of schizophrenia?

The symptoms of schizophrenia fall into three broad categories:

- Positive symptoms are unusual thoughts or perceptions, including hallucinations, delusions, thought disorder, and disorders of movement.
- Negative symptoms represent a loss or a decrease in the ability to initiate plans, speak, express emotion, or find pleasure in everyday life. These symptoms are harder to recognize as part of the disorder and can be mistaken for laziness or depression.
- Cognitive symptoms (or cognitive deficits) are problems with attention, certain types of memory, and the executive functions that allow us to plan and organize. Cognitive deficits can also be difficult to recognize as part of the disorder but are the most disabling in terms of leading a normal life.

Positive symptoms: Positive symptoms are easy-to-spot behaviors not seen in healthy people and usually involve a loss of contact with reality. They include hallucinations, delusions, thought disorder, and disorders of movement. Positive symptoms can come and go. Sometimes they are severe and at other times hardly noticeable, depending on whether the individual is receiving treatment.

- **Hallucinations:** A hallucination is something a person sees, hears, smells, or feels that no one else can see, hear, smell, or feel. "Voices" are the most common type of hallucination in schizophrenia. Many people with the disorder hear voices that may comment on their behavior, order them to do things, warn them of impending danger, or talk to each other (usually about the patient).They may hear these voices for a long time before family and friends notice that something is wrong. Other types of hallucinations include seeing people or objects that are not there, smelling odors that no one else detects (although this can also be a symptom of certain brain tumors), and feeling things like invisible fingers touching their bodies when no one is near.
- **Delusions:** Delusions are false personal beliefs that are not part of the person's culture and do not change, even when other people present proof that the beliefs are not true or logical. People with schizophrenia can have delusions that are quite bizarre, such as believing that neighbors can control their behavior with magnetic waves, people on television are directing special messages to them, or radio stations are broadcasting their thoughts aloud to others. They may also have delusions of grandeur and

think they are famous historical figures. People with paranoid schizophrenia can believe that others are deliberately cheating, harassing, poisoning, spying upon, or plotting against them or the people they care about. These beliefs are called delusions of persecution.

- **Thought disorder:** People with schizophrenia often have unusual thought processes. One dramatic form is disorganized thinking, in which the person has difficulty organizing his or her thoughts or connecting them logically. Speech may be garbled or hard to understand. Another form is "thought blocking," in which the person stops abruptly in the middle of a thought. When asked why, the person may say that it felt as if the thought had been taken out of his or her head. Finally, the individual might make up unintelligible words, or "neologisms."
- **Disorders of movement:** People with schizophrenia can be clumsy and uncoordinated. They may also exhibit involuntary movements and may grimace or exhibit unusual mannerisms. They may repeat certain motions over and over or, in extreme cases, may become catatonic. Catatonia is a state of immobility and unresponsiveness. It was more common when treatment for schizophrenia was not available; fortunately, it is now rare.

Negative symptoms: The term "negative symptoms" refers to reductions in normal emotional and behavioral states. These include the following:

- flat affect (immobile facial expression, monotonous voice);
- lack of pleasure in everyday life;
- diminished ability to initiate and sustain planned activity; and
- speaking infrequently, even when forced to interact.

People with schizophrenia often neglect basic hygiene and need help with everyday activities. Because it is not as obvious that negative symptoms are part of a psychiatric illness, people with schizophrenia are often perceived as lazy and unwilling to better their lives.

Cognitive symptoms: Cognitive symptoms are subtle and are often detected only when neuropsychological tests are performed. They include the following:

- poor "executive functioning" (the ability to absorb and interpret information and make decisions based on that information);
- inability to sustain attention; and
- problems with "working memory" (the ability to keep recently learned information in mind and use it right away).

Cognitive impairments often interfere with the patient's ability to lead a normal life and earn a living. They can cause great emotional distress.

When does it start and who gets it?

Psychotic symptoms (such as hallucinations and delusions) usually emerge in men in their late teens and early 20s and in women in their mid-20s to early 30s. They seldom occur after age 45 and only rarely before puberty, although cases of schizophrenia in children as young as 5 have been reported. In adolescents, the first signs can include a change of friends, a drop in grades, sleep problems, and irritability. Because many normal adolescents exhibit these behaviors as well, a diagnosis can be difficult to make at this stage. In young people who go on to develop the disease, this is called the "prodromal" period.

Research has shown that schizophrenia affects men and women equally and occurs at similar rates in all ethnic groups around the world.

Are people with schizophrenia violent?

People with schizophrenia are not especially prone to violence and often prefer to be left alone. Studies show that if people have no record of criminal violence before they develop schizophrenia and are not substance abusers, they are unlikely to commit crimes after they become ill. Most violent crimes are not committed by people with schizophrenia, and most people with schizophrenia do not commit violent crimes. Substance abuse always increases violent behavior, regardless of the presence of schizophrenia. If someone with paranoid schizophrenia becomes violent, the violence is most often directed at family members and takes place at home.

What about suicide?

People with schizophrenia attempt suicide much more often than people in the general population. About 10 percent (especially young adult males) succeed. It is hard to predict which people with schizophrenia are prone to suicide, so if someone talks about or tries to commit suicide, professional help should be sought right away.

What about substance abuse?

Some people who abuse drugs show symptoms similar to those of schizophrenia, and people with schizophrenia may be mistaken for people who are high on drugs. While most researchers do not believe that substance abuse causes schizophrenia, people who have schizophrenia abuse alcohol and/or drugs more often than the general population.

Substance abuse can reduce the effectiveness of treatment for schizophrenia. Stimulants (such as amphetamines or cocaine), PCP [phencyclidine], and marijuana may make the symptoms of schizophrenia worse, and substance abuse also makes it more likely that patients will not follow their treatment plan.

Schizophrenia and nicotine: The most common form of substance abuse in people with schizophrenia is an addiction to nicotine. People with schizophrenia are addicted to nicotine at three times the rate of the general population (75-90 percent vs. 25-30 percent).

Research has revealed that the relationship between smoking and schizophrenia is complex. People with schizophrenia seem to be driven to smoke, and researchers are exploring whether there is a biological basis for this need. In addition to its known health hazards, several studies have found that smoking interferes with the action of antipsychotic drugs. People with schizophrenia who smoke may need higher doses of their medication.

Quitting smoking may be especially difficult for people with schizophrenia since nicotine withdrawal may cause their psychotic symptoms to temporarily get worse. Smoking cessation strategies that include nicotine replacement methods may be better tolerated. Doctors who treat people with schizophrenia should carefully monitor their patient's response to antipsychotic medication if the patient decides to either start or stop smoking.

What causes schizophrenia?

Like many other illnesses, schizophrenia is believed to result from a combination of environmental and genetic factors. All the tools of modern science are being used to search for the causes of this disorder.

Can schizophrenia be inherited?

Scientists have long known that schizophrenia runs in families. It occurs in 1 percent of the general population but is seen in 10 percent of people with a first-degree relative (a parent, brother, or sister) with the disorder. People who have second-degree relatives (aunts, uncles, grandparents, or cousins) with the disease also develop schizophrenia more often than the general population. The identical twin of a person with schizophrenia is most at risk, with a 40 to 65 percent chance of developing the disorder.

Our genes are located on 23 pairs of chromosomes that are found in each cell. We inherit two copies of each gene, one from each parent. Several of these genes are thought to be associated with an increased risk of schizophrenia, but scientists believe that each gene has a very small effect and is not responsible for causing the disease by itself. It is still not possible to predict who will develop the disease by looking at genetic material.

Although there is a genetic risk for schizophrenia, it is not likely that genes alone are sufficient to cause the disorder. Interactions between genes and the environment are thought to be necessary for schizophrenia to develop. Many environmental factors have been suggested as risk factors, such as exposure to viruses or malnutrition in the womb, problems during birth, and psychosocial factors, like stressful environmental conditions. People with schizophrenia may be mistaken for people who are high on drugs.

Do people with schizophrenia have faulty brain chemistry?

It is likely that an imbalance in the complex, interrelated chemical reactions of the brain involving the neurotransmitters dopamine and glutamate (and possibly others) plays a role in schizophrenia. Neurotransmitters are substances that allow brain cells to communicate with one another. Basic knowledge about brain chemistry and its link to schizophrenia is expanding rapidly and is a promising area of research.

Do the brains of people with schizophrenia look different?

The brains of people with schizophrenia look a little different than the brains of healthy people, but the differences are small. Sometimes the fluid-filled cavities at the center of the brain, called ventricles, are larger in people with schizophrenia; overall gray matter volume is lower; and some areas of the brain have less or more metabolic activity. Microscopic studies of brain tissue after death have also revealed small changes in the distribution or characteristics of brain cells in people with schizophrenia. It appears that many of these changes were prenatal because they are not accompanied by glial cells, which are always present when a brain injury occurs after birth. One theory suggests that problems during brain development lead to faulty connections that lie dormant until puberty. The brain undergoes major changes during puberty, and these changes could trigger psychotic symptoms.

The only way to answer these questions is to conduct more research. Scientists in the United States and around the world are studying schizophrenia and trying to develop new ways to prevent and treat the disorder.

How is schizophrenia treated?

Because the causes of schizophrenia are still unknown, current treatments focus on eliminating the symptoms of the disease.

Antipsychotic medications: Antipsychotic medications have been available since the mid-1950s. They effectively alleviate the positive symptoms of schizophrenia. While these drugs have greatly improved the lives of many patients, they do not cure schizophrenia.

Everyone responds differently to antipsychotic medication. Sometimes several different drugs must be tried before the right one is found. People with schizophrenia should work in partnership with their doctors to find the medications that control their symptoms best with the fewest side effects.

The older antipsychotic medications include chlorpromazine (Thorazine®), haloperidol (Haldol®), perphenazine (Etrafon®, Trilafon®), and fluphenazine (Prolixin®).The older medications can cause extrapyramidal side effects, such as rigidity, persistent muscle spasms, tremors, and restlessness.

In the 1990s, new drugs, called atypical antipsychotics, were developed that rarely produced these side effects. The first of these new drugs was clozapine (Clozaril®). It treats psychotic symptoms effectively even in people who do not respond to other medications, but it can produce a serious problem called agranulocytosis, a loss of the white blood cells that fight infection. Therefore, patients who take clozapine must have their white blood cell counts monitored every week or two. The inconvenience and cost of both the blood tests and the medication itself has made treatment with clozapine difficult for many people, but it is the drug of choice for those whose symptoms do not respond to the other antipsychotic medications, old or new. Everyone responds differently to antipsychotic medication.

Some of the drugs that were developed after clozapine was introduced—such as risperidone (Risperdal®), olanzapine (Zyprexa®), quetiapine (Seroquel®), sertindole (Serdolect®),and ziprasidone (Geodon®)—are effective and rarely produce extrapyramidal symptoms and do not cause agranulocytosis; but they can cause weight gain and metabolic changes associated with an increased risk of diabetes and high cholesterol.

Aripiprazole (Abilify) is another atypical antipsychotic medication used to treat the symptoms of schizophrenia and manic or mixed (manic and depressive) episodes of bipolar I disorder. Aripiprazole is in tablet and liquid form. An injectable form is used in the treatment of symptoms of agitation in schizophrenia and manic or mixed episodes of bipolar I disorder.

People respond individually to antipsychotic medications, although agitation and hallucinations usually improve within days and delusions usually improve within a few weeks. Many people see substantial improvement in both types of symptoms by the sixth week of treatment. No one can tell beforehand exactly how a medication will affect a particular individual, and sometimes several medications must be tried before the right one is found.

When people first start to take atypical antipsychotics, they may become drowsy; experience dizziness when they change positions; have blurred vision; or develop a rapid heartbeat, menstrual problems, a sensitivity to the sun, or skin rashes. Many of these symptoms will go away after the first days of treatment, but people who are taking atypical antipsychotics should not drive until they adjust to their new medication.

If people with schizophrenia become depressed, it may be necessary to add an antidepressant to their drug regimen.

A large clinical trial funded by the National Institute of Mental Health (NIMH), known as CATIE (Clinical Antipsychotic Trials of Intervention Effectiveness), compared the effectiveness and side effects of five antipsychotic medications—both new and older antipsychotics—that are used to treat people with schizophrenia. For more information on CATIE, visit http://www.nimh.nih.gov/healthinformation/catie.cfm.

Length of treatment: Like diabetes or high blood pressure, schizophrenia is a chronic disorder that needs constant management. At the moment, it cannot be cured, but the rate of recurrence of psychotic episodes can be decreased significantly by staying on medication. Although responses vary from person to person, most people with schizophrenia need to take some type of medication for the rest of their lives as well as use other approaches, such as supportive therapy or rehabilitation.

Relapses occur most often when people with schizophrenia stop taking their antipsychotic medication because they feel better, or only take it occasionally because they forget or don't think taking it regularly is important. It is very important for people with schizophrenia to take their medication on a regular basis and for as long as their doctors recommend. If they do so, they will experience fewer psychotic symptoms.

No antipsychotic medication should be discontinued without talking to the doctor who prescribed it, and it should always be tapered off under a doctor's supervision rather than being stopped all at once.

There are a variety of reasons why people with schizophrenia do not adhere to treatment. If they don't believe they are ill, they may not think they need medication at all. If their thinking is too disorganized, they may not remember to take their medication every day. If they don't like the side effects of one medication, they may stop taking it without trying a different medication. Substance abuse can also interfere with treatment effectiveness. Doctors should ask patients how often they take their medication and be sensitive to a patient's request to change dosages or to try new medications to eliminate unwelcome side effects.

There are many strategies to help people with schizophrenia take their drugs regularly. Some medications are available in long-acting, injectable forms, which eliminate the need to take a pill every day. Medication calendars or pillboxes labeled with the days of the week can both help patients remember to take their medications and let caregivers know whether medication has been taken. Electronic timers on clocks or watches can be programmed to beep when people need to take their pills, and pairing medication with routine daily events, like meals, can help patients adhere to dosing schedules.

Medication interactions: Antipsychotic medications can produce unpleasant or dangerous side effects when taken with certain other drugs. For this reason, the doctor who prescribes the antipsychotics should be told about all medications (over-the-counter and prescription) and all vitamins, minerals, and herbal supplements the patient takes. Alcohol or other drug use should also be discussed.

Psychosocial treatment: Numerous studies have found that psychosocial treatments can help patients who are already stabilized on antipsychotic medication deal with certain aspects of schizophrenia, such as difficulty with communication, motivation, self-care, work, and establishing and maintaining relationships with others. Learning and using coping mechanisms to address these problems allows people with schizophrenia to attend school, work, and socialize. Patients who receive regular psychosocial treatment also adhere better to their medication schedule and have fewer relapses and hospitalizations. A positive relationship with a therapist or a case manager gives the patient a reliable source of information, sympathy, encouragement, and hope, all of which are essential for managing the disease. The therapist can help patients better understand and adjust to living with schizophrenia by educating them about the causes of the disorder, common symptoms or problems they may experience, and the importance of staying on medications.

Illness management skills: People with schizophrenia can take an active role in managing their own illness. Once they learn basic facts about schizophrenia and the principles of schizophrenia treatment, they can make informed decisions about their care. If they are taught how to monitor the early warning signs of relapse and make a plan to respond to these signs, they can learn to prevent relapses. Patients can also be taught more effective coping skills to deal with persistent symptoms.

Integrated treatment for co-occurring substance abuse: Substance abuse is the most common co-occurring disorder in people with schizophrenia, but ordinary substance abuse treatment programs usually do not address this population's special needs. Integrating schizophrenia treatment programs and drug treatment programs produces better outcomes.

Rehabilitation: Rehabilitation emphasizes social and vocational training to help people with schizophrenia function more effectively in their communities. Because people with schizophrenia frequently become ill during the critical career-forming years of life (ages 18 to 35) and because the disease often interferes with normal cognitive functioning, most patients do not receive the training required for skilled work. Rehabilitation programs can include vocational counseling, job training, money management counseling, assistance in learning to use public transportation, and opportunities to practice social and workplace communication skills.

Family education: Patients with schizophrenia are often discharged from the hospital into the care of their families, so it is important that family members know as much as possible about the disease to prevent relapses. Family members should be able to use different kinds of treatment adherence programs and have an arsenal of coping strategies and problem-solving skills to manage their ill relative effectively. Knowing where to find outpatient and family services that support people with schizophrenia and their caregivers is also valuable.

Cognitive behavioral therapy: Cognitive behavioral therapy is useful for patients with symptoms that persist even when they take medication. The cognitive therapist teaches people with schizophrenia how to test the reality of their thoughts and perceptions, how to "not listen" to their voices, and how to shake off the apathy that often immobilizes them. This treatment appears to be effective in reducing the severity of symptoms and decreasing the risk of relapse.

Self-help groups: Self-help groups for people with schizophrenia and their families are becoming increasingly common. Although professional therapists are not involved, the group members are a continuing source of mutual support and comfort for each other, which is also therapeutic. People in self-help groups know that others are facing the same problems they face and no longer feel isolated by their illness or the illness of their loved one. The networking that takes place in self-help groups can also generate social action. Families working together can advocate for research and more hospital and community treatment programs, and patients acting as a group may be able to draw public attention to the discriminations many people with mental illnesses still face in today's world. Support groups and advocacy groups are excellent resources for people with many types of mental disorders.

Section 43.2

Schizoaffective Disorder

Schizoaffective disorder is one of the more common, chronic, and disabling mental illnesses. As the name implies, it is characterized by a combination of symptoms of schizophrenia and an affective (mood) disorder. There has been a controversy about whether schizoaffective disorder is a type of schizophrenia or a type of mood disorder. Today, most clinicians and researchers agree that it is primarily a form of schizophrenia. Although its exact prevalence is not clear, it may range from two to five in a 1,000 people (i.e., 0.2% to 0.5%). Schizoaffective disorder may account for one-fourth or even one-third of all persons with schizophrenia.

To diagnose schizoaffective disorder, a person needs to have primary symptoms of schizophrenia (such as delusions, hallucinations, disorganized speech, disorganized behavior) along with a period of time when he or she also has symptoms of major depression or a manic episode. Accordingly, there may be two subtypes of schizoaffective disorder:

- Depressive subtype, characterized by major depressive episodes only, and
- Bipolar subtype, characterized by manic episodes with or without depressive symptoms or depressive episodes.

Differentiating schizoaffective disorder from schizophrenia and from mood disorder can be difficult. The mood symptoms in schizoaffective disorder are more prominent, and last for a substantially longer time than those in schizophrenia. Schizoaffective disorder may be distinguished from a mood disorder by the fact that delusions or hallucinations must be present in persons with schizoaffective disorder for at least 2 weeks in the absence of prominent mood symptoms.

The diagnosis of a person with schizophrenia or mood disorder may change later to that of schizoaffective disorder, or vice versa.

The most effective treatment for schizoaffective disorder is a combination of drug treatment and psychosocial interventions. The medications include antipsychotics along with antidepressants or mood stabilizers. The newer atypical antipsychotics such as clozapine, risperidone, olanzapine, quetiapine, ziprasidone, and aripiprazole are safer than the older typical or conventional antipsychotics such as haloperidol and fluphenazine in terms of parkinsonism and tardive dyskinesia. The newer drugs may also have better effects on mood symptoms. Nonetheless, these medications do have some side effects, especially at higher doses. The side effects may include excessive sleepiness, weight gain, and sometimes diabetes. Different antipsychotic drugs have somewhat different side effect profiles. Changing from one antipsychotic to another one may help if a person with schizoaffective disorder does not respond well or develops distressing side effects with the first medication. The same principle applies to the use of antidepressants or mood stabilizers.

There has been much less research on psychosocial treatments for schizoaffective disorder than there has been in schizophrenia or depression. However, the available evidence suggests that cognitive behavior therapy, brief psychotherapy, and social skills training are likely to have a beneficial effect. Most people with schizoaffective disorder require long-term therapy with a combination of medications and psychosocial interventions in order to avoid relapses and maintain an appropriate level of functioning and quality of life.

Section 43.3

Psychosis May Be Caused by Schizophrenia

Alternative Names

Psychotic

Definition

Psychosis is a loss of contact with reality, usually including false ideas about what is taking place or who one is (delusions) and seeing or hearing things that aren't there (hallucinations).

Causes

Psychosis is a severe mental condition in which there is a loss of contact with reality. There are many possible causes:

- Alcohol and certain drugs
- Brain tumors
- Dementia (including Alzheimer disease)
- Epilepsy
- Manic depression (bipolar disorder)
- Psychotic depression
- Schizophrenia
- Stroke

Symptoms

- Abnormal displays of emotion
- Confusion
- Depression and sometimes suicidal thoughts

- Disorganized thought and speech
- Extreme excitement (mania)
- False beliefs (delusions)
- Loss of touch with reality
- Mistaken perceptions (illusions)
- Seeing, hearing, feeling, or perceiving things that are not there (hallucinations)
- Unfounded fear/suspicion

Exams and Tests

Psychological evaluation and testing are used to diagnose the cause of the psychosis.

Laboratory and x-ray testing may not be needed, but sometimes can help pinpoint the exact diagnosis. Tests may include:

- Drug screens
- MRI [magnetic resonance imaging] of the brain
- Tests for syphilis

Treatment

Treatment depends on the cause of the psychosis. Care in a hospital is often needed to ensure the patient's safety.

Antipsychotic drugs, which reduce "hearing voices" (auditory hallucinations) and delusions, and control thinking and behavior are helpful. Group or individual therapy can also be useful.

Outlook (Prognosis)

How well a person will do depends on the specific disorder. Long-term treatment can control many of the symptoms.

Possible Complications

Psychosis can prevent people from functioning normally and caring for themselves. If the condition is left untreated, people can harm themselves or others.

When to Contact a Medical Professional

Call your health care provider or mental health professional if a member of your family acts as though they have lost contact with reality. If there is any concern about safety, immediately take the person to the nearest emergency room to be checked.

Prevention

Prevention depends on the cause. For example, avoiding alcohol abuse prevents alcohol-induced psychosis.

Section 43.4

Certain Antipsychotic Medications Warrant Extra Monitoring

From "Health Risks Associated with Certain Antipsychotics Warrant Extra Monitoring," from the National Institute of Mental Health (NIMH, www.nimh.nih.gov), part of the National Institutes of Health, July 24, 2008.

Some atypical antipsychotics may be more likely than others to cause metabolic and cardiovascular side effects, according to recent analyses using data from the NIMH-funded Clinical Antipsychotic Trials of Intervention Effectiveness (CATIE). The two studies were published recently in Schizophrenia Research.

Metabolic changes that lead to weight gain or signs of insulin resistance (e.g., elevated blood glucose or increased serum triglycerides) are known side effects of several antipsychotics. In addition, people with serious mental illnesses (SMIs) like schizophrenia are at higher risk for cardiovascular disease compared to people without SMI. Such risk may be associated with antipsychotic treatment or inadequate treatment of common conditions like high blood pressure. They may also result from lifestyle factors, such as smoking or limited exercise.

Participants of CATIE were randomly assigned to treatment with one of five antipsychotics—olanzapine, risperidone, ziprasidone, quetiapine, or perphenazine. All are atypical antipsychotics except the older medication perphenazine. Results from the CATIE trial have been previously reported.

Jonathan Meyer, M.D., of the University of California, San Diego, and colleagues compared baseline data with data collected 3 months later from 281 CATIE participants. They found that the prevalence of metabolic syndrome increased the most among those on olanzapine (from 35 percent to 44 percent), even if they had preexisting metabolic problems. The prevalence of metabolic syndrome decreased for those on ziprasidone from 38 percent to 30 percent, and remained about the same for risperidone, quetiapine, and perphenazine. Those on olanzapine and quetiapine gained the most weight—waist size increased an average 0.7 inches. Waist size of those taking risperidone grew an average 0.4 inches, while those taking ziprasidone showed no change in waist size, and those taking perphenazine lost a small amount of weight on average. Olanzapine also was associated with significant increases in fasting triglycerides, which are a marker of insulin resistance and potential for developing diabetes.

Meyer and colleagues then studied changes in nonfasting triglyceride levels, which are taken when a person has more than one meal in an 8-hour time frame. These levels also may be associated with cardiovascular risk. Using data from 246 different CATIE participants who had provided nonfasting triglyceride baseline and 3-month data, they found the greatest increase in levels among those taking quetiapine and olanzapine. Among those taking ziprasidone or perphenazine, there was no change in nonfasting triglyceride levels. Levels for those taking risperidone decreased.

The researchers conclude that the need for frequent and routine monitoring of metabolic and cardiovascular factors is crucial, especially if patients are taking olanzapine and quetiapine, and if they have preexisting metabolic issues.

Part Six

Getting Help for Mental Health Disorders

Chapter 44

Finding the Right Mental Health Care for You

If you or someone you know may benefit from a counselor or mental health center, here are some questions and guidelines to help you find the right care.

Where Can I Go for Help?

Where you go for help will depend on who has the problem (an adult or child) and the nature of the problem and/or symptoms. Often, the best place to start is your local Mental Health Association. Check your Yellow Pages for a listing or calling Mental Health America. Other suggested resources:

- Your local health department's Mental Health Division. These services are state funded and are obligated to first serve individuals who meet "priority population criteria" as defined by the state Mental Health Department. There may be waiting lists and not all individuals may be eligible for services. In some jurisdictions local funding is provided for additional services.
- Other mental health organizations

- Family physician
- Clergyperson
- Family services agencies, such as Catholic Charities, Family Services, or Jewish Social Services
- Educational consultants or school counselors
- Marriage and family counselors
- Child guidance counselors
- Psychiatric hospitals accredited by the Joint Commission on Accreditation of Health Care Organizations
- Hotlines, crisis centers, and emergency rooms (call 411 for Directory Assistance)

Which Mental Health Professional Is Right for Me?

There are many types of mental health professionals. Finding the right one for you may require some research. Often it is a good idea to first describe the symptoms and/or problems to your family physician or clergy. He or she can suggest the type of mental health professional you should call.

Types of Mental Health Professionals

- **Psychiatrist:** Medical doctor with special training in the diagnosis and treatment of mental and emotional illnesses. Like other doctors, psychiatrists are qualified to prescribe medication. Qualifications: should have a state license and be board eligible or certified by the American Board of Psychiatry and Neurology.
- **Child/Adolescent Psychiatrist:** Medical doctor with special training in the diagnosis and treatment of emotional and behavioral problems in children. Child/adolescent psychiatrists are qualified to prescribe medication. Qualifications: should have a state license and be board eligible or certified by the American Board of Psychiatry and Neurology.
- **Psychologist:** Psychologist with a doctoral degree in psychology from an accredited/designated doctoral program in psychology and two years of supervised professional experience, including a year long internship from an approved internship. Trained to

make diagnoses and provide individual and group therapy. Qualifications: for some psychologists, credentialing as a health service provider in psychology.

- **Clinical Social Worker:** Counselor with a master's degree in social work from an accredited graduate program. Trained to make diagnoses and provide individual and group counseling. Qualifications: state license; may be member of the Academy of Certified Social Workers.
- **Licensed Professional Counselor:** Counselor with a master's degree in psychology, counseling, or a related field. Trained to diagnose and provide individual and group counseling. Qualifications: state license.
- **Mental Health Counselor:** Counselor with a master's degree and several years of supervised clinical work experience. Trained to diagnose and provide individual and group counseling. Qualifications: certification by the National Academy of Certified Clinical Mental Health Counselors.
- **Certified Alcohol and Drug Abuse Counselor:** Counselor with specific clinical training in alcohol and drug abuse. Trained to diagnose and provide individual and group counseling. Qualifications: state license.
- **Nurse Psychotherapist:** A registered nurse who is trained in the practice of psychiatric and mental health nursing. Trained to diagnose and provide individual and group counseling. Qualifications: certification, state license.
- **Marital and Family Therapist:** A counselor with a master's degree, with special education and training in marital and family therapy. Trained to diagnose and provide individual and group counseling. Qualifications: state license.
- **Pastoral Counselor:** Clergy with training in clinical pastoral education. Trained to diagnose and provide individual and group counseling. Qualifications: Certification from American Association of Pastoral Counselors.

You Make the Call to the Mental Health Professional . . . Now What Do You Do?

Spend a few minutes talking with him or her on the phone, ask about their approach to working with patients, their philosophy, whether or not they have a specialty or concentration (some psychologists for instance specialize in family counseling, or child counseling, while others specialize in divorce or coping with the loss of a loved one.) If you feel comfortable talking to the counselor or doctor, the next step is to make an appointment.

On your first visit, the counselor or the doctor, will want to get to know you and why you called him or her. The counselor will want to know—what you think the problem is, about your life, what you do, where you live, with whom you live. It is also common to be asked about your family and friends. This information helps the professional to assess your situation and develop a plan for treatment.

If you don't feel comfortable with the professional after the first, or even several visits, talk about your feelings at your next meeting; Don't be afraid to contact another counselor. Feeling comfortable with the professional you choose is very important to the success of your treatment.

Types of Treatment

Psychotherapy is a method of talking face-to-face with a therapist. The following are a few of the types of available therapy:

- **Behavior therapy:** Includes stress management, biofeedback, and relaxation training to change thinking patterns and behavior.
- **Psychoanalysis:** Long-term therapy meant to "uncover" unconscious motivations and early patterns to resolve issues and to become aware of how those motivations influence present actions and feelings.
- **Cognitive therapy:** Seeks to identify and correct thinking patterns that can lead to troublesome feelings and behavior.
- **Family therapy:** Includes discussion and problem-solving sessions with every member of the family.
- **Movement/art/music therapy:** These methods include the use of movement, art, or music to express emotions. Effective for persons who cannot otherwise express feelings.
- **Group therapy:** Includes a small group of people who, with the guidance of a trained therapist, discuss individual issues and help each other with problems.
- **Drug therapy:** Drugs can be beneficial to some persons with mental or emotional disorders. The patient should ask about

risk, possible side effects and interaction with certain foods, alcohol, and other medications. Medication should be taken in the prescribed dosage and at prescribed intervals and should be monitored daily.

- **Electric convulsive treatment (ECT):** Used to treat some cases of major depression, delusions, and hallucinations, or life-threatening sleep and eating disorders that can not be effectively treated with drugs and/or psychotherapy. Discuss with your physician about the risks and side effects of ECT.

How Much Will Therapy Cost?

The cost of treatment depends on many factors including: the type of treatment, the therapist's training, where treatment takes place, and your insurance coverage. The following is a description of typical treatment costs:

- **Community mental health center:** Fees are determined on a sliding scale based on personal income and medical expenses. Fees range from $5 to $50 per hour. Families covered by medical assistance pay no fee.
- **Private clinics:** Established fees range from $50 to $100. Some non-profit agencies have a sliding scale system which may qualify individuals for a lower rate. Fees for group therapy may be lower than for individual therapy.
- **Private therapist:** Fees generally range from $60 to $125 per hour. Rates for psychologists and psychiatrists are higher than rates for social workers, counselors, and psychiatric nurses.
- **Hospitalization:** Fees for inpatient care range from $400 to $550 per day and vary depending on the setting.
- **Partial hospitalization:** Typically, day treatment programs are similar to hospital care. Fees range from $95 to $175 per day.

Am I Getting the Care I Need?

As you progress through the therapeutic process, you should begin to feel gradual relief from your distress, to develop self-assurance, and have a greater ability to make decisions and increased comfort in your relationship with others. Therapy may be painful and uncomfortable at times but episodes of discomfort occur during the most successful therapy sessions. Mental health treatment should help you cope with your feelings more effectively.

If you feel you are not getting results, it may be because the treatment you are receiving is not the one best suited to your specific needs. If you feel there are problems, discuss them with your therapist. A competent therapist will be eager to discuss your reactions to therapy and respond to your feeling about the process. If you are still dissatisfied, a consultation with another therapist may help you and your therapist evaluate your work together.

What about Self-Help/Support Groups?

Self-help support groups bring together people with common experiences. Participants share experiences, provide understanding and support, and help each other find new ways to cope with problems.

There are support groups for almost any concern including alcoholism, overeating, the loss of a child, co-dependency, grandparenting, various mental illnesses, cancer, parenting, and many, many others.

Chapter 45

Choosing the Right Therapist

Why is this choice so important?

Therapy is a collaborative process, so finding the right match—someone with whom you have a sense of rapport—is critical. After you find someone, keep in mind that therapy is work and sometimes can be painful. However, it also can be rewarding and life changing.

Can a therapist share what I have said during therapy?

You can rest assured that all mental health professionals are ethically bound to keep what you say during therapy confidential. However, therapists also are bound by law to report information such as threats to blow up a building or to harm another person, for example.

What are the steps for choosing a therapist?

1. See your primary care physician to rule out a medical cause of your problems. If your thyroid is "sluggish," for example, your symptoms—such as loss of appetite and fatigue—could be mistaken for depression.

"Choosing the Right Mental Health Therapist," by the Substance Abuse and Mental Health Services Administration (SAMHSA, mentalhealth.samhsa.gov), part of the U.S. Department of Health and Human Services, April 2003. Reviewed and revised by David A. Cooke, M.D., January 10, 2009.

2. After you know your problems are not caused by a medical condition, find out what the mental health coverage is under your insurance policy or through Medicaid/Medicare.

3. Get two or three referrals before making an appointment. Specify age, sex, race, or religious background if those characteristics are important to you.

4. Call to find out about appointment availability, location, and fees. Ask the receptionist:
   - Does the mental health professional offer a sliding-scale fee based on income?
   - Does he or she accept your health insurance or Medicaid/Medicare?

5. Make sure the therapist has experience helping people whose problems are similar to yours. You may want to ask the receptionist about the therapist's expertise, education, and number of years in practice.

6. If you are satisfied with the answers, make an appointment.

7. During your first visit, describe those feelings and problems that led you to seek help. Find out:
   - what kind of therapy/treatment program he or she recommends;
   - whether it has proven effective for dealing with problems such as yours;
   - what the benefits and side effects are;
   - how much therapy the mental health professional recommends; and
   - whether he or she is willing to coordinate your care with another practitioner if you are personally interested in exploring credible alternative therapies, such as acupuncture.

8. Be sure the psychotherapist does not take a "cookie cutter" approach to your treatment—what works for one person with major depression does not necessarily work for another. Different psychotherapies and medications are tailored to meet specific needs.

9. Although the role of a therapist is not to be a friend, rapport is a critical element of successful therapy. After your initial visit, take some time to explore how you felt about the therapist.

10. If the answers to these questions and others you come up with are "yes," schedule another appointment to begin the process of working together to understand and overcome your problems. If the answers to most of these questions are "no," call another mental health professional from your referral list and schedule another appointment.

What is the difference between psychiatrists and clinical social workers?

Two kinds of therapists warrant special note: psychiatrists and clinical social workers. Psychiatrists are medical doctors and can prescribe medication. Clinical social workers are trained in client-centered advocacy and can assist you with information, referral, and direct help in dealing with local, State, or Federal government agencies. As a result, they often serve as case managers to help people "navigate the system." Clinical social workers and many other mental health professionals cannot write prescriptions. However, nurse practitioners that specialize in psychiatry and mental health can prescribe medication in most states. New Mexico allows psychologists to prescribe medications after receiving special training, but at present this is the only state with such a program.

Chapter 46

Psychotherapies and Psychosocial Treatments for Mental Health Disorders

What Are Psychosocial Treatments?

Psychosocial treatments—including certain forms of psychotherapy (often called talk therapy) and social and vocational training—are helpful in providing support, education, and guidance to people with mental illnesses and their families. Studies tell us that psychosocial treatments for mental illnesses can help consumers keep their moods more stable, stay out of the hospital, and generally function better. A licensed psychiatrist (a doctor, who can prescribe medications), psychologist, social worker, or counselor typically provides these psychosocial therapies. The therapist and a psychiatrist may work together as the psychiatrist prescribes medications and the therapist monitors the consumer's progress. The number, frequency, and type of psychotherapy sessions a consumer has should be based on his or her individual treatment needs. As with medication, it is important to follow the treatment plan for psychosocial treatments to gain the greatest benefit.

Individual Psychotherapy

Individual psychotherapy involves regularly scheduled sessions between the patient and a mental health professional such as a

---

 Reviewed by Rex Cowdry, M.D. Medical Director, NAMI (April 2001). Reviewed by David A. Cooke, M.D., January 2, 2009. Dr. Cooke is not affiliated with NAMI.

psychiatrist, psychologist, psychiatric social worker, or psychiatric nurse. The goal of this treatment is to help consumers understand why they are acting and thinking in ways that are troubling or dangerous to themselves or others so they have more control over their behaviors and can correct them.

Talk-therapy sessions may focus on a consumer's current or past problems, experiences, thoughts, feelings, or relationships. By sharing experiences with a trained, knowledgeable, and understanding person—by talking about the consumer's world with someone outside it—people with mental illnesses may gradually understand more about themselves and their problems.

Individual psychotherapy is used successfully to treat emotional, behavioral, and social problems in people with schizophrenia, bipolar disorder, attention-deficit/hyperactivity disorder, depression, eating disorders, and anxiety disorders.

Psychoeducation

Psychoeducation involves teaching people about their illness, how to treat it, and how to recognize signs of relapse so that they can get necessary treatment before their illness worsens or occurs again. Family psychoeducation includes teaching coping strategies and problem-solving skills to families (and friends) of people with mental illnesses to help them deal more effectively with their ill relative. Family psychoeducation reduces distress, confusion, and anxieties within the family, which may help the consumer recover.

Psychoeducation in combination with medication has been used successfully to treat people with schizophrenia, bipolar disorder, attention-deficit/hyperactivity disorder (ADHD), and depression as well as to help their loved ones.

Self-Help and Support Groups

Self-help and support groups for people and families dealing with mental illnesses are becoming increasingly common. Although not led by a professional therapist, these groups may be therapeutic because members give each other ongoing support. These groups also are comforting because ill people learn that others have problems similar to theirs.

Members of support groups share frustrations and successes, referrals to qualified specialists and community resources, and information about what works best when trying to recover. They also share friendship and hope for themselves, their loved ones, and others in the group.

Groups may also help families work together to advocate for needed research and treatments and for better hospital and community programs. And when consumers act as a group rather than individually, they are often more effective in the fight against stigma and more successful at drawing public attention to abuses such as discrimination.

What Are Examples of Specific Psychotherapies?

Therapists offer several different types of psychotherapy. In general no one type of therapy is necessarily "better" than another type. When deciding which therapy (or therapies) will likely be the most successful treatment option for an individual consumer, a psychotherapist considers the nature of the problem to be treated and the consumer's personality, cultural and family background, and personal experiences. Note that a psychiatrist or psychotherapist (or both) may offer each of the following therapies to an individual, family, couple, or group.

Interpersonal Therapy

Interpersonal therapy focuses on the relationships a consumer has with others. The goal of interpersonal therapy is, of course, to improve interpersonal skills. The therapist actively teaches consumers to evaluate their interactions with others and to become aware of self-isolation and difficulties getting along with, relating to, or understanding others. He or she also offers advice and helps consumers make decisions about the best way to deal with other people.

Interpersonal therapy is a relatively new psychosocial treatment used most frequently to help people with bipolar disorder, attention-deficit/hyperactivity disorder (ADHD), depression, eating disorders, and generalized anxiety disorder.

Cognitive Behavioral Therapy

Cognitive behavioral therapy (CBT) helps people learn to change inappropriate or negative thought patterns and behaviors associated with their illness. The goal is to recognize negative thoughts or mindsets (mental processes such as perceiving, remembering, reasoning, decision making, and problem solving) and replace them with positive thoughts, which will lead to more appropriate and beneficial behavior. For instance, cognitive behavioral therapy tries to replace thoughts that lead to low self-esteem ("I can't do anything right") with positive expectations ("I can do this correctly"). Combined with effective medication, CBT can successfully treat people with schizophrenia, bipolar disorder, ADHD, depression, eating disorders, generalized anxiety disorder, and panic disorder.

Exposure Therapy

A type of behavioral therapy known as exposure therapy or exposure and response prevention is very useful for treating obsessive compulsive disorder (OCD) and post-traumatic stress disorder (PTSD). During exposure therapy, a consumer is deliberately exposed to whatever triggers the obsessive thoughts or reaction to a previous traumatic experience under controlled conditions. The consumer is then taught techniques to avoid performing the compulsive rituals or to work through the trauma.

Dialectical Behavior Therapy (DBT)

Dialectical behavior therapy (DBT) was developed to treat chronically suicidal individuals, but it has evolved into a treatment for multi-disordered consumers with borderline personality disorder (BPD) as one of their diagnoses. DBT has also been adapted for behavioral disorders involving emotion dysfunction (such as substance dependence in individuals with BPD and binge eating) and for treating people with severe depression and suicidal thoughts. DBT combines the basic strategies of behavior therapy with a philosophy that focuses on the idea that opposites may really not be opposite when looked at differently.

As a comprehensive treatment, DBT:

- improves destructive behaviors,
- improves motivation to change (by modifying inhibitions and providing positive reinforcement),
- ensures that new capabilities generalize to the natural environment,
- provides a treatment environment that emphasizes what consumers and therapist are best at when working together, and
- enhances the therapist's motivation and ability to treat consumers effectively.

In standard DBT, different types of psychosocial therapy—including individual psychotherapy, group skills training, and even phone consultations—are used to help consumers.

Chapter 47

Medications for Treating Mental Health Disorders

This information is designed to help mental health patients and their families understand how and why medications can be used as part of the treatment of mental health problems.

It is important for you to be well informed about medications you may need. You should know what medications you take and the dosage, and learn everything you can about them. Many medications now come with patient package inserts, describing the medication, how it should be taken, and side effects to look for. When you go to a new doctor, always take with you a list of all of the prescribed medications (including dosage), over-the-counter medications, and vitamin, mineral, and herbal supplements you take. The list should include herbal teas and supplements such as St. John's wort, echinacea, ginkgo, ephedra, and ginseng. Almost any substance that can change behavior can cause harm if used in the wrong amount or frequency of dosing, or in a bad combination. Drugs differ in the speed, duration of action, and in their margin for error. If you are taking more than one medication, and at different times of the day, it is essential that you take the correct dosage of each medication. An easy way to make sure you do this is to use a 7-day pillbox, available in any pharmacy, and to fill the box with the proper medication at the beginning of each week. Many pharmacies also have pillboxes with sections for medications that must be taken more than once a day.

Excerpted from "Medications," by the National Institute of Mental Health (NIMH, www.nimh.nih.gov), part of the National Institutes of Health, January 2007.

This information is intended to inform you, but it is not a "do-it-yourself" manual. Leave it to the doctor, working closely with you, to diagnose mental illness, interpret signs and symptoms of the illness, prescribe and manage medication, and explain any side effects. This will help you ensure that you use medication most effectively and with minimum risk of side effects or complications.

Anyone can develop a mental illness: you, a family member, a friend, or a neighbor. Some disorders are mild; others are serious and long-lasting. These conditions can be diagnosed and treated. Most people can live better lives after treatment. And psychotherapeutic medications are an increasingly important element in the successful treatment of mental illness.

Medications for mental illnesses were first introduced in the early 1950s with the antipsychotic chlorpromazine. Other medications have followed. These medications have changed the lives of people with these disorders for the better.

Psychotherapeutic medications also may make other kinds of treatment more effective. Someone who is too depressed to talk, for instance, may have difficulty communicating during psychotherapy or counseling, but the right medication may improve symptoms so the person can respond. For many patients, a combination of psychotherapy and medication can be an effective method of treatment.

Another benefit of these medications is an increased understanding of the causes of mental illness. Scientists have learned much more about the workings of the brain as a result of their investigations into how psychotherapeutic medications relieve the symptoms of disorders such as psychosis, depression, anxiety, obsessive-compulsive disorder, and panic disorder.

Relief from Symptoms

Just as aspirin can reduce a fever without curing the infection that causes it, psychotherapeutic medications act by controlling symptoms. Psychotherapeutic medications do not cure mental illness, but in many cases, they can help a person function despite some continuing mental pain and difficulty coping with problems. For example, drugs like chlorpromazine can turn off the "voices" heard by some people with psychosis and help them to see reality more clearly. And antidepressants can lift the dark, heavy moods of depression. The degree of response ranging from a little relief of symptoms to complete relief depends on a variety of factors related to the individual and the disorder being treated.

How long someone must take a psychotherapeutic medication depends on the individual and the disorder. Many depressed and anxious people may need medication for a single period perhaps for several months and then never need it again. People with conditions such as schizophrenia or bipolar disorder (also known as manic-depressive illness), or those whose depression or anxiety is chronic or recurrent, may have to take medication indefinitely.

Like any medication, psychotherapeutic medications do not produce the same effect in everyone. Some people may respond better to one medication than another. Some may need larger dosages than others do. Some have side effects, and others do not. Age, sex, body size, body chemistry, physical illnesses and their treatments, diet, and habits such as smoking are some of the factors that can influence a medication's effect.

Questions for Your Doctor

You and your family can help your doctor find the right medications for you. The doctor needs to know your medical history, other medications being taken, and life plans such as hoping to have a baby. After taking the medication for a short time, you should tell the doctor about favorable results as well as side effects. The Food and Drug Administration (FDA) and professional organizations recommend that the patient or a family member ask the following questions when a medication is prescribed:

- What is the name of the medication, and what is it supposed to do?
- How and when do I take it, and when do I stop taking it?
- What foods, drinks, or other medications should I avoid while taking the prescribed medication?
- Should it be taken with food or on an empty stomach?
- Is it safe to drink alcohol while on this medication?
- What are the side effects, and what should I do if they occur?
- Is a Patient Package Insert for the medication available?

Medications for Mental Illness

This text describes medications by their generic (chemical) names and by their trade names (brand names used by pharmaceutical companies). They are divided into four large categories: antipsychotic, antimanic, antidepressant, and antianxiety medications. Medications that specifically affect children, the elderly, and women during the reproductive years are discussed in a separate section.

Treatment evaluation studies have established the effectiveness of the medications described here, but much remains to be learned about them. The National Institute of Mental Health, other Federal agencies, and private research groups are sponsoring studies of these medications. Scientists are hoping to improve their understanding of how and why these medications work, how to control or eliminate unwanted side effects, and how to make the medications more effective.

Antipsychotic Medications

A person who is psychotic is out of touch with reality. People with psychosis may hear "voices" or have strange and illogical ideas (for example, thinking that others can hear their thoughts, or are trying to harm them, or that they are the President of the United States or some other famous person). They may get excited or angry for no apparent reason, or spend a lot of time by themselves, or in bed, sleeping during the day and staying awake at night. The person may neglect appearance, not bathing or changing clothes, and may be hard to talk to—barely talking or saying things that make no sense. They often are initially unaware that their condition is an illness.

These kinds of behaviors are symptoms of a psychotic illness such as schizophrenia. Antipsychotic medications act against these symptoms. These medications cannot "cure" the illness, but they can take away many of the symptoms or make them milder. In some cases, they can shorten the course of an episode of the illness as well.

There are a number of antipsychotic (neuroleptic) medications available. These medications affect neurotransmitters that allow communication between nerve cells. One such neurotransmitter, dopamine, is thought to be relevant to schizophrenia symptoms. All these medications have been shown to be effective for schizophrenia. The main differences are in the potency—that is, the dosage (amount) prescribed to produce therapeutic effects and the side effects. Some people might think that the higher the dose of medication prescribed, the more serious the illness; but this is not always true.

The first antipsychotic medications were introduced in the 1950s. Antipsychotic medications have helped many patients with psychosis lead a more normal and fulfilling life by alleviating such symptoms as hallucinations, both visual and auditory, and paranoid thoughts. However, the early antipsychotic medications often have unpleasant side effects, such as muscle stiffness, tremor, and abnormal movements, leading researchers to continue their search for better drugs.

The 1990s saw the development of several new drugs for schizophrenia, called "atypical antipsychotics." Because they have fewer side effects than the older drugs, today they are often used as a first-line treatment. The first atypical antipsychotic, clozapine (Clozaril), was introduced in the United States in 1990. In clinical trials, this medication was found to be more effective than conventional or "typical" antipsychotic medications in individuals with treatment-resistant schizophrenia (schizophrenia that has not responded to other drugs), and the risk of tardive dyskinesia (a movement disorder) was lower. However, because of the potential side effect of a serious blood disorder agranulocytosis (loss of the white blood cells that fight infection) patients who are on clozapine must have a blood test every 1 or 2 weeks. The inconvenience and cost of blood tests and the medication itself have made maintenance on clozapine difficult for many people. Clozapine, however, continues to be the drug of choice for treatment-resistant schizophrenia patients.

Several other atypical antipsychotics have been developed since clozapine was introduced. The first was risperidone (Risperdal), followed by olanzapine (Zyprexa), quetiapine (Seroquel), and ziprasidone (Geodon). Each has a unique side effect profile, but in general, these medications are better tolerated than the earlier drugs.

All these medications have their place in the treatment of schizophrenia, and doctors will choose among them. They will consider the person's symptoms, age, weight, and personal and family medication history.

Dosages and side effects: Some drugs are very potent and the doctor may prescribe a low dose. Other drugs are not as potent and a higher dose may be prescribed.

Unlike some prescription drugs, which must be taken several times during the day, some antipsychotic medications can be taken just once a day. In order to reduce daytime side effects such as sleepiness, some medications can be taken at bedtime. Some antipsychotic medications are available in "depot" forms that can be injected once or twice a month.

Most side effects of antipsychotic medications are mild. Many common ones lessen or disappear after the first few weeks of treatment. These include drowsiness, rapid heartbeat, and dizziness when changing position.

Some people gain weight while taking medications and need to pay extra attention to diet and exercise to control their weight. Other side effects may include a decrease in sexual ability or interest, problems with menstrual periods, sunburn, or skin rashes. If a side effect occurs, the doctor should be told. He or she may prescribe a different medication, change the dosage or schedule, or prescribe an additional medication to control the side effects.

Just as people vary in their responses to antipsychotic medications, they also vary in how quickly they improve. Some symptoms may diminish in days; others take weeks or months. Many people see substantial improvement by the sixth week of treatment. If there is no improvement, the doctor may try a different type of medication. The doctor cannot tell beforehand which medication will work for a person. Sometimes a person must try several medications before finding one that works. If a person is feeling better or even completely well, the medication should not be stopped without talking to the doctor. It may be necessary to stay on the medication to continue feeling well.

If, after consultation with the doctor, the decision is made to discontinue the medication, it is important to continue to see the doctor while tapering off medication. Many people with bipolar disorder, for instance, require antipsychotic medication only for a limited time during a manic episode until mood-stabilizing medication takes effect. On the other hand, some people may need to take antipsychotic medication for an extended period of time. These people usually have chronic (long-term, continuous) schizophrenic disorders, or have a history of repeated schizophrenic episodes, and are likely to become ill again. Also, in some cases a person who has experienced one or two severe episodes may need medication indefinitely. In these cases, medication may be continued in as low a dosage as possible to maintain control of symptoms. This approach, called maintenance treatment, prevents relapse in many people and removes or reduces symptoms for others.

Multiple medications: Antipsychotic medications can produce unwanted effects when taken with other medications. Therefore, the doctor should be told about all medicines being taken, including over-the-counter medications and vitamin, mineral, and herbal supplements, and the extent of alcohol use. Some antipsychotic medications interfere with antihypertensive medications (taken for high blood pressure), anticonvulsants (taken for epilepsy), and medications used for Parkinson's disease. Other antipsychotics add to the effect of alcohol and other central nervous system depressants such as antihistamines, antidepressants, barbiturates, some sleeping and pain medications, and narcotics.

Other effects: Long-term treatment of schizophrenia with one of the older, or "conventional," antipsychotics may cause a person to develop tardive dyskinesia (TD). Tardive dyskinesia is a condition characterized by involuntary movements, most often around the mouth. It may range from mild to severe. In some people, it cannot be reversed, while others recover partially or completely. Tardive dyskinesia is sometimes seen in people with schizophrenia who have never been treated with an antipsychotic medication; this is called "spontaneous dyskinesia." However, it is most often seen after long-term treatment with older antipsychotic medications. The risk has been reduced with the newer "atypical" medications. There is a higher incidence in women, and the risk rises with age. The possible risks of long-term treatment with an antipsychotic medication must be weighed against the benefits in each case. The risk for TD is 5 percent per year with older medications; it is less with the newer medications.

Antimanic Medications

Bipolar disorder is characterized by cycling mood changes: severe highs (mania) and lows (depression). Episodes may be predominantly manic or depressive, with normal mood between episodes. Mood swings may follow each other very closely, within days (rapid cycling), or may be separated by months to years. The "highs" and "lows" may vary in intensity and severity and can coexist in "mixed" episodes.

When people are in a manic "high," they may be overactive, overly talkative, have a great deal of energy, and have much less need for sleep than normal. They may switch quickly from one topic to another, as if they cannot get their thoughts out fast enough. Their attention span is often short, and they can be easily distracted. Sometimes people who are "high" are irritable or angry and have false or inflated ideas about their position or importance in the world. They may be very elated, and full of grand schemes that might range from business deals to romantic sprees. Often, they show poor judgment in these ventures. Mania, untreated, may worsen to a psychotic state.

In a depressive cycle the person may have a "low" mood with difficulty concentrating; lack of energy, with slowed thinking and movements; changes in eating and sleeping patterns (usually increases of both in bipolar depression); feelings of hopelessness, helplessness, sadness, worthlessness, guilt; and, sometimes, thoughts of suicide.

Lithium: The medication used most often to treat bipolar disorder is lithium. Lithium evens out mood swings in both directions from mania to depression, and depression to mania so it is used not just for manic attacks or flare-ups of the illness but also as an ongoing maintenance treatment for bipolar disorder.

Although lithium will reduce severe manic symptoms in about 5 to 14 days, it may be weeks to several months before the condition is fully controlled. Antipsychotic medications are sometimes used in the first several days of treatment to control manic symptoms until the lithium begins to take effect. Antidepressants may also be added to lithium during the depressive phase of bipolar disorder. If given in the absence of lithium or another mood stabilizer, antidepressants may provoke a switch into mania in people with bipolar disorder.

A person may have one episode of bipolar disorder and never have another, or be free of illness for several years. But for those who have more than one manic episode, doctors usually give serious consideration to maintenance (continuing) treatment with lithium.

Some people respond well to maintenance treatment and have no further episodes. Others may have moderate mood swings that lessen as treatment continues, or have less frequent or less severe episodes. Unfortunately, some people with bipolar disorder may not be helped at all by lithium. Response to treatment with lithium varies, and it cannot be determined beforehand who will or will not respond to treatment.

Regular blood tests are an important part of treatment with lithium. If too little is taken, lithium will not be effective. If too much is taken, a variety of side effects may occur. The range between an effective dose and a toxic one is small. Blood lithium levels are checked at the beginning of treatment to determine the best lithium dosage. Once a person is stable and on a maintenance dosage, the lithium level should be checked every few months. How much lithium people need to take may vary over time, depending on how ill they are, their body chemistry, and their physical condition.

Side effects of lithium: When people first take lithium, they may experience side effects such as drowsiness, weakness, nausea, fatigue, hand tremor, or increased thirst and urination. Some may disappear or decrease quickly, although hand tremor may persist. Weight gain may also occur. Dieting will help, but crash diets should be avoided because they may raise or lower the lithium level. Drinking low-calorie or no-calorie beverages, especially water, will help keep weight down. Kidney changes, increased urination and, in children, enuresis (bed wetting) may develop during treatment. These changes are generally manageable and are reduced by lowering the dosage. Because lithium may cause the thyroid gland to become underactive (hypothyroidism) or sometimes enlarged (goiter), thyroid function monitoring is a part of the therapy. To restore normal thyroid function, thyroid hormone may be given along with lithium.

Because of possible complications, doctors either may not recommend lithium or may prescribe it with caution when a person has thyroid, kidney, or heart disorders, epilepsy, or brain damage. Women of childbearing age should be aware that lithium increases the risk of congenital malformations in babies. Special caution should be taken during the first 3 months of pregnancy.

Anything that lowers the level of sodium in the body reduced intake of table salt, a switch to a low-salt diet, heavy sweating from an unusual amount of exercise or a very hot climate, fever, vomiting, or diarrhea may cause a lithium buildup and lead to toxicity. It is important to be aware of conditions that lower sodium or cause dehydration and to tell the doctor if any of these conditions are present so the dose can be changed.

Lithium, when combined with certain other medications, can have unwanted effects. Some diuretics—substances that remove water from the body—increase the level of lithium and can cause toxicity. Other diuretics, like coffee and tea, can lower the level of lithium. Signs of lithium toxicity may include nausea, vomiting, drowsiness, mental dullness, slurred speech, blurred vision, confusion, dizziness, muscle twitching, irregular heartbeat, and, ultimately, seizures. A lithium overdose can be life-threatening. People who are taking lithium should tell every doctor who is treating them, including dentists, about all medications they are taking.

With regular monitoring, lithium is a safe and effective drug that enables many people, who otherwise would suffer from incapacitating mood swings, to lead normal lives.

Anticonvulsants: Some people with symptoms of mania who do not benefit from or would prefer to avoid lithium have been found to respond to anticonvulsant medications commonly prescribed to treat seizures.

The anticonvulsant valproic acid (Depakote, divalproex sodium) is the main alternative therapy for bipolar disorder. It is as effective in non-rapid-cycling bipolar disorder as lithium and appears to be superior to lithium in rapid-cycling bipolar disorder. Although valproic acid can cause gastrointestinal side effects, the incidence is low. Other adverse effects occasionally reported are headache, double vision, dizziness, anxiety, or confusion. Because in some cases valproic acid has caused liver dysfunction, liver function tests should be performed before therapy and at frequent intervals thereafter, particularly during the first 6 months of therapy.

Other anticonvulsants used for bipolar disorder include carbamazepine (Tegretol), lamotrigine (Lamictal), gabapentin (Neurontin), and topiramate (Topamax). The evidence for anticonvulsant effectiveness is stronger for acute mania than for long-term maintenance of bipolar disorder. Some studies suggest particular efficacy of lamotrigine in bipolar depression. At present, the lack of formal FDA [Food and Drug Administration] approval of anticonvulsants other than valproic acid for bipolar disorder may limit insurance coverage for these medications.

Most people who have bipolar disorder take more than one medication. Along with the mood stabilizer lithium and/or an anticonvulsant they may take a medication for accompanying agitation, anxiety, insomnia, or depression. It is important to continue taking the mood stabilizer when taking an antidepressant because research has shown that treatment with an antidepressant alone increases the risk that the patient will switch to mania or hypomania, or develop rapid cycling. Sometimes, when a bipolar patient is not responsive to other medications, an atypical antipsychotic medication is prescribed. Finding the best possible medication, or combination of medications, is of utmost importance to the patient and requires close monitoring by a doctor and strict adherence to the recommended treatment regimen.

Antidepressant Medications

Major depression, the kind of depression that will most likely benefit from treatment with medications, is more than just “the blues.” It is a condition that lasts 2 weeks or more, and interferes with a person’s ability to carry on daily tasks and enjoy activities that previously brought pleasure. Depression is associated with abnormal functioning of the brain. An interaction between genetic tendency and life history appears to determine a person’s chance of becoming depressed. Episodes of depression may be triggered by stress, difficult life events, side effects of medications, or medication/substance withdrawal, or even viral infections that can affect the brain.

Depressed people will seem sad, or “down,” or may be unable to enjoy their normal activities. They may have no appetite and lose weight (although some people eat more and gain weight when depressed). They may sleep too much or too little, have difficulty going to sleep, sleep restlessly, or awaken very early in the morning. They may speak of feeling guilty, worthless, or hopeless; they may lack energy or be jumpy and agitated. They may think about killing themselves and may even make a suicide attempt. Some depressed people have delusions (false, fixed ideas) about poverty, sickness, or sinfulness that are related to their depression. Often feelings of depression are worse at a particular time of day, for instance, every morning or every evening.

Not everyone who is depressed has all these symptoms, but everyone who is depressed has at least some of them, coexisting, on most days. Depression can range in intensity from mild to severe. Depression can co-occur with other medical disorders such as cancer, heart disease, stroke, Parkinson disease, Alzheimer disease, and diabetes. In such cases, the depression is often overlooked and is not treated. If the depression is recognized and treated, a person's quality of life can be greatly improved.

Antidepressants are used most often for serious depressions, but they can also be helpful for some milder depressions. Antidepressants are not "uppers" or stimulants, but rather take away or reduce the symptoms of depression and help depressed people feel the way they did before they became depressed.

The doctor chooses an antidepressant based on the individual's symptoms. Some people notice improvement in the first couple of weeks; but usually the medication must be taken regularly for at least 6 weeks and, in some cases, as many as 8 weeks before the full therapeutic effect occurs. If there is little or no change in symptoms after 6 or 8 weeks, the doctor may prescribe a different medication or add a second medication such as lithium, to augment the action of the original antidepressant. Because there is no way of knowing beforehand which medication will be effective, the doctor may have to prescribe first one and then another. To give a medication time to be effective and to prevent a relapse of the depression once the patient is responding to an antidepressant, the medication should be continued for 6 to 12 months, or in some cases longer, carefully following the doctor's instructions. When a patient and the doctor feel that medication can be discontinued, withdrawal should be discussed as to how best to taper off the medication gradually. Never discontinue medication without talking to the doctor about it. For those who have had several bouts of depression, long-term treatment with medication is the most effective means of preventing more episodes.

Dosage of antidepressants varies, depending on the type of drug and the person's body chemistry, age, and, sometimes, body weight. Traditionally, antidepressant dosages are started low and raised gradually over time until the desired effect is reached without the appearance of troublesome side effects. Newer antidepressants may be started at or near therapeutic doses.

Early antidepressants: From the 1960s through the 1980s, tricyclic antidepressants (named for their chemical structure) were the first line of treatment for major depression. Most of these medications affected two chemical neurotransmitters, norepinephrine and serotonin. Though the tricyclics are as effective in treating depression as the newer antidepressants, their side effects are usually more unpleasant; thus, today tricyclics such as imipramine, amitriptyline, nortriptyline, and desipramine are used as a second- or third-line treatment. Other antidepressants introduced during this period were monoamine oxidase inhibitors (MAOIs). MAOIs are effective for some people with major depression who do not respond to other antidepressants. They are also effective for the treatment of panic disorder and bipolar depression. MAOIs approved for the treatment of depression are phenelzine (Nardil), tranylcypromine (Parnate), and isocarboxazid (Marplan). Because substances in certain foods, beverages, and medications can cause dangerous interactions when combined with MAOIs, people on these agents must adhere to dietary restrictions. This has deterred many clinicians and patients from using these effective medications, which are in fact quite safe when used as directed.

The past decade has seen the introduction of many new antidepressants that work as well as the older ones but have fewer side effects. Some of these medications primarily affect one neurotransmitter, serotonin, and are called selective serotonin reuptake inhibitors (SSRIs). These include fluoxetine (Prozac), sertraline (Zoloft), fluvoxamine (Luvox), paroxetine (Paxil), and citalopram (Celexa).

The late 1990s ushered in new medications that, like the tricyclics, affect both norepinephrine and serotonin but have fewer side effects. These new medications include venlafaxine (Effexor) and nefazodone (Serzone).

Other newer medications chemically unrelated to the other antidepressants are the sedating mirtazapine (Remeron) and the more activating bupropion (Wellbutrin). Wellbutrin has not been associated with weight gain or sexual dysfunction but is not used for people with, or at risk for, a seizure disorder.

Each antidepressant differs in its side effects and in its effectiveness in treating an individual person, but the majority of people with depression can be treated effectively by one of these antidepressants.

Side effects of antidepressant medications: Antidepressants may cause mild, and often temporary, side effects (sometimes referred to as adverse effects) in some people. Typically, these are not serious. However, any reactions or side effects that are unusual, annoying, or that interfere with functioning should be reported to the doctor immediately. The most common side effects of tricyclic antidepressants, and ways to deal with them, are as follows:

- *Dry mouth:* It is helpful to drink sips of water; chew sugarless gum; brush teeth daily.
- *Constipation*: Bran cereals, prunes, fruit, and vegetables should be in the diet.
- *Bladder problems:* Emptying the bladder completely may be difficult, and the urine stream may not be as strong as usual. Older men with enlarged prostate conditions may be at particular risk for this problem. The doctor should be notified if there is any pain.
- *Sexual problems:* Sexual functioning may be impaired; if this is worrisome, it should be discussed with the doctor.
- *Blurred vision:* This is usually temporary and will not necessitate new glasses. Glaucoma patients should report any change in vision to the doctor.
- *Dizziness:* Rising from the bed or chair slowly is helpful.
- *Drowsiness:* As a daytime problem this usually passes soon. A person who feels drowsy or sedated should not drive or operate heavy equipment. The more sedating antidepressants are generally taken at bedtime to help sleep and to minimize daytime drowsiness.
- *Increased heart rate:* Pulse rate is often elevated. Older patients should have an electrocardiogram (EKG) before beginning tricyclic treatment.

The newer antidepressants, including SSRIs, have different types of side effects, as follows:

- *Sexual problems:* Fairly common, but reversible, in both men and women. The doctor should be consulted if the problem is persistent or worrisome.
- *Headache:* This will usually go away after a short time.

- *Nausea:* May occur after a dose, but it will disappear quickly.
- *Nervousness and insomnia (trouble falling asleep or waking often during the night):* These may occur during the first few weeks; dosage reductions or time will usually resolve them.
- *Agitation (feeling jittery):* If this happens for the first time after the drug is taken and is more than temporary, the doctor should be notified.

Any of these side effects may be amplified when an SSRI is combined with other medications that affect serotonin. In the most extreme cases, such a combination of medications (e.g., an SSRI and an MAOI) may result in a potentially serious or even fatal "serotonin syndrome," characterized by fever, confusion, muscle rigidity, and cardiac, liver, or kidney problems.

The small number of people for whom MAOIs are the best treatment need to avoid taking decongestants and consuming certain foods that contain high levels of tyramine, such as many cheeses, wines, and pickles. The interaction of tyramine with MAOIs can bring on a sharp increase in blood pressure that can lead to a stroke. The doctor should furnish a complete list of prohibited foods that the individual should carry at all times. Other forms of antidepressants require no food restrictions. MAOIs also should not be combined with other antidepressants, especially SSRIs, due to the risk of serotonin syndrome.

Medications of any kind—prescribed, over-the-counter, or herbal supplements—should never be mixed without consulting the doctor; nor should medications ever be borrowed from another person. Other health professionals who may prescribe a drug such as a dentist or other medical specialist should be told that the person is taking a specific antidepressant and the dosage. Some drugs, although safe when taken alone, can cause severe and dangerous side effects if taken with other drugs. Alcohol—(wine, beer, and hard liquor)—or street drugs may reduce the effectiveness of antidepressants and their use should be minimized or, preferably, avoided by anyone taking antidepressants. Some people who have not had a problem with alcohol use may be permitted by their doctor to use a modest amount of alcohol while taking one of the newer antidepressants. The potency of alcohol may be increased by medications since both are metabolized by the liver; one drink may feel like two.

Although not common, some people have experienced withdrawal symptoms when stopping an antidepressant too abruptly. Therefore, when discontinuing an antidepressant, gradual withdrawal is generally advisable.

Questions about any antidepressant prescribed, or problems that may be related to the medication, should be discussed with the doctor and/or the pharmacist.

Antianxiety Medications

Everyone experiences anxiety at one time or another—"butterflies in the stomach" before giving a speech or sweaty palms during a job interview are common symptoms. Other symptoms include irritability, uneasiness, jumpiness, feelings of apprehension, rapid or irregular heartbeat, stomachache, nausea, faintness, and breathing problems.

Anxiety is often manageable and mild, but sometimes it can present serious problems. A high level or prolonged state of anxiety can make the activities of daily life difficult or impossible. People may have generalized anxiety disorder (GAD) or more specific anxiety disorders such as panic, phobias, obsessive-compulsive disorder (OCD), or posttraumatic stress disorder (PTSD).

Both antidepressants and antianxiety medications are used to treat anxiety disorders. The broad-spectrum activity of most antidepressants provides effectiveness in anxiety disorders as well as depression. The first medication specifically approved for use in the treatment of OCD was the tricyclic antidepressant clomipramine (Anafranil). The SSRIs, fluoxetine (Prozac), fluvoxamine (Luvox), paroxetine (Paxil), and sertraline (Zoloft), have now been approved for use with OCD. Paroxetine has also been approved for social anxiety disorder (social phobia), GAD, and panic disorder; and sertraline is approved for panic disorder and PTSD. Venlafaxine (Effexor) has been approved for GAD.

Antianxiety medications include the benzodiazepines, which can relieve symptoms within a short time. They have relatively few side effects: drowsiness and loss of coordination are most common; fatigue and mental slowing or confusion can also occur. These effects make it dangerous for people taking benzodiazepines to drive or operate some machinery. Other side effects are rare.

Benzodiazepines vary in duration of action in different people; they may be taken two or three times a day, sometimes only once a day, or just on an "as-needed" basis. Dosage is generally started at a low level and gradually raised until symptoms are diminished or removed. The dosage will vary a great deal depending on the symptoms and the individual's body chemistry.

It is wise to abstain from alcohol when taking benzodiazepines, because the interaction between benzodiazepines and alcohol can lead to serious and possibly life-threatening complications. It is also important to tell the doctor about other medications being taken.

People taking benzodiazepines for weeks or months may develop tolerance for and dependence on these drugs. Abuse and withdrawal reactions are also possible. For these reasons, the medications are generally prescribed for brief periods of time days or weeks and sometimes just for stressful situations or anxiety attacks. However, some patients may need long-term treatment.

It is essential to talk with the doctor before discontinuing a benzodiazepine. A withdrawal reaction may occur if the treatment is stopped abruptly. Symptoms may include anxiety, shakiness, headache, dizziness, sleeplessness, loss of appetite, or in extreme cases, seizures. A withdrawal reaction may be mistaken for a return of the anxiety because many of the symptoms are similar. After a person has taken benzodiazepines for an extended period, the dosage is gradually reduced before it is stopped completely. Commonly used benzodiazepines include clonazepam (Klonopin), alprazolam (Xanax), diazepam (Valium), and lorazepam (Ativan).

The only medication specifically for anxiety disorders other than the benzodiazepines is buspirone (BuSpar). Unlike the benzodiazepines, buspirone must be taken consistently for at least 2 weeks to achieve an antianxiety effect and therefore cannot be used on an "as-needed" basis.

Beta blockers, medications often used to treat heart conditions and high blood pressure, are sometimes used to control "performance anxiety" when the individual must face a specific stressful situation a speech, a presentation in class, or an important meeting. Propranolol (Inderal, Inderide) is a commonly used beta blocker.

Chapter 48

Understanding Antidepressant Medications

Depression affects about 121 million people worldwide and is a leading cause of disability, according to the World Health Organization (WHO).

"In my experience as a practicing psychiatrist, I've seen that many people with depression don't realize that they have the condition or that it's treatable," says Mitchell Mathis, M.D., deputy director of the Division of Psychiatry Products at the Food and Drug Administration (FDA).

Some who suffer from depression don't recognize the symptoms, or they attribute them to lack of sleep or a poor diet. Others realize they are depressed, but they feel too fatigued or ashamed to seek help.

Not all depression requires treatment with medication.

"Studies have shown that the best way to treat a patient with the more severe form of major depressive disorder is through both therapy and prescribed antidepressant medication," Mathis says. "They work best in combination with one another."

Diagnosing the Disease

Medical professionals generally base a diagnosis of major depressive disorder on the presence of certain symptoms listed in the American Psychiatric Association's *Diagnostic and Statistical Manual of Mental Disorders, Fourth Edition*. Diagnosis depends on the number, severity, and duration of these symptoms:

From the U.S. Food and Drug Administration (FDA, www.fda.gov), January 9, 2009.

- depressed mood
- loss of interest or pleasure in almost all activities
- changes in appetite or weight
- disturbed sleep
- slowed or restless movements
- fatigue, loss of energy
- feelings of worthlessness or excessive guilt
- trouble in thinking, concentrating, or making decisions
- recurring thoughts of death or suicide

Types of Antidepressants

Antidepressants work to normalize naturally occurring brain chemicals called neurotransmitters—primarily serotonin, norepinephrine, and dopamine. Scientists have found that these particular chemicals are involved in regulating a person's mood.

There are several different classifications of antidepressants:

- **Selective serotonin reuptake inhibitors (SSRIs):** Examples are Prozac (fluoxetine), Celexa (citalopram), and Paxil (paroxetine).
- **Serotonin and norepinephrine reuptake inhibitors (SNRIs):** Examples are Effexor (venlafaxine) and Cymbalta (duloxetine).
- **Tricyclic antidepressants (TCAs):** Examples are Elavil (amitriptyline), Tofranil (imipramine), and Pamelor (nortriptyline).
- **Monoamine oxidase inhibitors (MAOIs):** Examples are Nardil (phenelzine) and Parnate (tranylcypromine).

There are other antidepressants that don't fall into any of these classifications and are considered unique, such as:

- Remeron (mirtazapine)
- Wellbutrin (bupropion)

The antidepressant medications in each classification affect different neurotransmitters in particular ways. For example, SSRIs increase the production of serotonin in the brain. MAOIs block monoamine oxidase, an enzyme that breaks down neurotransmitters. Blocking their breakdown means that neurotransmitters remain active in the brain. Research is ongoing to determine antidepressants' exact mechanism of action on a person's brain.

Selecting Antidepressants

So how does a physician determine which antidepressant to prescribe? Doctors typically use a patient history and a mental status exam. With this information, the doctor can evaluate symptoms, rule out medical causes of depression, and decide if the criteria are met for major depressive disorder.

"In my opinion, it's best when antidepressant medications are personalized," says Mathis. "For example, some depressed people have difficulty sleeping. So they would benefit from a more sedating antidepressant at night. Other people with depression sleep too much and would benefit from a more activating antidepressant in the morning."

It's important to communicate how you are feeling so that your physician can evaluate the medication's effectiveness.

Effectiveness of Antidepressants

Approximately 60 to 70 percent of patients respond to the first antidepressant that is prescribed or to an increased dosage of that drug, according to Mathis.

But patients must take regular doses of a prescribed antidepressant for at least 3 to 4 weeks before they are likely to experience the full therapeutic effect. And if patients start to feel better, they should not stop taking the antidepressant.

"Even if you start to feel better, you may be in between episodes," says Mathis. "Depression tends to be chronic and requires everyday treatment just like high blood pressure."

If you get used to an antidepressant and just quit it, you may experience some withdrawal symptoms such as anxiety and irritability. Worst of all, depression may recur.

Patients should continue taking an antidepressant for 6 to 12 months, or in some cases longer, according to the National Institute of Mental Health (NIMH). This gives medication time to be effective and can help prevent a relapse of the depression. Patients should carefully follow their doctor's instructions.

Mathis estimates that about 10 percent of depressions are treatment resistant and won't respond to prescribed antidepressants.

That means that 20 to 30 percent of patients may not respond to the first antidepressant that is prescribed for them. NIMH-funded research has shown that patients who did not get well after taking a first medication increased their chances of becoming symptom-free after they switched to a different medication or added another medication to their existing one.

With appropriate treatment, many people with depression experience improvement of their symptoms and return to living normal and productive lives.

Managing Side Effects

All antidepressants come with Medication Guides. These guides provide FDA-approved information for patients, families, and caregivers that could help improve monitoring of a drug's effects. Medication Guides are intended to be distributed at the pharmacy with each prescription or refill of a medication.

Many people who take antidepressants have at least one side effect. Side effects can include:

- headache;
- nausea;
- sexual problems;
- constipation.
- night sweats;
- agitation;
- dry mouth; and/or

Side effects are the most common reason people stop taking antidepressants. It's recommended that you don't stop taking your antidepressants or reduce the dosage without talking to your doctor or mental health professional first.

And there are coping strategies for the most common side effects of antidepressants. For a more complete list of side effects and suggested coping strategies, visit www.nimh.nih.gov/health/publications/medications/antidepressant-medications.shtml

Serious Risks

Suicidal thinking: In October 2004, FDA directed manufacturers to add a boxed warning to the labeling of all antidepressant medications to alert the public about the increased risk of suicidal thinking or suicide attempts by children and adolescents taking antidepressants.

A boxed warning is the most serious type of warning used on prescription drug labeling. In May 2007, FDA directed that the warning should be extended to include young adults up through age 24.

More detailed analysis by FDA of antidepressant clinical trials showed an increased risk of suicidality—suicidal thoughts or behavior. "There weren't more actual suicides, but more people under 24 were thinking or talking about it," explains Mathis. "This occurs most often within the first 30 days of an adolescent or young adult starting on an antidepressant."

Mania: When people are in a manic "high," they may be overactive, overly talkative, have a great deal of energy, and need less sleep than normal.

There are two different types of mood disorders, both of which are cyclical. One is unipolar disorder, in which the cycle is that a person feels normal and then feels depressed. The other type is bipolar disorder, in which the person's mood cycles from depressed to normal to manic.

"The doctor needs to screen patients for a bipolar history," said Mathis. If an antidepressant is prescribed to a person with bipolar disorder, it can cause mania. And the person can even become psychotic if the mania is severe.

Birth defects: In December 2005, FDA changed Paxil (paroxetine) from a pregnancy risk category of C to D. With a Category C drug, fetal risk can't be ruled out. With a Category D drug, positive evidence of fetal risk exists. FDA chooses a medicine's letter category based on what is known about the medicine when used in pregnant women and animals.

High blood pressure: It can be much more difficult for patients to take one of the MAOIs for depression because of the many dietary and medicinal restrictions that must be followed. People taking MAOIs must avoid certain foods that contain high levels of the chemical tyramine, which is found in many cheeses, wines, and pickles, and some medications including decongestants. MAOIs interact with tyramine in such a way that may cause a sharp increase in blood pressure, which could lead to a stroke or other complications.

Chapter 49

Is Hospitalization Necessary for Mental Health Disorders?

Of the 5.4 million people who sought mental health treatment in 1990, less than 7% required hospitalization. More than half of those who needed inpatient-care had schizophrenia, one of the most severe forms of mental illness. If you or someone you know may have a mental illness, the chances are that you will not need hospitalization. But, if you do, the following information will help assure you of the best care possible.

Questions to Ask

- Has the person been professionally evaluated? By whom? Do I understand the diagnosis?
- If the patient has not been evaluated, why am I seeking admission for the person? a) A doctor's recommendation? b) Need to have patient removed from family situation? Why? Because of behavioral problems? c) What are they? Because family cannot care for him or her? Why? d) What symptoms is the patient exhibiting which cause concern?

The Hospital/Treatment Center at Check-In

- Does your facility treat patients only for this specific diagnosis?
- If the patient has other health or emotional problems will he/she receive treatment for these problems also?
- Does your facility require tests when admitted? If so, what are they?
- Who will perform these tests?
- Who will evaluate the patient when he/she is admitted?
- What are the person's qualifications/title?
- Will this person continue to treat the patient?
- Will the patient be seen by this professional on a regular basis?
- When will the initial evaluation take place?

During the Patient's Stay

- When can I (or another family member) talk to the therapist or doctor?
- Will we be able to discuss treatment with the doctor or therapist? When? How often?
- When can family members visit? For how long?
- Will the patient be allowed to receive phone calls?
- Will the patient have a daily schedule of activities or treatments? If so, what activities will the patient be involved in?
- Is therapy group or private and is it part of the treatment plan?
- What clothes should the patient bring?
- How long will the patient be at the facility?
- Who makes this decision?
- Will the family be advised of changes in treatment?
- Who will make the evaluation for discharging the patient? When will this happen?

Leaving the Hospital

- Will someone advise the patient and family about adjustment concerns such as the need for further counseling or a medication schedule?
- What can we expect when the patient is discharged?
- Will he/she be on medications? Which ones?
- How will these medications help? Are they habit-forming? What are the side effects? What is the dosage?
- How long will the patient have to take this medication?
- If the patient leaves the hospital without permission how will the hospital handle this?
- If this occurs, what is the parent or family's responsibility?
- Will the patient be able to continue school work while in the hospital? Or how soon after he or she is discharged?
- If classes are offered to patients, what are they and who teaches them?
- What follow-up treatment or support group options should the family and patient consider?

Financial and Insurance Issues

Ask the treatment center and/or insurance company the following questions:

- Does the hospital accept this type of insurance? If not, what are the alternatives? If it does, what is covered?
- Can coverage be reviewed with a member of the staff?
- Are there separate charges and how much are they for physicians, therapists, or caretakers? What may these separate charges be?
- How are fees assessed?
- When will billing occur?
- If insurance only covers part of the cost, what other arrangements can be made for payments?

- Is there other assistance available? Will the facility accept partial payments or payments on a schedule?

Ask the Therapist

- What can the patient and family expect during the treatment process?
- What can be the expected reactions/behaviors of the patient?
- How should the family respond?
- How can the patient and family prepare for unexpected behavior and possible setbacks?

Chapter 50

Deep Brain Stimulation

Deep brain stimulation (DBS) was associated with a decrease in depressive symptoms in patients with treatment-resistant depression, according to results of a 6-month pilot study reported by Helen Mayberg, M.D., at the 161st Annual Meeting of the American Psychiatric Association. This novel therapeutic approach, developed by Dr. Mayberg and colleagues at the University of Toronto, was modeled after high-frequency DBS for Parkinson's disease, which has been shown to dramatically improve motor symptoms, she said. Functional imaging studies of depressed patients and antidepressant treatment effects provided the foundation for the specific brain region targeted for depressed patients.

Stimulation of Brodmann Area 25

Dr. Mayberg, Professor of Neurology and Psychiatry at Emory University in Atlanta, and colleagues at the University of Toronto selected six patients with treatment-resistant depression to undergo DBS; all had been treated unsuccessfully with at least four antidepressant medications and cognitive behavioral therapy, and five had been treated unsuccessfully with electroshock therapy. Dr. Mayberg summarized the results of the initial pilot study, which was published

---

"Deep Brain Stimulation: A Novel Therapeutic Approach for Treatment-Resistant Depression," by Andrew Wilner, M.D., *Neuropsychiatry Reviews,* July 2008.

in *Neuron* in 2005, and presented new data on an expanded patient sample with long-term follow-up.

"Our best available treatment, electroshock therapy, may get patients well temporarily but will not keep them well if they have already failed more than four medications," Dr. Mayberg commented.

It is not clear which neuroanatomic region is best suited for DBS to relieve depressive symptoms, she said. In the past, surgical approaches for depression have included subcaudate tractotomy, cingulotractotomy, anterior capsulotomy, and cingulotomy. Because previous neuroimaging studies have suggested that Brodmann area 25, the subgenual cingulate region, is consistently hyperactive in patients with depression, Dr. Mayberg and colleagues selected this area for DBS. Area 25 has many connections, including direct projections to the medial hypothalamus, dorsal raphe, periaqueductal gray, amygdala, and the nucleus accumbens.

"Area 25 appears to be a critical hub in this network and is uniquely positioned to influence behaviors affected in major depression, including stress responses, circadian regulation, motivation and drive, and emotion," said Dr. Mayberg.

The initial pilot study enrolled three men and three women (mean age, 46; mean age at onset of major depression, 29.5). Five patients had unipolar depression, and one had bipolar depression. All patients were on disability due to depression. Quadripolar electrodes were implanted stereotactically through the skull in area 25 bilaterally. Each electrode was 1.2 cm long, 1 mm wide, and had four contacts. A pulse generator was implanted in the chest wall, and the mean stimulation parameters at six months were 4 V, 60-μs pulse width, and a frequency of 130 Hz. During the 6-month study, baseline medications were not changed, and patients underwent PET [positron emission tomography] scans and neuropsychologic testing. The study has since been expanded to 20 patients with results from 1-year follow-up now in press in the *Journal of Biological Psychiatry*.

Patient Reports after DBS

Patients remained awake during the surgical procedure, related Dr. Mayberg. She reported that several patients had dramatic responses as soon as the stimulation began. One patient said, "I suddenly feel a sense of quiet, relief, lightness." This was followed 10 to 15 seconds later by an increase in interest, energy, awareness, attention, motor speed, spontaneous speech, sense of connectedness, social engagement, visual perception (colors, clarity, brightness, and details), and positive affect, and less psychomotor retardation. There were no autonomic, motor, or overt mood changes.

One patient reported, "It is as if instead of being in the Grand Canyon, you are up on a ledge, no longer in a pit. You look around, and you know it is still 80 feet to where you want to be, but you are not in a hole anymore. Now it comes down to you."

Another patient observed, "The most fundamental change that I can see is that it isn't like something has been added; no, something has been taken away. That heavy sinking vortex feeling was always there in some form or another, and now it is gone."

Neuroimaging and Neuropsychologic Testing

After 3 months of stimulation, PET scans revealed a decrease in local cerebral blood flow in area 25 and the adjacent orbital frontal cortex. Patients who were long-term responders also had cerebral blood flow decreases in the hypothalamus, anterior insula, and medial frontal cortex, as well as cerebral blood flow increases in the dorsolateral prefrontal, dorsal anterior and posterior cingulate, premotor, and parietal regions.

Neuropsychologic testing revealed significant improvements in the four responders at 6 months. The Hamilton Depression Rating Scale (HDRS) 17 score decreased from 27.3 preoperatively to 7.8 during DBS; the HDRS 24 score decreased from 35.7 preoperatively to 11.3 during DBS; the Montgomery-Asberg Depression Rating Scale score decreased from 33.8 preoperatively to 9.7 during DBS; and the Clinical Global Impressions Scale score decreased from 6.3 preoperatively to 3 during DBS.

Four subjects had normalization of early morning sleep disturbance in the first week of chronic DBS. Patients also reported increased energy, interest, and psychomotor speed. However, all patients still reported feeling "moderately depressed" for several weeks after the beginning of stimulation. Progressive improvement occurred over 4 to 6 weeks, with responders differentiated from nonresponders by 3 months. Ongoing follow-up of these patients has shown sustained response for more than 4 years.

Adverse Effects and Limitations

Two patients had wound infections related to the connector cable at the scalp or chest, and another patient had skin erosion over the hardware. All were treated with antibiotics.

Dr. Mayberg noted that the device costs $10,000 to $15,000, and hospital charges are approximately $50,000 for the procedure. Limitations of the study included the small sample size, short follow-up, and lack of sham surgery or placebo arm.

"DBS for treatment-refractory depression will have to show that it is efficacious and that people are functional and the effect is sustained, if it is to be worthwhile," she said. "The next steps in this research are to refine electrode placement and contact selection and improve our understanding of the dysfunctional neural networks in depression. We are fundamentally getting closer to learning about the core areas that are critical to mood modulation," Dr. Mayberg concluded.

Mayberg HS, Lozano AM, Voon V, et al. Deep brain stimulation for treatment-resistant depression. *Neuron.* 2005;45(5):651–660.

Chapter 51

Transcranial Magnetic Stimulation

What is rTMS?

Transcranial magnetic stimulation (TMS) is a technique for gently stimulating the brain. It utilizes a specialized electromagnet placed on the patient's scalp that generates short magnetic pulses, roughly the strength of an MRI [magnetic resonance imaging] scanner's magnetic field but much more focused. The magnetic pulses pass easily through the skull just like the MRI scanner fields do, but because they are short pulses and not a static field, they can stimulate the underlying cerebral cortex (brain). Low frequency (once per second) TMS has been shown to induce reductions in brain activation while stimulation at higher frequencies (> 5 pulses per second) has been shown to increase brain activation. It has also been shown that these changes can last for periods of time after stimulation is stopped. TMS was first developed in 1985, and has been studied significantly since 1995. [Editor's Note: rTMS stands for repetitive transcranial magnetic stimulation.]

What disorders has TMS been shown to be useful for?

TMS is currently being investigated as a potential treatment for patients with major depression, patients who experience hallucinated "voices" and a variety of other psychiatric and neurological disorders. Over 1500 patients have been studied with TMS. For patients with major depression, many, but by no means all studies have shown clinical improvement following TMS. Recent studies that have used newer technology and stronger stimulation have shown much improved results. These pilot studies have taught researchers about how to better use TMS for depression. This information is now being used in a large pivotal clinical trial which, if successful, will be used to support Food and Drug Administration (FDA) clearance of TMS thus making it available to the general public.

For patients reporting auditory hallucinations (voices), research has not been as extensive but initial results have been promising and suggest that low frequency TMS administered to parts of the brain underlying speech perception may reduce these voices.

The Food and Drug Administration has not approved TMS for any psychiatric treatment at this time. Therefore TMS is only available as a research procedure. TMS has been approved in Canada and Israel as a treatment of depression for patients who have not responded to medications and who might ordinarily be considered for a trial of electroconvulsive therapy (ECT).

What does it feel like to receive TMS?

Generally TMS produces a slight knocking or tapping sensation on the head. This is also associated with a tapping sound produced by the TMS device. When administered at some stimulation sites it can cause contraction of the muscles of the scalp and occasionally the jaw. Mild headache and transient lightheadedness may sometimes result from TMS. These symptoms usually resolve by themselves shortly after the treatment is over.

Do you need to get anesthetized for TMS?

No. TMS is an outpatient procedure and does not require anesthesia or an IV [intravenous]. It can be administered in a physician's office or clinic.

Does it hurt?

Approximately 5-10% of patients experience discomfort at the site of stimulation. In general this has not been a problem when administering TMS to patients volunteering for research studies.

How long does a treatment session last?

It depends on the research protocol, but generally each session takes about a half an hour.

How many times do you need to receive TMS?

Research protocols vary in the treatment duration, but most require at least two weeks of daily stimulation given five times per week, some require up to 6 weeks.

Are there any side-effects or risks associated with rTMS?

Yes. The main risk of TMS is inducing a seizure, though with close monitoring this complication has been very rare. No seizures have been reported in the scientific literature since safety guidelines have been implemented. For stimulation at low frequency (once per second) there have been no reports of seizures.

Insofar as the brain is directly stimulated by TMS, there is a potential risk of disturbing the brain's normal functions. However, in depression studies reported so far, no cognitive side-effects like loss of memory, negative changes in concentration and other cognitive capacities have been reported. This is in stark contrast to the well known cognitive side effects associated with electroconvulsive therapy (ECT).

Is TMS widely available to patients in the United States?

No, not at this time. Because TMS is not yet FDA [U.S. Food and Drug Administration] cleared, it is only available at a limited number of research centers in the United States.

Why are researchers evaluating TMS?

TMS has some very unique properties. It is non-invasive (does not break the skin and can be delivered in a physician's office), can easily be focused on small areas of the brain, and can change brain activity. This makes it particularly well suited for treating the brain, while minimizing side effects typical with other psychiatric treatments which affect areas of the brain and body not involved in the disorder.

Specifically for major depression, researchers understand there are a significant number of patients suffering from this disorder that are not helped by the available medications and other therapies, only receive partial benefit, or are not able to take medications at all. TMS offers hope that, if proven effective, many of these patients may be able to experience symptom relief.

Chapter 52

Electroconvulsive Therapy

What is ECT?

Electroconvulsive therapy (ECT) is a procedure in which a brief application of electric stimulus is used to produce a generalized seizure. It is not known how or why ECT works or what the electrically stimulated seizure does to the brain. In the United States during the 1940s and 50s, the treatment was administered mostly to people with severe mental illnesses. During the last few decades, researchers have been attempting to identify the effectiveness of ECT, to learn how and why it works, to understand its risks and adverse side effects, and to determine the best treatment technique. Today, ECT is administered to an estimated 100,000 people a year, primarily in general hospital psychiatric units and in psychiatric hospitals. It is generally used in treating patients with severe depression, acute mania, and certain schizophrenic syndromes. ECT is also used with some suicidal patients, who cannot wait for antidepressant medication to take effect.

How is it administered?

ECT treatment is generally administered in the morning, before breakfast. Prior to the actual treatment, the patient is given general

---

anesthesia and a muscle relaxant. Electrodes are then attached to the patient's scalp and an electric current is applied which causes a brief convulsion. Minutes later, the patient awakens confused and without memory of events surrounding the treatment. This treatment is usually repeated three times a week for approximately 1 month. The number of treatments varies from six to 12. It is often recommended that the patient maintain a regimen of medication, after the ECT treatments, to reduce the chance of relapse.

To maximize the benefits of ECT, it is crucial that the patient's illness be accurately diagnosed and that the risks and adverse side effects be weighed against those of alternative treatments. The risks and side effects involved with the use of ECT are related to the misuse of equipment, ill-trained staff, incorrect methods of administration, persistent memory loss, and transient post-treatment confusion.

Why is ECT so controversial?

After 60 years of use, ECT is still the most controversial psychiatric treatment. Much of the controversy surrounding ECT revolves around its effectiveness vs. the side effects, the objectivity of ECT experts, and the recent increase in ECT as a quick and easy solution, instead of long-term psychotherapy or hospitalization.

Because of the concern about permanent memory loss and confusion related to ECT treatment, some researchers recommend that the treatment only be used as a last resort. It is also unclear whether or not ECT is effective. In some cases, the numbers are extremely favorable, citing 80 percent improvement in severely depressed patients, after ECT. However, other studies indicate that the relapse is high, even for patients who take medication after ECT. Some researchers insist that no study proves that ECT is effective for more than 4 weeks.

During the last decade, the "typical" ECT patient has changed from low-income males under 40, to middle-income women over 65. This coincides with changing demographics: The increase in the elderly population and Medicare, and the push by insurance companies to provide fast, "medical" treatment rather than talk therapy. Unfortunately, concerns have been raised concerning inappropriate and even dangerous treatment of elderly patients with heart conditions, and the administration of ECT without proper patient consent.

Is ECT an option?

The patient and physician should discuss all options available before deciding on any treatment. If ECT is recommended, the patient should be given a complete medical examination including a history, physical, neurological examination, EKG [electrocardiogram], and laboratory test. Medications need to be noted and monitored closely, as should cardiac conditions and hypertension. The patient and family should be educated and informed about the procedure via videos, written material, discussion, and any other means available before a written consent is signed.

The procedure should be administered by trained health professionals with experience in ECT administration as well as a specifically trained and certified anesthesiologist to administer the anesthesia. The seizure initiated by the electrical stimulus varies from person to person and should be monitored carefully by the administration team. Monitoring should be done by an EEG [electroencephalogram] or "cuff" technique.

The nature of ECT, its history of abuse, unfavorable medical and media reports, and testimony from former patients all contribute to the debate surrounding its use. Research should continue, and techniques should be refined to maximize the efficacy and minimize the risks and side effects resulting from ECT.

Chapter 53

Assertive Community Treatment

What Is ACT?

ACT is a service-delivery model that provides comprehensive, locally based treatment to people with serious and persistent mental illnesses. Unlike other community-based programs, ACT is not a linkage or brokerage case-management program that connects individuals to mental health, housing, or rehabilitation agencies or services. Rather, it provides highly individualized services directly to consumers. ACT recipients receive the multidisciplinary, round-the-clock staffing of a psychiatric unit, but within the comfort of their own home and community. To have the competencies and skills to meet a client's multiple treatment, rehabilitation, and support needs, ACT team members are trained in the areas of psychiatry, social work, nursing, substance abuse, and vocational rehabilitation. The ACT team provides these necessary services 24 hours a day, seven days a week, 365 days a year.

How Did ACT Begin?

Now in its 26th year, the ACT model evolved out of work led by Arnold Marx, M.D., Leonard Stein, M.D., and Mary Ann Test, Ph.D.,

---

 The text that follows this document under the heading "*Health Reference Series* Medical Advisor's Notes and Updates" was provided to Omnigraphics, Inc. by David A. Cooke, M.D., January 2, 2009. Dr. Cooke is not affiliated with NAMI.

on an inpatient research unit of Mendota State Hospital, Madison, Wisconsin, in the late 1960s. Noting that the gains made by clients in the hospital were often lost when they moved back into the community, they hypothesized that the hospital's round-the-clock care helped alleviate clients' symptoms and that this ongoing support and treatment was just as important—if not more so—following discharge. In 1972, the researchers moved hospital-ward treatment staff into the community to test their assumption and, thus, launched ACT.

What Are the Primary Goals of ACT?

ACT strives to lessen or eliminate the debilitating symptoms of mental illness each individual client experiences and to minimize or prevent recurrent acute episodes of the illness, to meet basic needs and enhance quality of life, to improve functioning in adult social and employment roles, to enhance an individual's ability to live independently in his or her own community, and to lessen the family's burden of providing care.

What Are the Key Features of ACT?

Treatment

- psychopharmacologic treatment, including new atypical antipsychotic and antidepressant medications
- individual supportive therapy
- mobile crisis intervention
- hospitalization
- substance abuse treatment, including group therapy (for clients with a dual diagnosis of substance abuse and mental illness)

Rehabilitation

- behaviorally oriented skill teaching (supportive and cognitive-behavioral therapy), including structuring time and handling activities of daily living
- supported employment, both paid and volunteer work
- support for resuming education

Support Services

- support, education, and skill-teaching to family members
- collaboration with families and assistance to clients with children
- direct support to help clients obtain legal and advocacy services, financial support, supported housing, money-management services, and transportation

Who Benefits from the ACT Model?

The ACT model is indicated for individuals in their late teens to their elderly years who have a severe and persistent mental illness causing symptoms and impairments that produce distress and major disability in adult functioning (e.g., employment, self-care, and social and interpersonal relationships). ACT participants usually are people with schizophrenia, other psychotic disorders (e.g., schizoaffective disorder), and bipolar disorder (manic-depressive illness); those who experience significant disability from other mental illnesses and are not helped by traditional outpatient models; those who have difficulty getting to appointments on their own as in the traditional model of case management; those who have had bad experiences in the traditional system; or those who have limited understanding of their need for help.

What Is the Difference between ACT and Traditional Care?

Most individuals with severe mental illnesses who are in treatment are involved in a linkage or brokerage case-management program that connects them to services provided by multiple mental health, housing, or rehabilitation agencies or programs in the community. Under this traditional system of care, a person with a mental illness is treated by a group of individual case managers who operate in the context of a case-management program and have primary responsibility only for their own caseloads. In contrast, the ACT multidisciplinary staff work as a team. The ACT team works collaboratively to deliver the majority of treatment, rehabilitation, and support services required by each client to live in the community. A psychiatrist is a member of, not a consultant to, the team. The consumer is a client of the team, not of an individual staff member. Individuals with the most severe mental illnesses are typically not served well by the traditional outpatient model that directs patients to various services that they then must navigate on their own. ACT goes to the consumer whenever and wherever needed. The consumer is not required to adapt to or follow prescriptive rules of a treatment program.

Is There a Difference between ACT and PACT?

There is no difference between the PACT (Program of Assertive Community Treatment) model and the ACT (Assertive Community Treatment) model. Not only does NAMI use ACT and PACT interchangeably, but ACT or PACT is also known by other names across the country. For example, in Wisconsin, ACT programs are called Community Support Programs, or CSP. In Florida, ACT programs are called FACT (Florida Assertive Community Treatment); in Rhode Island and Delaware ACT programs are called Mobile Treatment Teams (MTT), while Virginia uses PACT for its assertive community treatment teams.

While the official name that a state, county, or locality uses for ACT varies widely, there is only one set of standards that NAMI sets forth for all programs of assertive community treatment.

How Do ACT Clients Compare with Those Receiving Hospital Treatment?

ACT clients spend significantly less time in hospitals and more time in independent living situations, have less time unemployed, earn more income from competitive employment, experience more positive social relationships, express greater satisfaction with life, and are less symptomatic. In one study, only 18 percent of ACT clients were hospitalized the first year compared to 89 percent of the non-ACT treatment group. For those ACT clients that were rehospitalized, stays were significantly shorter than stays of the non-ACT group. ACT clients also spend more time in the community, resulting in less burden on family. Additionally, the ACT model has shown a small economic advantage over institutional care. However, this finding does not factor in the significant societal costs of lack of access to adequate treatment (i.e., hospitalizations, suicide, unemployment, incarceration, homelessness, etc.).

How Available Are ACT Programs?

Despite the documented treatment success of ACT, only a fraction of those with the greatest needs have access to this uniquely effective program. Only six states (DE, ID, MI, RI, TX, WI) currently have statewide ACT programs. Nineteen states have at least one or more ACT pilot programs in their state. In the United States, adults with severe and persistent mental illnesses constitute one-half to one percent of the adult population. It is estimated that 20 percent to 40 percent of this group could be helped by the ACT model if it were available.

Health Reference Series *Medical Advisor's Notes and Updates*

Since the original publication of this article, the number of states with ACT programs has increased to eighteen. The availability of ACT continues to grow, although it is still far from universal.

Chapter 54

After Your Mental Health Diagnosis: Finding Information and Support

Five Basic Steps

This text describes five basic steps to help you cope with your diagnosis, make decisions, and get on with your life.

- **Step 1: Take the time you need.** Do not rush important decisions about your health. In most cases, you will have time to carefully examine your options and decide what is best for you.
- **Step 2: Get the support you need.** Look for support from family and friends, people who are going through the same thing you are, and those who have "been there." They can help you cope with your situation and make informed decisions.

  Your medical care might come from a doctor, nurse, physician assistant, or another kind of clinician or health care practitioner. To keep it simple, in this text we use the term "doctor" to refer to any of these professionals with whom you might interact.
- **Step 3: Talk with your doctor.** Good communication with your doctor can help you feel more satisfied with the care you receive. Research shows it can even have a positive effect on

---

Excerpted from "Next Steps After Your Diagnosis: Finding Information and Support," a booklet from the Agency for Healthcare Research and Quality (AHRQ, www.ahrq.gov), July 2005.

things such as symptoms and pain. Getting a "second opinion" may help you feel more confident about your care.

- **Step 4: Seek out information.** When learning about your health problem and its treatment, look for information that is based on a careful review of the latest scientific findings published in medical journals.
- **Step 5: Decide on a treatment plan.** Work with your doctor to decide on a treatment plan that best meets your needs.

As you take each step, remember this: Research shows that patients who are more involved in their health care tend to get better results and be more satisfied.

Step 1: Take the Time You Need

A diagnosis can change your life in an instant. Like so many other people in your situation, you might be feeling one or more of the following emotions after getting your diagnosis:

- Afraid
- Alone
- Angry
- Anxious
- Ashamed
- Confused
- Depressed
- Helpless
- In denial
- Numb
- Overwhelmed
- Panicky
- Powerless
- Relieved (that you finally know what's wrong)
- Sad
- Shocked
- Stressed

It is perfectly normal to have these feelings. It is also normal, and very common, to have trouble taking in and understanding information after you receive the news—especially if the diagnosis was a surprise. And it can be even harder to make decisions about treating or managing your disease or condition.

Take time to make your decisions. No matter how the news of your diagnosis has affected you, do not rush into a decision. In most cases, you do not need to take action right away. Ask your doctor how much time you can safely take.

Taking the time you need to make decisions can help you:

- feel less anxious and stressed;
- avoid depression;
- cope with your condition;
- feel more in control of your situation; and
- play a key role in decisions about your treatment.

Step 2: Get the Support You Need

You do not have to go through it alone. Sometimes the emotional side of illness can be just as hard to deal with as the physical side. You may have fears or concerns. You may feel overwhelmed. No matter what your situation, having other people to turn to will help you know you are not alone.

Here are the kinds of support you might want to seek.

Family and friends: Talking to family and friends you feel close to can help you cope with your illness or condition. Just knowing that someone is there can be a comfort.

Sometimes it is hard to ask for help. And sometimes your family and friends want to help, but they do not want to intrude, or they do not know how to ask or what to offer. Think about specific ways people can help you. One idea is to ask someone to come with you to a doctor's appointment to help ask questions, take notes, and talk with you afterward.

If you do not have family or friends who can provide support, other people or groups can.

Support or self-help groups: Support groups are made up of people with the same disease or condition who get together to share information and concerns and to help one another.

Support groups may or may not be led by experts. Self-help groups are similar to support groups but usually are led by the participants. The names "support group" and "self-help group" sometimes are used to refer to either kind.

Research on support groups shows that participants feel less anxious, experience less depression, have a better quality of life, and have more success coping with their disease or condition. Similar findings have been reported for self-help groups.

Online support or self-help groups: The internet has support or self-help groups for people whose concerns and situations may be similar to yours. You can also find "message boards," where you can post questions and get answers. These online communities can help you connect with people who can give you support and provide information.

But be careful. Not every idea or treatment you come across in these groups will be scientifically proven to be safe and effective. If you read about something interesting and new, check it out with your doctor.

Counselor or therapist: A good counselor or therapist can help you cope with sadness, depression, and feelings of being overwhelmed. If you think this kind of help might be right for you, ask your doctor or other health care professional to recommend someone in your area.

People like you: You might want to meet and talk with someone in your own situation. Someone who has "been there" can talk about the real-life outcomes of their treatment choices as well as how they have learned to live with their disease or condition. Some advocacy or support groups can help you make this kind of contact.

Step 3: Talk with Your Doctor

Your doctor is your partner in health care. You probably have many questions about your disease or condition. The first person to ask is your doctor.

It is fine to seek more information from other sources; in fact, it is important to do so. But consider your doctor your partner in health care—someone who can discuss your situation with you, explain your options, and help you make decisions that are right for you.

It is not always easy to feel comfortable around doctors. But research has shown that good communication with your doctor can actually be good for your health. It can help you to:

- feel more satisfied with the care you receive; and
- have better outcomes (end results), such as reduced pain and better recovery from symptoms.

Being an active member of your health care team also helps to reduce your chances of medical mistakes, and it helps you get high-quality care.

Of course, good communication is a two-way street. Here are some ways to help make the most of the time you spend with your doctor.

Prepare for your visit:

- Think about what you want to get out of your appointment. Write down all your questions and concerns.
- Prepare and bring to your doctor visit a list of all the medicines you take.
- Consider bringing along a trusted relative or friend. This person can help ask questions, take notes, and help you remember and understand everything once you leave the doctor's office.

Give information to your doctor:

- Do not wait to be asked.
- Tell your doctor everything he or she needs to know about your health—even the things that might make you feel embarrassed or uncomfortable.
- Tell your doctor how you are feeling—both physically and emotionally.
- Tell your doctor if you are feeling depressed or overwhelmed.

Get information from your doctor:

- Ask questions about anything that concerns you. Keep asking until you understand the answers. If you do not, your doctor may think you understand everything that is said.
- Ask your doctor to draw pictures if that will help you understand something.
- Take notes.
- Tape record your doctor visit, if that will be helpful to you. But first ask your doctor if this is okay.
- Ask your doctor to recommend resources such as websites, booklets, or tapes with more information about your disease or condition.

Do not hesitate to seek a second opinion:

- A second opinion is when another doctor examines your medical records and gives his or her views about your condition and how it should be treated.

- You might want a second opinion to:
  - be clear about what you have;
  - know all of your treatment choices; and
  - have another doctor look at your choices with you.

It is not pushy or rude to want a second opinion. Most doctors will understand that you need more information before making important decisions about your health.

Check to see whether your health plan covers a second opinion. In some cases, health plans require second opinions.

Here are some ways to find a doctor for a second opinion:

- Ask your doctor. Request someone who does not work in the same office, because doctors who work together tend to share similar views.
- Contact your health plan or your local hospital, medical society, or medical school.
- Use the Doctor Finder online service of the American Medical Association at www.ama-assn.org.

Get information about next steps:

- Get the results of any tests or procedures. Discuss the meaning of these results with your doctor.
- Make sure you understand what will happen if you need surgery.
- Talk with your doctor about which hospital is best for your health care needs.

Finally, if you are not satisfied with your doctor, you can do two things: (1) talk with your doctor and try to work things out, and/or (2) switch doctors, if you are able to. It is very important to feel confident about your care.

Ten important questions to ask your doctor after a diagnosis: These 10 basic questions can help you understand your disease or condition, how it might be treated, and what you need to know and do before making treatment decisions.

1. What is the technical name of my disease or condition, and what does it mean in plain English?

2. What is my prognosis (outlook for the future)?
3. How soon do I need to make a decision about treatment?
4. Will I need any additional tests, and if so what kind and when?
5. What are my treatment options?
6. What are the pros and cons of my treatment options?
7. Is there a clinical trial (research study) that is right for me?
8. Now that I have this diagnosis, what changes will I need to make in my daily life?
9. What organizations do you recommend for support and information?
10. What resources (booklets, websites, audiotapes, videos, DVDs, etc.) do you recommend for further information?

Step 4: Seek out Information

Now that you know your treatment options, you can learn which ones are backed up by the best scientific evidence. "Evidence-based" information—that is, information that is based on a careful review of the latest scientific findings in medical journals—can help you make decisions about the best possible treatments for you.

Evidence-based information comes from research on people like you. Evidence-based information about treatments generally comes from two major types of scientific studies:

- Clinical trials are research studies on human volunteers to test new drugs or other treatments. Participants are randomly assigned to different treatment groups. Some get the research treatment, and others get a standard treatment or may be given a placebo (a medicine that has no effect), or no treatment. The results are compared to learn whether the new treatment is safe and effective.

- Outcomes research looks at the impact of treatments and other health care on health outcomes (end results) for patients and populations. End results include effects that people care about, such as changes in their quality of life.

Step 5: Decide on a Treatment Plan

At this point, you have learned about your disease or condition and how it can be treated or managed. Your information may have come from the following sources:

- your doctor;
- second opinions from one or more other doctors;
- other people who are or were in the same situation as you; and
- information sources such as websites, health or medical libraries, and nonprofit groups.

Work with your doctor to make decisions. When you are ready to make treatment decisions, you and your doctor can discuss:

- which treatments have been found to work well, or not work well, for your particular condition; and
- the pros and cons of each treatment option.

Make sure that your doctor knows your preferences and feelings about the different treatments—for example, whether you prefer medicine over surgery.

Once you and your doctor decide on one or more treatments that are right for you, you can work together to develop a treatment plan. This plan will include everything that will be done to treat or manage your disease or condition—including what you need to do to make the plan work.

Remember, being an active member of your health care team helps to reduce your chances of medical mistakes, and it helps you get high-quality care.

Take another deep breath. You have taken important steps to cope with your diagnosis, make decisions, and get on with your life. Remember two things:

- Call on others for support as you need it.
- Make use of evidence-based information for any future health decisions.

Chapter 55

How Spirituality Can Help Mental Health Problems

Spirituality—an abiding belief or interest in the metaphysical—can be an important tool in the effort to achieve recovery. In a 2001 *International Review of Psychiatry* study, researchers found that spirituality helped residents of a mental health facility cope with stressful situations while providing needed emotional support and enhancing their sense of well-being. In a study published in 1995 in the *Psychosocial Rehabilitation Journal*, 83 percent of those surveyed who were receiving treatment for mental illnesses said that spiritual beliefs offered comfort and feelings of being cared for, and helped them feel less alone. And at the first National Summit of Mental Health Consumers and Survivors—organized in 1999 by the National Mental Health Consumers' Self-Help Clearinghouse to develop consensus around the issues of greatest concern to people with psychiatric histories and to create action plans—participants identified spirituality as one of the values most important to recovery. At the same time, some researchers have found that spirituality may at times be "pathologic" in people with severe mental illnesses.

Recovery and Spirituality

The Reverend Bob Dell became acutely aware of mental illness when his brother-in-law committed suicide in 1958. "Figuratively

---

"Focus on Spirituality," © 2008 National Mental Health Consumers' Self-Help Clearinghouse (www.mhselfhelp.org). Reprinted with permission.

speaking, that was the Dark Ages in terms of what we knew about treatment for depression—well before the advent of psychotropic medications. But when we're talking about a person as a whole, we have to look at mind, body and spirit," he says. He saw an opportunity for the church to help, and that experience now inspires his work as chair and acting executive director of Pathways to Promise, based in St. Louis, Missouri. Pathways to Promise is the education and publication arm of a national cooperative of faith groups that build connections between mental health treatment and spirituality.

Organizations and individuals representing a broad spectrum of faiths are recognizing the nexus between spirituality and recovery, offering resources for people with mental illnesses and improving awareness about mental illness in faith communities. For example, NAMI [National Alliance on Mental Illness] FaithNet facilitates support within religious communities for people with mental illnesses through education, advocacy, and outreach activities. Craig Rennebohm, a Universal Church of Christ minister who has struggled with serious depression, founded the Seattle-based Mental Health Chaplaincy in 1987, offering community outreach, companionship, and training.

In San Diego, Methodist minister Susan Gregg-Schroeder directs the Mental Health Ministries, which she founded after enduring her own bout with depression and anxiety in the early years of her ministry. "At that time I was suicidal and I was admitted to the hospital. That began a very long, humbling journey, and over time I started to speak out about my experience," she recalls. Gregg-Schroeder wrote a book about her personal experience; she also started consulting as well as creating workshops and multimedia resources that address the role of spirituality in recovery and work to erase stigma and discrimination.

How Spirituality Can Help

Spiritual leaders who work with people with mental illnesses agree that a person need not have a deep religious faith or even a strong spiritual orientation in order to gain the benefits that spirituality can bring to the recovery process. "Faith is a subjective judgment," Dell says. "We're all on a spiritual journey and we don't raise a bar that a person has to be on a certain part of that journey. We would walk with that person from whatever point they start at."

Indeed, acceptance within faith communities is one of the benefits of increasing involvement in a spiritual life. A chaplain or fellow congregants can help create connections and engender trust. "It's the role of the chaplain and the community of faith to attend to spiritual issues that arise in the course of mental illness," Rennebohm writes. "It's our responsibility to affirm God's love, ever active in the face of illness, and provide a full range of resources to support healing: medical, psychological, social, and spiritual." Rennebohm has established a "companionship" model for healing. He first helps someone acknowledge and understand the symptoms of her illness. He then helps her find practical treatment and support—a healthcare clinic, a shelter for the night—before helping to engage her in spiritual healing and, finally, to come to some acceptance of the illness.

A Supplement to Treatment

As community organizations with strong networks, churches, synagogues, mosques, and temples can provide an important supplement to more traditional treatment. "The current medical model allows very little to no room for incorporating a person's spirituality. Faith communities can do things in partnership with community-based groups—they can provide more holistic treatment, they can provide interfaith shelters—all kinds of things that are needed," Gregg-Schroeder says. Belief in recovery is also a critical component of the recovery process, whether it manifests itself in daily thought, prayer practice, the reading of sacred texts, observing ceremonies, or attending services. "Hope is what sustains people, and it is an important factor in recovery," she says.

Hope and deep spirituality helped Gregg-Schroeder in her own recovery. "For me, having depression was a journey of self-discovery. I learned more about myself and I was transformed by the experience. As painful as it is, it forces you to go inward and downward. It's about care more than a magic cure."

Limits of Spirituality

Yet even as some research has established that spirituality can play an important and therapeutic role in recovery, there is still much resistance from both the religious and medical establishments to the idea of addressing mental health issues within a spiritual context. "If you read the anecdotal evidence, there has been lots of support from religious organizations, which is good news," Dell says. "On the other hand, there is still much work to be done, places where we still have stigma against mental illness—and that's a tragedy."

Part of the problem is that religions often treat illness, both physical and mental, as a moral or spiritual failing. (And, as Rennebohm points out in his book *Souls in the Hands of a Tender God,* many pastors will visit the bedside of a person who has suffered a heart attack before they will even acknowledge a person grappling with schizophrenia.) There is a notion in some religious communities that prayer can heal all and that the existence of illness is evidence of a person's lack of devotion. Such blaming attitudes can be self-destructive for a person with mental illness, who may already suffer from feelings of guilt, doubt, and low self-esteem.

A 2004 paper in *Swiss Medical Weekly* acknowledges that religion may become part of the problem as well as part of the recovery: "Some patients are helped by their faith community, uplifted by spiritual activities, comforted, and strengthened by their beliefs. Other patients are rejected by their faith community, burdened by spiritual activities, disappointed, and demoralized by their beliefs."

Susan Gregg-Schroeder relates that, during her own mental health crisis, she wrestled with the possibility of bias and discrimination against people with mental illnesses in the church. "I was deeply afraid of losing my job," she says. "The stigma is strong in faith communities. What happens is, people tend to just drop off, they stop coming to church. Families struggle in silence. You hear horror stories of what people have gone through—some have been kicked out of their churches." Individuals who find themselves rejected from their faith community risk greater isolation, and in some cases the experience can exacerbate the symptoms of their illness.

Ignorance can be a significant barrier. Because mental illness is largely viewed as a medical issue, clergy often don't feel equipped to provide care and counsel to people with mental illness. "Clergy have shown themselves to be the least effective in making appropriate referrals, partly because we did not receive education in seminary," Gregg-Schroeder says. "In my own case, I didn't know what was happening to me. But studies have shown that a person will often go to their faith leader first before a mental health professional."

Similarly, there is some skepticism—which, according to some research, may be well-founded—in the mental health treatment community about spirituality and religion. A 2007 study in the *American Journal of Psychiatry* found that while the majority of surveyed psychiatrists recognized the positive impact that spirituality could have on health, psychiatrists were more likely than other doctors to recognize that religion or spirituality could also be a "pathologic" element and cause emotional suffering for individuals in treatment. For example, a 2002 study published in *Social Psychiatry and Psychiatric Epidemiology* concluded that people with schizophrenia commonly experience religious delusions, and that those who did have such delusions seemed to be more severely ill and functioned less well than a control group of people who also had schizophrenia but did not experience such delusions. In addition, studies have found that religious delusions may lead some individuals to commit acts of violence.

Some practitioners view spiritual matters as highly personal and don't want to intrude on their patients' personal lives by "prescribing" prayer. "You rarely see matters of faith brought into the medical model, though we are now seeing some medical professionals starting to conduct spiritual assessments and acknowledge that it can be a key support for people," Gregg- Schroeder says.

Working toward Recovery in a Faith Community

While there are many programs for people with mental illnesses within faith communities, some congregations and faith-based organizations don't offer recovery-focused resources. Mental health consumers who are already active in a faith community can take an active role in making their community more healing for people with mental illnesses. One way is by serving as an advocate: Being honest and candid about mental illness can help break down barriers among people who are simply uninformed. "Speaking out about mental illness can help to erase the stigma. After I shared my story, it was just amazing how many other people opened up. No one, clergy or anyone else, is immune to having depression or mental illness," Gregg-Schroeder says.

Other ways to create awareness about the issue are scheduling a speaker, establishing a counseling program or creating a religious study group focused on mental health issues. Individual congregations can reach out to members with mental illnesses by offering transportation to services, volunteer or employment opportunities, wellness resources, logistical and financial assistance, and regular companionship.

Resources

- Episcopal Mental Illness Network, www.eminnews.com
- *Faith and Mental Health: Religious Resources for Healing,* by Harold G. Koenig (Templeton Foundation Press, 2005)
- The Jewish Association for the Mentally Ill, www.jamiuk.org
- *Mental Health and Hindu Psychology,* by Swami Akhilananda (Munshiram Manoharlal Publishers, 2005)

- The Mental Health Chaplaincy, www.mentalhealthchaplain.org
- Mental Health Ministries, www.mentalhealthministries.net
- *Mindfulness and Mental Health,* by Chris Mace (Routledge, 2007)
- Muslim Mental Health, www.muslimmentalhealth.com
- NAMI FaithNet, www.nami.org/faithnet
- National Catholic Partnership on Disability, www.ncpd.org
- Pathways to Promise, www.pathways2promise.org
- Presbyterian Serious Mental Illness Network, www.pcusa.org/phewa/psmin.htm
- *Souls in the Hands of a Tender God,* by Craig Rennebohm, (Beacon, 2008)
- United Church of Christ Mental Illness Network, www.min-ucc.org
- Virginia Interfaith Committee on Mental Illness Ministries, www.vaumc.org/gm/micom.htm

Chapter 56

Alternative Approaches to Mental Health Care

What Are Alternative Approaches to Mental Health Care?

An alternative approach to mental health care is one that emphasizes the interrelationship between mind, body, and spirit. Although some alternative approaches have a long history, many remain controversial. Most of these therapies have not been studied scientifically, and claims for their effectiveness are often based on individual testimonials and word-of-mouth. It is crucial, however, to consult with your health care providers about the approaches you are using to achieve mental wellness. Although many of these therapies are likely to be harmless at worst, it is important to ensure they do not interfere with other forms of treatment you may be receiving. For example, some herbal remedies can cause life-threatening reactions if combined with some prescription medications.

Self-Help

Many people with mental illnesses find that self-help groups are an invaluable resource for recovery and for empowerment. Self-help generally refers to groups or meetings that:

Excerpted from "Alternative Approaches to Mental Health Care," from the Substance Abuse and Mental Health Services Administration (SAMHSA, mentalhealth.samhsa.gov), part of the U.S. Department of Health and Human Services, April 2003. Reviewed and revised by David A. Cooke, M.D., January 25, 2009.

- involve people who have similar needs;
- are facilitated by a consumer, survivor, or other layperson;
- assist people to deal with a "life-disrupting" event, such as a death, abuse, serious accident, addiction, or diagnosis of a physical, emotional, or mental disability, for oneself or a relative;
- are operated on an informal, free-of-charge, and nonprofit basis;
- provide support and education; and
- are voluntary, anonymous, and confidential.

Diet and Nutrition

Adjusting both diet and nutrition may help some people with mental illnesses manage their symptoms and promote recovery. For example, some practitioners claim that eliminating milk and wheat products can reduce the severity of symptoms for some people who have schizophrenia and some children with autism. Similarly, some holistic/natural physicians use herbal treatments, B-complex vitamins, riboflavin, magnesium, and thiamine to treat anxiety, autism, depression, drug-induced psychoses, and hyperactivity.

Pastoral Counseling

Some people prefer to seek help for mental health problems from their pastor, rabbi, or priest, rather than from therapists who are not affiliated with a religious community. Counselors working within traditional faith communities increasingly are recognizing the need to incorporate psychotherapy and/or medication, along with prayer and spirituality, to effectively help some people with mental disorders.

Animal Assisted Therapies

Working with an animal (or animals) under the guidance of a health care professional may benefit some people with mental illness by facilitating positive changes, such as increased empathy and enhanced socialization skills. Animals can be used as part of group therapy programs to encourage communication and increase the ability to focus. Developing self-esteem and reducing loneliness and anxiety are just some potential benefits of individual-animal therapy.

Expressive Therapies

Art therapy: Drawing, painting, and sculpting help many people to reconcile inner conflicts, release deeply repressed emotions, and foster self-awareness, as well as personal growth. Some mental health providers use art therapy as both a diagnostic tool and as a way to help treat disorders such as depression, abuse-related trauma, and schizophrenia. You may be able to find a therapist in your area who has received special training and certification in art therapy.

Dance/movement therapy: Some people find that their spirits soar when they let their feet fly. Others—particularly those who prefer more structure or who feel they have "two left feet"—gain the same sense of release and inner peace from the Eastern martial arts, such as Aikido and Tai Chi. Those who are recovering from physical, sexual, or emotional abuse may find these techniques especially helpful for gaining a sense of ease with their own bodies. The underlying premise to dance/movement therapy is that it can help a person integrate the emotional, physical, and cognitive facets of "self."

Music/sound therapy: It is no coincidence that many people turn on soothing music to relax or snazzy tunes to help feel upbeat. Research suggests that music stimulates the body's natural "feel good" chemicals (opiates and endorphins). This stimulation results in improved blood flow, blood pressure, pulse rate, breathing, and posture changes. Music or sound therapy has been used to treat disorders such as stress, grief, depression, schizophrenia, and autism in children, and to diagnose mental health needs.

Culturally Based Healing Arts

Traditional Oriental medicine (such as acupuncture, shiatsu, and Reiki), Indian systems of health care (such as Ayurveda and yoga), and Native American healing practices (such as the Sweat Lodge and Talking Circles) all incorporate the beliefs that:

- wellness is a state of balance between the spiritual, physical, and mental/emotional "selves";
- an imbalance of forces within the body is the cause of illness; and
- herbal/natural remedies, combined with sound nutrition, exercise, and meditation/prayer, will correct this imbalance.

Acupuncture: The Chinese practice of inserting needles into the body at specific points manipulates the body's flow of energy to balance the endocrine system. This manipulation regulates functions such as heart rate, body temperature, and respiration, as well as sleep patterns and emotional changes. Acupuncture has been used in clinics to assist people with substance abuse disorders through detoxification; to relieve stress and anxiety; to treat attention deficit and hyperactivity disorder in children; to reduce symptoms of depression; and to help people with physical ailments.

Ayurveda: Ayurvedic medicine is described as "knowledge of how to live." It incorporates an individualized regimen—such as diet, meditation, herbal preparations, or other techniques—to treat a variety of conditions, including depression, to facilitate lifestyle changes, and to teach people how to release stress and tension through yoga or transcendental meditation.

Yoga/meditation: Practitioners of this ancient Indian system of health care use breathing exercises, posture, stretches, and meditation to balance the body's energy centers. Yoga is used in combination with other treatment for depression, anxiety, and stress-related disorders.

Native American traditional practices: Ceremonial dances, chants, and cleansing rituals are part of Indian Health Service programs to heal depression, stress, trauma (including those related to physical and sexual abuse), and substance abuse.

Cuentos: Based on folktales, this form of therapy originated in Puerto Rico. The stories used contain healing themes and models of behavior such as self-transformation and endurance through adversity. Cuentos is used primarily to help Hispanic children recover from depression and other mental health problems related to leaving one's homeland and living in a foreign culture.

Relaxation and Stress Reduction Techniques

Biofeedback: Learning to control muscle tension and "involuntary" body functioning, such as heart rate and skin temperature, can be a path to mastering one's fears. It is used in combination with, or as an alternative to, medication to treat disorders such as anxiety, panic, and phobias. For example, a person can learn to "retrain" his or her breathing habits in stressful situations to induce relaxation and decrease hyperventilation. Some preliminary research indicates it may offer an additional tool for treating schizophrenia and depression.

Guided imagery or visualization: This process involves going into a state of deep relaxation and creating a mental image of recovery and wellness. Physicians, nurses, and mental health providers occasionally use this approach to treat alcohol and drug addictions, depression, panic disorders, phobias, and stress.

Massage therapy: The underlying principle of this approach is that rubbing, kneading, brushing, and tapping a person's muscles can help release tension and pent-up emotions. It has been used to treat trauma-related depression and stress. A highly unregulated industry, certification for massage therapy varies widely from state to state. Some states have strict guidelines, while others have none.

Technology-Based Applications

The boom in electronic tools at home and in the office makes access to mental health information just a telephone call or a "mouse click" away. Technology is also making treatment more widely available in once-isolated areas.

Telemedicine: Plugging into video and computer technology is a relatively new innovation in health care. It allows both consumers and providers in remote or rural areas to gain access to mental health or specialty expertise. Telemedicine can enable consulting providers to speak to and observe patients directly. It also can be used in education and training programs for generalist clinicians.

Telephone counseling: Active listening skills are a hallmark of telephone counselors. These also provide information and referral to interested callers. For many people telephone counseling often is a first step to receiving in-depth mental health care. Research shows that such counseling from specially trained mental health providers reaches many people who otherwise might not get the help they need. Before calling, be sure to check the telephone number for service fees; a 900 area code means you will be billed for the call, an 800 or 888 area code means the call is toll-free.

Electronic communications: Technologies such as the internet, bulletin boards, and electronic mail lists provide access directly to consumers and the public on a wide range of information. Online consumer groups can exchange information, experiences, and views on mental health, treatment systems, alternative medicine, and other related topics.

Radio psychiatry: Another relative newcomer to therapy, radio psychiatry was first introduced in the United States in 1976. Radio psychiatrists and psychologists provide advice, information, and referrals in response to a variety of mental health questions from callers. The American Psychiatric Association and the American Psychological Association have issued ethical guidelines for the role of psychiatrists and psychologists on radio shows.

This text does not cover every alternative approach to mental health. A range of other alternative approaches—psychodrama, hypnotherapy, recreational, and Outward Bound-type nature programs—offer opportunities to explore mental wellness. Before jumping into any alternative therapy, learn as much as you can about it. In addition to talking with your health care practitioner, you may want to visit your local library, book store, health food store, or holistic health care clinic for more information. Also, before receiving services, check to be sure the provider is properly certified by an appropriate accrediting agency.

Chapter 57

Dietary Supplements Used to Improve Mental Health Disorders

Chapter Contents

Section 57.1

Omega-3 Fatty Acids and Mental Health

Excerpted from "Effects of Omega-3 Fatty Acids on Mental Health Summary of Evidence Report/Technology Assessment, No. 116," by the Agency for Healthcare Research and Quality (AHRQ, www.ahrq.gov), July 2005. For the full report and references, see www.ahrq.gov.

Introduction

The purpose of this study was to conduct a systematic review of the scientific-medical literature to identify, appraise, and synthesize the human evidence for the effects of omega-3 fatty acids on mental health.

The mechanism by which diet may affect health, including depression or cardiovascular disease, has been thought to involve low levels of omega-3 fatty acid content in biomarkers (e.g., red blood cells [RBCs]). An omega-3 fatty acid deficiency hypothesis of depression has been put forward, which has helped justify treatment with omega-3 fatty acid supplementation. The membrane phospholipid hypothesis of schizophrenia has been proposed in an attempt to develop a model explaining its etiology. It describes the presumed biochemical dynamics underpinning a neurodevelopmental theory. Some of the evidence used to support this perspective suggests the existence of phospholipid and PUFA metabolic abnormalities in schizophrenia. It has been posited that modifications to diet could mitigate or even aggravate an underlying abnormality of phospholipid metabolism.

However, the present review was not conducted to test these hypotheses. Rather, the rationale for this 2-year project investigating the possible health benefits of omega-3 fatty acids was to systematically review the evidence to aid in the development of a research agenda. Nevertheless, these emerging models regarding depression and schizophrenia do suggest plausible bases for the use of omega-3 fatty acids to treat or prevent these psychiatric disorders.

Results

Inconsistent results, in addition to too few studies exhibiting sound methodologies or research designs that are ideally suited to investigate this question (e.g., prospective, controlled, with subject-level data), suggest that it is too early to conclude whether or not the intake of omega-3 fatty acids protects against the onset of depressive disorders or symptomatology.

The same issues prevent us from concluding whether or not the intake of omega-3 fatty acids protects against the onset of suicidal ideation or behavior. Given the inability of any cross-national ecological analysis to provide meaningful subject-level data, and the failure to control for key confounders (i.e., socioeconomic status, urban/rural ratio, educational level, marital status, alcohol consumption, smoker status or family history), we cannot conclude anything about the value of seafood consumption as protection against the onset of bipolar disorder.

Two RCTs failed to clarify the protective value of omega-3 fatty acid intake with respect to the onset of symptoms, not disorders, of anxiety. However, these small studies do not constitute optimal tests of this potential. Based on one cross-sectional study, which controlled for age, income, smoking, alcohol consumption and eating patterns, mental health difficulties were more prevalent in those consuming no fish. However, this design precludes inferring a causal link between fish consumption and the onset of mental health difficulties.

Four RCTs, three of which enrolled healthy volunteers, one single population cross-sectional survey and one cross-national ecological analysis studied the possible association between omega-3 fatty acid intake and the onset of tendencies or behavior with the potential to harm others. Overall, their findings are too inconsistent and involve too few research designs permitting the drawing of causal inferences or too many different definitions of the exposure, population or outcome to permit us to draw a consistent, individual/patient-level conclusion regarding the value of omega-3 fatty acid intake to protect against tendencies or behavior with the potential to harm others.

Research designs were not identified which—due to their prospective and controlled nature—are most appropriate for addressing the question of the possible relationship between intake of omega-3 fatty acids (e.g., via breastfeeding) and the onset of schizophrenia. Five case-control designs, one single prospective cohort and three cross-national ecological analyses were found. The only prospective study was not controlled, and its followup was very short. Moreover, failures to control for confounders were common (e.g., maternal feeding patterns, sex of children, maternal age, socioeconomic status, early mother-infant contact). Thus, nothing definitive can be asserted about a reliable association between omega-3 fatty acid intake and the onset of schizophrenia.

Discussion

A notable safety profile (i.e., beyond occasional and mild discomfort) for any type or dose of omega-3 fatty acid supplementation was not observed. Overall, other than for the topics of schizophrenia and depression, few studies were identified.

Only with respect to the supplemental treatment of schizophrenia is the evidence even somewhat suggestive of omega-3 fatty acids' potential as short-term intervention. However, these meta-analytic results exclusively pertaining to 2 g/d EPA require replication using design and methods refinements. Additional research might reveal the short-term or long-term therapeutic value of omega-3 fatty acids.

One study demonstrating a significant placebo-controlled clinical effect related to 1 g/d E-EPA given, over 12 weeks, to 17 patients with depressive symptoms—rather than depressive disorders—cannot be taken to support the view of the utility of this exposure as a supplemental treatment for depressive symptomatology or disorders.

Nothing can yet be concluded concerning the clinical utility of omega-3 fatty acids as supplemental treatment for any other psychiatric disorder or condition, or as a primary treatment for all psychiatric disorders or conditions examined in our review. Primary treatment studies were rare.

Much more research, implementing design and methods improvements, is needed before we can begin to ascertain the possible utility of (foods or supplements containing) omega-3 fatty acids as primary prevention for psychiatric disorders or conditions. Studies of omega-3 fatty acids' primary protective potential in mental health could be "piggybacked" onto longitudinal studies of their impact on general health and development.

Overall, almost nothing is known about the therapeutic or preventive potential of each source, type, dose, or combination of omega-3 fatty acids. Likewise, limitations within the evidence base prevented us from identifying the influence of key covariables (e.g., smoking, alcohol use, psychotropic medication) on the relationship between omega-3 fatty acid content and clinical outcomes.

Because of limited study designs, little is known about the relationship between PUFA [polyunsaturated fatty acid] biomarker profiles and the onset of any psychiatric disorder or condition. Studies examining the possible association between the intake of omega-3 fatty acids, or the PUFA content of biomarkers, and the continuation or recurrence of psychiatric disorders or conditions were virtually nonexistent.

If future research is going to produce data that are unequivocally applicable to North Americans, it will likely need to enroll either North American populations or populations exhibiting a high omega-6/ omega-3 fatty acid intake ratio similar to what has been observed in the diet of North Americans.

Furthermore, if a reasonable view is that omega-3 fatty acids may play a role in mental health, then given the observed or proposed interrelationships among omega-3 and omega-6 fatty acid contents both in the human diet and metabolism, it may behoove researchers to investigate the possible therapeutic or preventive value of the dietary omega-6/omega-3 fatty acid intake ratio.

Section 57.2

St. John's Wort and Depression

Excerpted from the fact sheet "St. John's Wort," by the National Center for Complementary and Alternative Medicine (NCCAM, nccam.nih.gov), part of the National Institutes of Health, December 2007.

This text provides basic information about the herb St. John's wort—common names, uses, and potential side effects. St. John's wort is a plant with yellow flowers whose medicinal uses were first recorded in ancient Greece. The name St. John's wort apparently refers to John the Baptist, as the plant blooms around the time of the feast of St. John the Baptist in late June.

- **Common names:** St. John's wort, hypericum, Klamath weed, goat weed
- **Latin name:** *Hypericum perforatum*

What It Is Used For

St. John's wort has been used for centuries to treat mental disorders and nerve pain.

St. John's wort has also been used as a sedative and a treatment for malaria, as well as a balm for wounds, burns, and insect bites.

Today, St. John's wort is used by some for depression, anxiety, and/or sleep disorders.

How It Is Used

The flowering tops of St. John's wort are used to prepare teas and tablets containing concentrated extracts.

What the Science Says

There is some scientific evidence that St. John's wort is useful for treating mild to moderate depression. However, two large studies, one sponsored by NCCAM, showed that the herb was no more effective than placebo in treating major depression of moderate severity.

NCCAM is studying the use of St. John's wort in a wider spectrum of mood disorders, including minor depression.

Side Effects and Cautions

St. John's wort may cause increased sensitivity to sunlight. Other side effects can include anxiety, dry mouth, dizziness, gastrointestinal symptoms, fatigue, headache, or sexual dysfunction.

Research shows that St. John's wort interacts with some drugs. The herb affects the way the body processes or breaks down many drugs; in some cases, it may speed or slow a drug's breakdown. Drugs that can be affected include:

- antidepressants;
- birth control pills;
- cyclosporine, which prevents the body from rejecting transplanted organs;
- digoxin, which strengthens heart muscle contractions;
- indinavir and possibly other drugs used to control HIV [human immunodeficiency virus] infection;

- irinotecan and possibly other drugs used to treat cancer; and
- warfarin and related anticoagulants.

When combined with certain antidepressants, St. John's wort may increase side effects such as nausea, anxiety, headache, and confusion.

St. John's wort is not a proven therapy for depression. If depression is not adequately treated, it can become severe. Anyone who may have depression should see a health care provider. There are effective proven therapies available.

Tell your health care providers about any complementary and alternative practices you use. Give them a full picture of what you do to manage your health. This will help ensure coordinated and safe care.

Section 57.3

S-Adenosyl-L-Methionine for Treatment of Depression

Excerpted from "S-Adenosyl-L-Methionine for Treatment of Depression, Osteoarthritis, and Liver Disease: Summary of Evidence Report/Technology Assessment, No. 64," by the Agency for Healthcare Research and Quality (AHRQ, www.ahrq.gov), August 2002. Reviewed by David A. Cooke, M.D., January 10, 2009.

Researchers conducted a search of the published literature on the use of S-adenosyl-L-methionine (SAMe) for the treatment of osteoarthritis, depression, and liver disease; and, on the basis of that search, evaluated the evidence for the efficacy of SAMe. A broad search revealed sufficient literature to support a detailed review of the use of SAMe for three conditions: depression, osteoarthritis, and cholestasis of pregnancy and intrahepatic cholestasis associated with liver disease.

About depression: Depression will affect 10 to 25 percent of women and 5 to 12 percent of men in the United States during their lifetimes.

Approximately 10 to 15 million people experience clinical depression in any given year. The annual cost for treatment and lost wages is estimated at $43.7 to $52.9 billion.

Reporting the Evidence

Searches of the literature yielded 1,624 titles, of which 294 were selected to review; the latter included meta-analyses, clinical trials, and reports that contained supplemental information on SAMe.

Ninety-nine articles, representing 102 individual studies, met the screening criteria. They focused on SAMe treatment for depression, osteoarthritis, or liver disease and presented data from clinical trials on humans. Of these 102 studies, 47 focused on depression, 14 focused on osteoarthritis, and 41 focused on liver disease (all conditions).

Findings

Researchers identified 102 relevant studies in the three selected areas: 47 studies for depression, 14 studies for osteoarthritis, and 41 studies for liver disease. The majority of the studies enrolled small numbers of patients, and the quality of the studies varied greatly. After removal of duplicate studies, the distribution of studies across the three selected areas was as follows:

Out of 39 unique studies considered, 28 studies were included in a meta-analysis of the efficacy of SAMe to decrease symptoms of depression.

Compared to placebo, treatment with SAMe was associated with an improvement of approximately 6 points in the score of the Hamilton Rating Scale for Depression measured at 3 weeks. This degree of improvement is statistically as well as clinically significant and is equivalent to a partial response to treatment. Too few studies were available for which a risk ratio could be calculated for either a 25 percent or 50 percent improvement in the Hamilton Rating Scale for Depression. Therefore a pooled analysis could not be done, but the results generally favored SAMe compared to placebo.

Compared to treatment with conventional antidepressant pharmacology, treatment with SAMe was not associated with a statistically significant difference in outcomes.

Chapter 58

Exercise and Sleep: How They Improve Symptoms of Mental Health Disorders

Chapter Contents

Section 58.1

Exercise Helps Keep Your Psyche Fit

Exercise is an effective, cost-effective treatment for depression and may help in the treatment of other mental disorders.

Findings

You know that exercise is good for your body. Among other facts, exercise decreases the risk of coronary heart disease and stroke and related factors, decreases the risk of various cancers, lowers blood pressure, improves metabolism, reduces problems related to diabetes, assists in the maintenance of bone density, and improves your immune system.

But did you know that exercise is also good for your head? The most common treatments for depression, for example, are psychotherapy or medication. Psychologists have found that exercise is a third successful alternative. In a 1990 meta-analysis (an analysis that statistically summarized 80 studies of exercise and depression), a research team that included psychologist Penny McCullagh, Ph.D., reached the following conclusions:

- Exercise was a beneficial antidepressant both immediately and over the long term.
- Although exercise decreased depression among all populations studied, it was most effective in decreasing depression for those most physically and/or psychologically unhealthy at the start of the exercise program.
- Although exercise significantly decreased depression across all age categories, the older people were (the ages ranged from 11 to 55), the greater the decrease in depression with exercise.

- Exercise was an equally effective antidepressant for both genders.
- Walking and jogging were the most frequent forms of exercise that had been researched, but all modes of exercise examined, anaerobic as well as aerobic, were effective in lessening depression at least to some degree.
- The greater the length of the exercise program and the larger the total number of exercise sessions, the greater the decrease in depression with exercise.
- The most powerful antidepressant effect occurred with the combination of exercise and psychotherapy.

How does exercise compare with medication for the treatment of depression? Research regarding this question has only recently been explored. Psychologist James Blumenthal, Ph.D., and colleagues at Duke University have conducted a number of systematic studies of patients diagnosed with major depressive disorder using the two treatment conditions of exercise and medication. They have compared patients' response to aerobic exercise only, psychotropic medication only (Zoloft, an SSRI [selective serotonin reuptake inhibitor]), or a combination of the two. After 4 1/2 months of treatment, patients receiving any of these treatments were significantly less depressed. About two-thirds were no longer depressed (Blumenthal et al. 1999). In a follow-up study by psychologist Michael Babyak, Ph.D., and colleagues, these same patients were contacted 6 months after the original study. They found that patients who had been in the exercise group were more likely to be partially or fully recovered than those who were in the medication or medication plus exercise group (Babyak et al. 2000).

Significance

Both individual experiments and general findings repeatedly point to the power of exercise in the treatment of clinical depression. Other studies indicate that exercise can be important in the treatment of various types of anxiety; issues of self-esteem; weight loss and weight loss management; and addictions. Research is emerging on the effectiveness of exercise in the maintenance of cognitive or mental functioning and the treatment of serious mental illness.

Practical Application

Evidence of the antidepressant benefits of exercise is being used by psychotherapists and other health practitioners who are increasingly recommending exercise to their patients as part of a treatment program. This research is also now being applied in books and articles that guide people toward happier living. In her 2002 book, *Move your body, tone your mood,* psychologist Kate Hays, Ph.D., suggests that if you are depressed and are considering exercise, the following are advisable:

- Review your health status with your health care provider and obtain clearance to exercise.
- Begin exercise gradually and set reasonable goals for yourself.
- There is no one form of exercise guaranteed to lift depression. For many people, walking, running, or swimming is helpful, but some people value yoga and others feel emotionally as well as physically strengthened by weight lifting. This is an opportunity for personal experimentation.
- Exercise may be an opportunity to increase contact with other people, especially if depression has resulted in decreased connection with others. Many people find that they can stick to their exercise plan if they work out with a friend who has similar goals.
- Pay attention even to minor changes in your mood to evaluate what form of exercise or exercise intensity is most helpful to you.

Cited Research

Babyak, M. A., Blumenthal, J. A., Herman, S., Khatri, P., Doraiswamy, P. M., Moore, K. A., Craighead, W. E., Baldewicz, T. T., & Krishnan, K. R. (2000). Exercise treatment for major depression: Maintenance of therapeutic benefit at 10 months. *Psychosomatic Medicine,* Vol. 62. pp. 633-638.

Blumenthal, J. A., Babyak, M.A., Moore, K. A., Craighead, W. E., Herman, S., Khatri, P., Waugh, R., Napolitano, M. A., Forman, L. M., Appelbaum, M., Doraiswamy, P. M., & Krishnan, K. R. (1999). Effects of exercise training on older patients with major depression. *Archives of Internal Medicine,* Vol. 159 pp. 2349-2356.

North, T. C., P. McCullagh, and Z. V. Tran. (1990). Effect of exercise on depression. *Exercise and Sport Sciences Reviews* Vol. 18 pp. 379-415.

Additional Sources

Hays, K. F. (1999). *Working it Out: Using Exercise in Psychotherapy.* Washington, DC: APA.

Hays, K. F. (2002). *Move your body, tone your mood.* Oakland, CA: New Harbinger.

Johnsgard, K. W. (2004). *Conquering Depression and Anxiety Through Exercise.* New York: Prometheus.

Leith, L. M. (1998). *Exercising your way to better mental health.* Morgantown, WV: Fitness Information Technology.

Section 58.2

Exercise Reduces Depression Symptoms

"The latest research on depression and exercise," reprinted with permission from the American Federation for Aging Research, © 2003. For further information, visit www.infoaging.org. The American Federation for Aging Research considers this information updated and current.

During the last 15 years, several hundred studies have looked at the effects of exercise on depression and found that exercise increases self-esteem, improves mood, reduces anxiety levels, increases the ability to handle stress, and improves sleep patterns. While getting older (and indeed all) adults to stay on a regular exercise regimen can be a challenge, recent research suggests that it may be an effective antidote to major depression.

A small study done at Harvard of 32 depressed people over the age of 60 compared the effects of resistance training to no training. The resistance-trained group showed significant gains in social functioning, vitality, and mood, and they also increased their strength by 33%. A Norwegian study of depressed patients enrolled in an exercise program found that more than half of them stayed in the exercise segment a full year after the rest of their treatment finished. Many of them rated the exercise as the most important part of their program.

Duke researchers recently confirmed these findings in a single site clinical trial, testing 156 outpatients 50 and older who met the criteria for a major depressive disorder. Subjects received SSRI [selective serotonin reuptake inhibitor] antidepressant medication, performed supervised exercise sessions (a 10-minute warm-up and biking, walking, or jogging) or did both (medication + exercise). After 4 months and evaluations by psychiatrists, the three groups' rate of major depression were relatively similar. Six months following the treatment, however, only 30% of those in the exercise group were diagnosed with major depression, compared to 52% in the medication group and 55% in the exercise + medication group. Also, among patients diagnosed in remission from their depression after 4 months, those doing just exercise were less likely to relapse into major depression than the other two groups. After that Duke study was completed, the researchers re-interviewed and re-examined the study participants. They found that 4 months after the completion of the study, all three groups of patients—exercise alone, medication alone, and the combination of medication and exercise—had similar rates of remission and relapse of depression. Ten months after the completion of the study, the exercise alone group demonstrated the lowest rate of relapse, and those who continued to exercise afterward on their own also had a reduced likelihood of being still diagnosed as depressed after the completion of the study.

A study conducted at Northeastern University in Boston looked at the effect of exercise on overweight women. Obesity can contribute to poor self-esteem, one characteristic of depression. Eight women who were overweight enrolled in an exercise program. Five of the eight had scores on a depression screening test that indicated they were suffering mild to moderate depressive symptoms. At the end of the 6-month exercise program, only one of those women still scored mild depression on the screening tests—yet none of the women experienced any significant weight loss. Thus, exercise alone reduced the depressive symptoms in the study subjects.

For older people, exercise apparently may do more than fight depression—it may also improve your mind. A Swedish study randomly assigned 40 men and women with an average age of 66 to either exercise three times a week or to serve as controls. At the end of 3 months, the exercise group had significantly higher scores on performing complex tasks. A larger study, undertaken at the Prince of Wales Medical Research Institute in Sydney, Australia, enrolled 187 older women in either an exercise group or a control group. After a year, the exercisers had improved reaction time, muscle strength, and memory span. Their mood scores were also much improved by the end of the study.

For older adults, it seems that exercise may not only be good for the body, it may be good for the mind.

Section 58.3

Sleep and Mental Health Problems

"Ask the Sleep Expert: Sleep Hygiene, Insomnia and Mental Health," by Michael Perlis, Ph.D. Reprinted with permission. For additional information, visit www.drowsydriving.org. Reviewed by David A. Cooke, M.D., January 23, 2009. Dr. Cooke is not affiliated with the National Sleep Foundation.

What psychiatric/mental health conditions involve insomnia?

Substance abuse, mood, anxiety, and psychotic disorders are a few of the many conditions that involve insomnia. It is unknown why insomnia is such a common symptom among these illnesses.

Why is it important for a person with mental health problems to treat their insomnia?

Insomnia may not only be a symptom of some psychiatric diseases, it may also contribute to these disorders. Depending on the person, it may be important to get targeted treatment for insomnia, especially when the treatment of the primary disorder(s) does not improve the patient's sleep.

Does insomnia lead to these conditions or is it only a symptom?

If you asked this question 20 years ago, the answer would have been "insomnia is a symptom." Over the years, this perspective has changed. It is now recognized that insomnia may occur and not be associated with acute psychiatric or medical illness. This is called Primary Insomnia (or Psychophysiologic Insomnia). The question now is whether such a disorder represents a risk factor for, or a sign of, psychiatric and/or medical illness. While the jury is out regarding insomnia and medical illness, the evidence with respect to psychiatric illness is clear and compelling. Patients with persistent and untreated insomnia are at between 2 and 10 times the risk for new onset or recurrent episodes of major depression. There is also good evidence that insomnia is a risk factor for the development and/or recurrence of anxiety disorders and substance abuse.

If a person is experiencing insomnia, what should he or she do about it?

If the insomnia is acute (less than approximately 14 days), there are two viable options. First, do nothing. If one does not compensate for sleep loss (does not go to bed earlier, get out of bed later, stay in bed waiting for sleep, nap, etc.), it is likely that "the ship will right itself." When adopting this strategy (the "tough-it-out" approach), the one thing you can do is judiciously use caffeine to maintain daytime function. Second, visit your doctor, who may prescribe a sedative.

At what point should someone seek out treatment?

While it is unknown precisely when acute insomnia becomes chronic, a good rule of thumb would be 2 to 4 weeks. The bottom line is: getting treatment earlier rather than later can only be a good thing. There will be less personal suffering. It may also be true that the disorder is easier to treat when it is dealt with early and that early treatment may reduce your risk for the development of other disorders.

Michael Perlis, PhD, is Associate Professor, Department of Psychiatry, and Director of the UR Sleep Research Laboratory & Behavioral Sleep Medicine Service at the University of Rochester in Rochester, NY.

Chapter 59

Paying for Mental Health Treatment

Chapter Contents

Section 59.1

How to Pay for Mental Health Care

From "How to Pay for Mental Health Services," by the Substance Abuse and Mental Health Services Administration (SAMHSA, www.mentalhealth.samhsa.gov), part of the U.S. Department of Health and Human Services, April 2003. Reviewed and revised by David A. Cooke, M.D., January 10, 2009.

Why are payment methods important?

The high cost of health care makes treatment out of reach for many people. Those who do not have health insurance—more than 45 million Americans—often avoid treatment entirely, because costs can be staggering.

What is private insurance?

The majority of working Americans are covered under employer-provided health insurance plans. One type of plan is a standard indemnity policy, which gives people freedom to visit a health care provider of their choice and pay out of pocket for their treatment. The insurance plan reimburses members for some portion of the cost. The other common plan is a managed care plan. Under this plan, medically necessary care is provided in the most cost-effective, or least expensive, way available. Plan members must visit health care providers chosen by the managed care plan. Generally, a co-payment is charged to the patient, but sometimes all care received from providers within the plan is covered. Managed care companies provide services in many states for low-income Medicare and Medicaid beneficiaries. Both types of private health coverage may offer some coverage for mental health treatment. However, this treatment often is not paid for at the same rate as other health care costs.

The Mental Health Parity Act of 2008 prevents insurers from placing greater limits on mental health care than other types of medical treatment. This law will take effect in 2010, and it is hoped this will broadly improve access and coverage for mental health care.

What are some resources for the uninsured?

- **Community-based resources:** Many communities have community mental health centers (CMHCs). These centers offer a range of mental health treatment and counseling services, usually at a reduced rate for low-income people. CMHCs generally require you to have a private insurance plan or to be a recipient of public assistance.

- **Pastoral counseling:** Most religious organizations can put you in touch with a pastoral counseling program. Certified pastoral counselors, who are ministers in a recognized religious body, have advanced degrees in pastoral counseling, as well as professional counseling experience. Pastoral counseling is often provided on a sliding-scale fee basis.

- **Self-help groups:** Another option is to join a self-help or support group. Such groups give people a chance to learn about, talk about, and work on their common problems, such as alcoholism, substance abuse, depression, family issues, and relationships. Self-help groups are generally free and can be found in virtually every community in America. Many people find them to be effective.

- **Public assistance:** People with severe mental illness may be eligible for several forms of public assistance, both to meet the basic costs of living and to pay for health care. Examples of such programs are Social Security, Medicare, and Medicaid.

    - **Social Security** has two types of programs to help individuals with disabilities. Social Security Disability Insurance provides benefits for those individuals who have worked for a required length of time and have paid Social Security taxes. Supplemental Security Income provides benefits to individuals based on their economic needs (Social Security Administration, 2002).

    - **Medicare** is America's primary federal health insurance program for people who are 65 or older and for some with disabilities who are under 65. It provides basic protection for the cost of health care. Two programs exist to help people with low incomes receive benefits: the Qualified Medicare Beneficiary (QMB) and the Specified Low-Income Medicare Beneficiary (SLMB) programs.

- **Medicaid** pays for some health care costs for America's poorest and most vulnerable people. More information about Medicaid and eligibility requirements is available at local welfare and medical assistance offices. Although there are certain federal requirements, each state also has its own rules and regulations for Medicaid.

Section 59.2

Medicare and Your Mental Health Benefits

Excerpted from the booklet "Medicare and Your Mental Health Benefits," by the Centers for Medicare and Medicaid Services, www.medicare.gov, September 2007.

Mental health care includes services and programs to help diagnose and treat mental health conditions. These services and programs may be given in outpatient and inpatient settings. Medicare helps cover outpatient and inpatient mental health care, as well as prescription drugs. This text gives you information about mental health benefits in the Original Medicare Plan.

If you get your Medicare benefits through a Medicare Health Plan, other than the Original Medicare Plan, check your plan's membership materials and call the plan for details about how the plan provides your Medicare-covered mental health benefits.

How Mental Health Benefits Are Paid in the Original Medicare Plan

Medicare Part B (Medical Insurance) helps cover mental health services that you would generally get outside a hospital, including visits with a doctor, psychiatrist or other doctor, visits with a clinical psychologist, or clinical social worker, and lab tests ordered by your doctor. Medicare Part B may also pay for partial hospitalization services, if you need intensive coordinated outpatient care.

Medicare Part A (Hospital Insurance) helps cover mental health care if you are a hospital inpatient. Medicare Part A covers your room, meals, nursing, and other related services and supplies.

Medicare Part D (Medicare prescription drug coverage) helps cover prescription drugs you may need to treat a mental health condition.

Section 1: Outpatient Mental Health Care and Professional Services

What the Original Medicare Plan Covers

If you are in the Original Medicare Plan and have Medicare Part B (Medical Insurance), Medicare helps cover visits with these types of health professionals:

- a psychiatrist or other doctor;
- clinical psychologist;
- clinical social worker;
- clinical nurse specialist;
- nurse practitioner; and
- physician's assistant.

It's important to know that Medicare only covers these visits when they are given by a health care professional who accepts Medicare payment. To further reduce the amount you have to pay, you should also ask your health professional if they accept assignment before you schedule an appointment.

Medicare Part B helps cover outpatient mental health services. This includes services that are usually given outside a hospital (like in a clinic, or doctor's or therapist's office), and those that are given in a hospital's outpatient department. Medicare helps cover the following services:

- individual and group therapy with doctors or certain other licensed professionals allowed by the state to give these services;
- family counseling if the main purpose is to help with your treatment;
- testing to help find out if you are getting the right services and if your treatment is helping;
- psychiatric evaluation;

- medication management;
- occupational therapy that is part of your mental health treatment;
- certain prescription drugs that aren't usually self-administered, like some injections;
- individual patient training and education about your condition;
- diagnostic tests;
- a screening for mental health conditions during the one-time "Welcome to Medicare" physical exam (Note: This physical exam is only covered if you have it within the first 6 months you have Medicare Part B.); and
- partial hospitalization may be covered.

What You Have to Pay

After you pay your yearly Medicare Part B deductible ($135 in 2008), the amount of coinsurance you pay for mental health services will depend on the kind of service you get. For visits to a doctor to diagnose a mental health condition, or to monitor or change your drug prescription for mental health conditions, you will generally pay 20% of the Medicare-approved amount. For outpatient treatment of your mental health condition (such as therapy), you will have to pay about 50% of the Medicare-approved amount. Medicare will send you a notice showing what you owe. Talk to your doctor or other health care provider if you need help understanding your outpatient mental health benefits.

If you get your services in a hospital outpatient clinic, or in an outpatient department of a hospital, you will have to pay a separate copayment or coinsurance amount to the hospital. This amount will vary depending on the service provided, but won't exceed 40% of the Medicare-approved amount.

Getting treatment from a doctor or provider who is enrolled with Medicare and who accepts "assignment" can reduce your out-of-pocket costs. If a doctor or provider accepts assignment, they agree to the following conditions:

- to be paid by Medicare;
- to accept only the amount Medicare approves for their services; and

- to only charge you, or other insurance you may have, the Medicare deductible or coinsurance amount.

Partial Hospitalization May Be Covered

Partial hospitalization is a structured program of mental health care that is more intense than the care you get in a doctor's or therapist's office. This type of treatment is provided during the day and doesn't require an overnight stay. These programs are given through hospital outpatient departments and local community mental health centers.

Your doctor or therapist may think that you could get help from a partial hospitalization program. Under certain conditions, Medicare helps cover this kind of care. For a partial hospitalization program to be covered, a doctor must say that you would otherwise need inpatient treatment. To be covered, your doctor and the program must accept Medicare payment.

Section 2: Inpatient Mental Health Care

What the Original Medicare Plan Covers

If you are in the Original Medicare Plan and have Medicare Part A (Hospital Insurance), Medicare helps pay for mental health services given in a hospital that require you to be admitted as an inpatient. These services can be given in a general hospital, or in a psychiatric hospital that only provides care for people with mental health conditions. Regardless of which type of hospital you choose, Medicare Part A will cover mental health services.

If you are in a psychiatric hospital (instead of a general hospital), Medicare Part A only pays for up to 190 days of inpatient psychiatric hospital services care during your lifetime.

Section 3: Medicare Prescription Drug Coverage (Medicare Part D)

About Medicare Prescription Drug Coverage

Medicare offers prescription drug coverage for everyone with Medicare. Medicare prescription drug coverage gives you access to drugs that you may need to stay physically and mentally healthy. To get Medicare prescription drug coverage, you must join a Medicare drug plan. Medicare drug plans are run by insurance companies and other private companies approved by Medicare. Each Medicare drug plan can vary in cost and drugs covered.

Medicare Drug Plans Have Special Rules

The formulary: Almost all Medicare drug plans have a list of drugs that the plan covers. This list is called a formulary. In general, Medicare drug plans are not required to cover every drug, as long as they cover all drugs that are medically necessary. However, all Medicare drug plans are required to cover all or almost all antidepressant, anticonvulsant, and antipsychotic medications, which may be necessary to keep you mentally healthy. Medicare reviews each plan's formulary to make sure it contains a wide range of medically necessary drugs and that it doesn't discriminate against certain groups (like people with disabilities or mental health conditions).

There are certain drugs that Medicare drug plans aren't required to cover, such as benzodiazepines, barbiturates, or drugs for weight loss or gain. Some Medicare drug plans may choose to pay for these drugs as an added benefit. Also, some states may cover these drugs if you have Medicaid. In addition, Medicare drug plans generally aren't allowed to cover over-the-counter drugs. Be sure to ask your doctor and your plan any questions you may have about the drugs you need.

The formulary can change. A Medicare drug plan can make some changes to its formulary during the year according to guidelines set by Medicare. If you are currently taking a drug and the plan's formulary changes, you will be notified before the change is made and the drug would usually be covered for you for the rest of the plan year. The cost of a drug can also change during the year, but established copayments should remain the same.

What if my doctor thinks I need a certain drug that my plan doesn't cover? If you belong to a Medicare drug plan, you have the right to:

- Get a written explanation (called a "coverage determination") from your Medicare drug plan if your plan won't cover or pay for a certain prescription drug you need, or if you are asked to pay more than you think you should pay for a drug.

- Ask your Medicare drug plan for an exception which is a type of coverage determination. If you ask for an exception, your doctor must give your drug plan a supporting statement that says why you need the drug you are requesting. You can ask for an exception if:

- You or your doctor believe you need a drug that isn't on your drug plan's list of covered drugs.
- You or your doctor believe that a coverage rule (such as prior authorization) should be waived.
- You believe you should get a drug you need at a lower copayment because you can't take any of the drugs on the drug plan's list of preferred drugs.

You or your doctor must contact your plan to ask for a coverage determination. If your network pharmacy can't fill a prescription as written, the pharmacist will give or show you a notice that explains how to contact your Medicare drug plan so you can make your request.

A standard request for a coverage determination (including an exception) must be made in writing (unless your plan accepts requests by phone). You or your doctor can also call or write your plan for an expedited (fast) request. If you are requesting an exception, your prescribing doctor must provide a statement explaining the medical reason for the request (such as why similar drugs covered by your plan won't work or may be harmful to you).

Once your Medicare drug plan gets your request for a coverage determination or your doctor's statement (if you are requesting an exception), the Medicare drug plan has 72 hours (for a standard request) or 24 hours (for an expedited request) to notify you of its decision.

If you disagree with your Medicare drug plan's coverage determination or exception decision, you have the right to appeal the decision. The plan's written decision will explain how to file an appeal. You should read this decision carefully.

Your Rights as a Person with Medicare

As a person with Medicare, you have certain guaranteed rights. Your rights include the right to participate in treatment decisions, to know your treatment choices, and to have your personal and health information kept private. You also have the right to appeal decisions about your Medicare services. These rights and protections are described in your "Medicare & You" handbook or the "Your Medicare

Rights and Protections" booklet. You can view or download these booklets by visiting www.medicare.gov on the web. Under "Search Tools," select "Find a Medicare Publication." Or, call 800-MEDICARE (800-633-4227). TTY users should call 877-486-2048.

Section 59.3

Social Security Disability Benefits for People with Mental Health Disorders

"Social Security Benefits," © 2007 NAMI: The Nation's Voice on Mental Illness (www.nami.org). Reprinted with permission.

Are you or your relative entitled to Social Security Disability Benefits?

Mental illness, like a physical illness, can be disabling. Persons with a serious mental illness are just as entitled to disability payments as persons with a serious physical illness. If you or your relative has a mental illness such as schizophrenia, obsessive-compulsive disorder, manic depression, or another disabling brain disorder (mental illness), you may be entitled to benefits from the Social Security Administration. For all inquiries, call the Social Security Administration at 1-800-772-1213 or visit their website at www.ssa.gov.

What are Social Security Disability Benefits?

The benefits include cash payment that averages $900 per month. In most states, Social Security Disability Insurance comes with Medicare and Supplemental Security Income with Medicaid, although some states have different names or slightly different programs. Often the Social Security Disability benefit is the most important benefit because many states tie a Social Security Disability finding to eligibility for local programs.

Who receives disability payments?

Millions of Americans receive Social Security Disability benefits each year, and each year more that 2.5 million new applications are filed. The Social Security Administration defines disability in terms of ability to work. Persons who cannot work for a year or more, or whose condition is likely to result in death, may qualify for benefits. Disability examiners at state agencies, consulting with SSA doctors, determine disability based on clinical evidence and examinations. Unfortunately, these examiners do not meet the applicants.

What specific disability program might I be eligible for?

You could be entitled to receive payments from one, or both, of two Social Security programs: Supplemental Security Income (SSI) and Social Security Disability Insurance (SSDI). SSI is for persons who are disabled, poor, and unable to work. SSDI is for persons who are disabled and unable to work, but who have worked in the past, or whose parents have worked and paid into the social security trust fund. The most SSI will pay for 2007 is $623 a month for an individual. About half the states supplement SSI, which increases cash benefits. The amount you may be entitled to from SSDI can be much larger, depending on work history, but the average payment is about $900 per month.

How do I apply for Social Security benefits?

All disability claims start with an application to Social Security. This may be done in person, or electronically over the internet at www.ssa.gov. Or call any local Social Security office or the national toll free number: 1-800-772-1213. Family members or guardians should call SSA to find out what procedures they should follow.

If it's clear I have a disability, will I automatically receive benefits?

No. The Social Security Administration has four basic standards for determining disability:

1. **Earnings:** Generally, if you make $900 a month or more in 2007, you will not be considered disabled. Some expenses directly related to your and that enable you to go to work may be deducted.

2. **Severity:** If your condition does not interfere with basic work-related activities, your claim will be denied. SSA must consider all your severe medical problems in combination, so make sure you tell them about each medical problem that affects your ability to work.

3. **Checklist:** If your condition(s), either individually or in combination, meet or equal the medical criteria on a list of disabling impairments maintained by Social Security, SSA will usually decide your case fairly quickly.

4. **Type of work:** If you cannot do the work you did in the 15 years before you became disabled, SSA looks to see if you can do any other kind of work, taking into account your age, education, past experience, and skills. If you cannot sustain work, at a competitive pace, day after day, you may be found disabled.

What does an application involve?

A claim representative will conduct an in-depth interview in person or over the telephone with the applicant and ask you to complete a variety of application forms. The representative will ask about the applicant's disability, medical history, leisure time activities, and financial status. This process can be difficult particularly if the applicant is experiencing symptoms or if the interviewer is not skilled. You may want a relative or friend, or a representative or lawyer, to accompany you to provide support and assistance.

After the interview is complete, what's the next step?

A caseworker from SSA and a caseworker from the state Disability Determination Service (DDS) share responsibility for determining eligibility for disability programs. The SSA caseworker will focus on financial eligibility while the DDS caseworker will focus on medical and functional information. A decision should be reached within three months from the application date. This happens rarely, however. The process will more likely take six months. It's a good idea to call and check on the status of the application. The DDS caseworker will NOT meet with you.

What are the chances of receiving benefits?

Good, if you are willing to be persistent. Two out of three persons who apply for disability benefits are initially rejected, although the rejection rate varies widely from state to state. These applications are often rejected for what appear to be arbitrary reasons. If you appeal an initial rejection until you get a hearing with a judge—and most persons do not appeal—your chances of obtaining benefits improve. In 2004, over 60% of disability cases that were appealed to an administrative law judge were won by beneficiaries.

If the application for benefits is turned down, what can I do?

There are four levels of appeal. You can:

1. Ask for reconsideration by another decision maker to determine whether the initial decision was proper. More than 90% of all reconsideration requests are denied.
2. Ask for an administrative hearing, which is a formal but private hearing before an administrative law judge. You may request a hearing before a judge if you disagree with the reconsideration decision. Such judges try hard to remain objective. In 2004, 64% of disability cases appealed to these judges were decided in favor of beneficiaries.
3. Ask for a review by the SSA Appeals Council. This council reviews decisions by administrative law judges. The council usually leaves judges' decisions unchanged about 70% of the time. Note that SSA has begun to do away with this appeal step, starting in the New England region on August 1, 2006. Those applicants will have to go to federal court.
4. Appeal a denial of disability benefits to a U.S. Federal District Court. Although relatively few cases get to federal court, almost 50% of applicants got some positive relief.

What if I was denied benefits in the past?

You can reapply. In some cases, you can reapply while an earlier unfavorable decision is on appeal. There may even be ways to "reopen" an old unfavorable decision; usually expert help is necessary to do this.

If I have other questions, where do I go for answers?

Call the Social Security Hotline at 1-800-772-1213 between 7 a.m. and 7 p.m. EST weekdays. The best times to call are early in the morning and early in the evening, in the middle of the week, and in the middle of the month. It may be worthwhile to call more than once and get a second opinion, or to consult with an attorney.

Two national groups have referral lists of representatives who can help you with your claim: The National Association of Disability Representatives (NADR) at 202-822-2155, or the National Organization of Social Security Claimants' Representatives (NOSSCR), at 201-567-4228.

Section 59.4

Getting Help with Paying for Prescriptions

Some pharmaceutical companies offer prescription assistance programs to individuals and families with financial needs. These programs typically require a doctor's consent and proof of your financial status. They may also require that you have either no health insurance or no prescription drug benefit through your health insurance.

In addition, there are county, state, and national prescription programs for which you may qualify and special drug discount cards offered by some pharmaceutical companies.

Beginning January 1, 2006, Medicare began a new program to help pay for prescription drugs for people who receive Medicare benefits and people who currently have both Medicare and Medicaid. Mental Health America has developed written materials to explain this new program, also called Medicare Rx, Part D [http://www.mentalhealthamerica.net/go/medicare], or the prescription drug benefit, to help consumers, their family and friends better understand this new benefit and what steps they need to take to get this benefit. RX assist [http://www.rxassist.org/patients/resources.cfm] has developed a section for Medicare Part D participants that provides information about prescription assistance programs that may help Medicare Part D beneficiaries.

Partnership for Prescription Assistance [https://www.pparx.org/Intro.php] is an interactive site designed to help you find patient prescription drug assistance programs for which you may qualify. You can use the on-line application wizard, view and read about prescription assistance programs offered by the drug manufacturers, and search for prescription drug assistance programs in your state. You can also contact the Partnership for Prescription Assistance by calling 1-888-4PPA-NOW (1-888-477-2669).

Your local and/or state Mental Health America office [http://www.mentalhealthamerica.net/go/searchMHA] is a resource for information about state and local prescription assistance programs.

Your state Medicaid office [http://www.nasmd.org/links/state_medicaid_links.asp] may offer information about prescription assistance and drug discount programs available in your state.

Medicare Rights Center [http://www.medicarerights.org] offers information about state and national prescription assistance programs, drug discount cards, mail order and internet discount pharmacies, and prescription drug price comparison web sites. This information is not only for Medicare Part D plan participants but for anyone needing information about help paying for their prescription drugs. Use the "Help Paying for Prescription Drugs" option on the left-hand side of the page to access this information.

211 [http://www.211.org] is an Information and Referral service to help people connect with important community services and help them find help in their community more easily. 211 is available in many states and, if available in your area, can help you find organizations that may assist with a broad range of needs including help paying for medications, financial assistance with other essential needs such as food, clothing, rent and utility assistance, child care, employment supports, services for older adults, etc.

RX Hope [https://www.rxhope.com] has program descriptions and downloadable applications for prescription assistance programs for specific medications including psychotropic medications.

RX Assist [http://www.rxassist.org/patients/resources.cfm] offers a patient assistance program directory along with information about a variety of programs including drug discount cards, prescription assistance programs for generic medications, programs that help with medication copays, programs that provide free and low cost health care, as well as information for Medicare Part D beneficiaries.

Needy Meds [http://www.needymeds.org] has a searchable list of disease-specific assistance programs (primarily for other medical conditions) with program description and contact information (Use link under "Additional Programs" on left-hand side of home page.) Some of these programs provide a broad range of financial assistance including help with other necessary expenses such as utility bills. They also have a list of state sponsored programs which can be accessed from the link under "Government Programs" also on the left-hand side of the home page. Once you have identified programs, you can contact the Partnership for Prescription Assistance at 1-888-4PPA-NOW (1-888-477-2669) for free assistance in applying for these programs.

There are a variety of organizations that offer prescription assistance for medications used to treat specific medical conditions. While these organizations do not offer assistance in covering the cost of psychotropic medications, they may be helpful if you have other health problems. Some of these programs offer financial assistance for those who have insurance but have high co-pays. Some also offer assistance with insurance premiums.

- Patient Advocate Foundation [http://www.copays.org] Co-Pay Relief at 1-866-512-3861
- National Organization for Rare Diseases [http://www.rarediseases.org/programs/medication] (NORD) at 1-800-999-NORD
- Patient Services Inc. [http://www.uneedpsi.org/cms400min/index.aspx] at 1-800-366-7741
- HealthWell Foundation [http://www.healthwellfoundation.org/faq.aspx] at 1-800-675-8416
- Patient Access Network Foundation [https://www.patientaccessnetwork.org] at 1-866-316-7263

Part Seven

Living with Mental Health Disorders

Chapter 60

Staying Well When You Have a Mental Health Disorder

Chapter Contents

Section 60.1

How to Deal with Grief and Loss

From "How to Deal with Grief," by the Substance Abuse and Mental Health Services Administration (SAMHSA, mentalhealth.samhsa.gov), part of the U.S. Department of Health and Human Services. This document is undated.

What is grief?

Grief is the normal response of sorrow, emotion, and confusion that comes from losing someone or something important to you. It is a natural part of life. Grief is a typical reaction to death, divorce, job loss, a move away from friends and family, or loss of good health due to illness.

How does grief feel?

Just after a death or loss, you may feel empty and numb, as if you are in shock. You may notice physical changes such as trembling, nausea, trouble breathing, muscle weakness, dry mouth, or trouble sleeping and eating.

You may become angry—at a situation, a particular person, or just angry in general. Almost everyone in grief also experiences guilt. Guilt is often expressed as "I could have, I should have, and I wish I would have" statements.

People in grief may have strange dreams or nightmares, be absent-minded, withdraw socially, or lack the desire to return to work. While these feelings and behaviors are normal during grief, they will pass.

How long does grief last?

Grief lasts as long as it takes you to accept and learn to live with your loss. For some people, grief lasts a few months. For others, grieving may take years.

The length of time spent grieving is different for each person. There are many reasons for the differences, including personality, health, coping style, culture, family background, and life experiences. The time spent grieving also depends on your relationship with the person lost and how prepared you were for the loss.

How will I know when I'm done grieving?

Every person who experiences a death or other loss must complete a four-step grieving process:

1. Accept the loss;
2. Work through and feel the physical and emotional pain of grief;
3. Adjust to living in a world without the person or item lost; and
4. Move on with life.

The grieving process is over only when a person completes the four steps.

Section 60.2

Tips for Taking Care of Yourself

When you have a mental health condition, you may not realize how important your overall health is to your recovery. Having poor overall health can get in the way and make recovery harder. Finding ways to take care of your health can aid your recovery and help you feel better overall. Here are some things you can do.

Connect with Others

Spending time with positive, loving people you care about and trust can ease stress, help your mood, and improve the way you feel overall.

They may be family members, close friends, members of a support group, or a counselor at the local drop-in center. Many communities even have warm lines you can call to talk to someone.

Advocate for Yourself

You deserve good health care. All too often, people with mental illnesses develop other health conditions, such as heart disease and diabetes, because their health is overlooked. If your doctor is not asking about your overall health, let him know that it's important to you and essential to your recovery.

Get the Care You Need

Get routine check-ups and visit your doctor when you're not feeling well. It may be due to your medicine or a symptom of your mental illness. But it could also be a different health problem.

Plan Your Sleep Schedule

Sleep can affect your mood and your body and is important to your recovery. Not getting the right amount of sleep can make day-to-day functioning and recovery harder. For tips on how to sleep better, contact the National Sleep Foundation at 202-347-3471 or visit www.sleepfoundation.org.

Watch What You Eat

Sometimes, medicine can cause you to gain weight. Other times, eating unhealthy foods can cause weight gain. Foods high in calories and saturated or "bad" fats can raise your blood pressure and cholesterol. This can increase you chances of gaining weight and having other health problems, like heart disease and diabetes. Here are some shortcuts you can take to healthy eating.

- If fresh vegetables are too costly, buy frozen vegetables. They can cost less and last a long time in your freezer.
- If you eat at fast food restaurants, many now offer healthy foods such as salads or grilled chicken.
- Talk to your doctor to learn more about how to have a healthy diet.

Manage Stress

Everyone has stress. It is a normal part of life. You can feel stress in your body when you have too much to do or when you haven't slept well. You can also feel stress when you worry about your job, money, relationships, or a friend or family member who is ill or in crisis. Stress can make you feel run down. It can also cause your mind to race and make it hard to focus on the things you need to do. If you have a mental illness, lots of stress can make you feel worse and make it harder to function. If you are feeling stressed, there are steps you can take to feel better:

- Slow down and take one thing at a time. If you feel like you have too much to do, make a list and work on it one task at a time.
- Know your limits. Let others know them too. If you're overwhelmed at home or work, or with friends, learn how to say "no." It may be hard at first, so practice saying no with the people you trust most.
- Practice stress reduction techniques. There are a lot of things you can do to make your life more peaceful and calm. Do something you enjoy, exercise, connect with others, or meditate.
- Know your triggers. What causes stress in your life? If you know where stress is coming from, you will be able to manage it better.
- Talk to someone. You don't have to deal with stress on your own. Talking to a trusted friend, family member, support group, or counselor can make you feel better. They also may help you figure out how to better manage stress in your life.

Exercise

Along with a healthy diet, exercise can improve your health and well-being. Exercising regularly can increase your self-esteem and confidence; reduce your feelings of stress, anxiety, and depression; improve your sleep; and help you maintain a healthy weight.

Find a type of exercise that you enjoy and talk to your doctor. You might enjoy walking, jogging, or even dancing. You don't have to go to a gym or spend money to exercise. Here are some things you can start doing now to get active:

- Check out your local community center for free, fun activities.
- Take a short walk around the block with family, friends, or co-workers.
- Take the stairs instead of the elevator. Make sure the stairs are well lit.
- Turn on some music and dance.

Do Something You Enjoy

During the week, find time—30 minutes, a couple of hours, or whatever you can fit in—to do something you enjoy. Read a book or magazine, go for a walk, or spend time with friends. Taking time for yourself to have fun and laugh can help you relax, ease stress, and improve the way you feel.

Substance Abuse

If you find yourself drinking or using drugs to cope, it is time to seek help. Although using drugs and alcohol may seem to help you cope, substance abuse can make your symptoms worse, delay your treatment, and complicate recovery. It can also cause abuse or addiction problems. To find help now, call 800-662-HELP or visit www.findtreatment.samhsa.gov.

Smoking

If you smoke, talk to your doctor about quitting. Smoking puts you at risk for problems like heart disease and cancer. For more information about quitting, call 800-QUIT-NOW or visit www.becomeanex.org.

For help finding treatment, support groups, medication information, help paying for your medications, your local Mental Health America affiliate, and other mental health-related services in your community, please access our Frequently Asked Questions and Answers (http://www.mentalhealthamerica.net/go/faqs). If you or someone you know is in crisis now, seek help immediately. Call 800-273-TALK (8255) to reach a 24 hour crisis center or dial 911 for immediate assistance.

Chapter 61

Stigma and Mental Illness

Anti-Stigma: Do You Know the Facts?

Stigma is not just a matter of using the wrong word or action. Stigma is about disrespect. It is the use of negative labels to identify a person living with mental illness. Stigma is a barrier. Fear of stigma, and the resulting discrimination, discourages individuals and their families from getting the help they need. An estimated 22 to 23 percent of the U.S. population experience a mental disorder in any given year, but almost half of these individuals do not seek treatment (U.S. Department of Health and Human Services, 2002; U.S. Surgeon General, 2001).

The educational information in this text encourages the use of positive images to refer to people with mental illness and underscores the reality that mental illness can be successfully treated.

- Do you know that an estimated 44 million Americans experience a mental disorder in any given year?
- Do you know that stigma is not a matter of using the wrong word or action?

This chapter contains text from "Anti-Stigma: Do You Know the Facts?" from the Substance Abuse and Mental Health Administration (SAMHSA, www.mentalhealth.samhsa.gov), part of the U.S. Department of Health and Human Services, February 2003. It also contains text from "Before You Label People, Look at Their Contents," by SAMHSA, 1996. Both documents were reviewed by David A. Cooke, M.D., January 10, 2009.

- Do you know that stigma is about disrespect and using negative labels to identify a person living with mental illness?
- Do you know that stigma is a barrier that discourages individuals and their families from seeking help?
- Do you know that many people would rather tell employers they committed a petty crime and served time in jail, than admit to being in a psychiatric hospital?
- Do you know that stigma can result in inadequate insurance coverage for mental health services?
- Do you know that stigma leads to fear, mistrust, and violence against people living with mental illness and their families?
- Do you know that stigma can cause families and friends to turn their backs on people with mental illness?
- Do you know that stigma can prevent people from getting access to needed mental health services?

Dos

- Do use respectful language.
- Do emphasize abilities, not limitations.
- Do tell someone if they express a stigmatizing attitude.

Don'ts

- Don't portray successful persons with disabilities as super human.
- Don't use generic labels such as retarded or the mentally ill.
- Don't use terms like crazy, lunatic, manic depressive, or slow functioning.

Before You Label People, Look at Their Contents

When mental illnesses are used as labels—depressed, schizophrenic, manic, or hyperactive—these labels hurt.

Labels lead to stigma—a word that means branding and shame. And stigma leads to discrimination. Everyone knows why it is wrong to discriminate against people because of their race, religion, culture, or appearance. They are less aware of how people with mental illnesses are discriminated against. Although such discrimination may not always be obvious, it exists—and it hurts.

Words Can Be Poison

The stigma of mental illness is real, painful, and damaging to the lives of people with mental illness. Stigma prevents them from getting the treatment and support they need to lead healthy, normal lives.

Stigma discourages people from getting help. At any given time, one in four adults and one in five children experience a mental health problem. Early and appropriate services can be the best way to prevent an illness from getting worse. Many people don't seek such services because they don't want to be labeled as "mentally ill" or "crazy."

Stigma keeps people from getting good jobs and advancing in the workplace. Some employers are reluctant to hire people who have mental illnesses. Thanks to the Americans with Disabilities Act (ADA), such discrimination is illegal. But it still happens.

Stigma leads to fear, mistrust, and violence. Even though the majority of people who have mental illnesses are no more violent than anyone else, the average television viewer sees three people with mental illnesses each week—and most of them are portrayed as violent. Such inaccurate portrayals lead people to fear those who have mental illnesses.

Stigma results in prejudice and discrimination. Many individuals try to prevent people who have mental illnesses from living in their neighborhoods.

Stigma results in inadequate insurance coverage. Many insurance plans do not cover mental health services to the same degree as other illnesses. When mental illnesses are covered, coverage may be limited, inappropriate, or inadequate.

Words Can Heal

Here are six steps you can follow to help end the stigma which surrounds mental illness:

- **Learn more.** Many organizations sponsor nationwide programs about mental health and mental illness.
- **Insist on accountable media.** Sometimes the media portray people who have mental illnesses inaccurately, and this makes stereotypes harder to change.

- **Obey the laws in the Americans with Disabilities Act (ADA).** The ADA prohibits discrimination against people with disabilities in all areas of public life, including housing, employment, and public transportation. Mental illnesses are considered a disability covered under the ADA.
- **Recognize and appreciate the contributions to society** made by people who have mental illnesses. People who have mental illnesses are major contributors to American life—from the arts to the sciences, from medicine to entertainment to professional sports.
- **Treat people with the dignity and respect we all deserve.** People who have mental illnesses may include your friends, your neighbors, and your family.
- **Think about the person**—the contents behind the label. Avoid labeling people by their diagnosis. Instead of saying, "She's a schizophrenic," say, "She has a mental illness." Never use the term "mentally ill."

Chapter 62

Anger Management Strategies for People with Mental Health Disorders

The Problem of Anger

In the most general sense, anger is a feeling or emotion that ranges from mild irritation to intense fury and rage. Anger is a natural response to those situations where we feel threatened, we believe harm will come to us, or we believe that another person has unnecessarily wronged us. We may also become angry when we feel another person, like a child or someone close to us, is being threatened or harmed. In addition, anger may result from frustration when our needs, desires, and goals are not being met. When we become angry, we may lose our patience and act impulsively, aggressively, or violently.

People often confuse anger with aggression. Aggression is behavior that is intended to cause harm to another person or damage property. This behavior can include verbal abuse, threats, or violent acts. Anger, on the other hand, is an emotion and does not necessarily lead to aggression. Therefore, a person can become angry without acting aggressively.

A term related to anger and aggression is hostility. Hostility refers to a complex set of attitudes and judgments that motivate aggressive behaviors. Whereas anger is an emotion and aggression is a

---

Excerpted from "Anger Management for Substance Abuse and Mental Health Clients," by the Substance Abuse and Mental Health Services Administration (SAMHSA, mentalhealth.samhsa.gov), part of the U.S. Department of Health and Human Services, 2003. Reviewed by David A. Cooke, M.D., January 23, 2009.

behavior, hostility is an attitude that involves disliking others and evaluating them negatively.

When Does Anger Become a Problem?

Anger becomes a problem when it is felt too intensely, is felt too frequently, or is expressed inappropriately. Feeling anger too intensely or frequently places extreme physical strain on the body. During prolonged and frequent episodes of anger, certain divisions of the nervous system become highly activated. Consequently, blood pressure and heart rate increase and stay elevated for long periods. This stress on the body may produce many different health problems, such as hypertension, heart disease, and diminished immune system efficiency. Thus, from a health standpoint, avoiding physical illness is a motivation for controlling anger.

Another compelling reason to control anger concerns the negative consequences that result from expressing anger inappropriately. In the extreme, anger may lead to violence or physical aggression, which can result in numerous negative consequences, such as being arrested or jailed, being physically injured, being retaliated against, losing loved ones, being terminated from a substance abuse treatment or social service program, or feeling guilt, shame, or regret.

Even when anger does not lead to violence, the inappropriate expression of anger, such as verbal abuse or intimidating or threatening behavior, often results in negative consequences. For example, it is likely that others will develop fear, resentment, and lack of trust toward those who subject them to angry outbursts, which may cause alienation from individuals, such as family members, friends, and coworkers.

Payoffs and Consequences

The inappropriate expression of anger initially has many apparent payoffs. One payoff is being able to manipulate and control others through aggressive and intimidating behavior; others may comply with someone's demands because they fear verbal threats or violence. Another payoff is the release of tension that occurs when one loses his or her temper and acts aggressively.

The individual may feel better after an angry outburst, but everyone else may feel worse. In the long term, however, these initial payoffs lead to negative consequences. For this reason they are called "apparent" payoffs because the long-term negative consequences far outweigh the short-term gains. For example, consider a father who persuades his children to comply with his demands by using an angry tone of voice and threatening gestures. These behaviors imply to the children that they will receive physical harm if they are not obedient. The immediate payoff for the father is that the children obey his commands. The long-term consequence, however, may be that the children learn to fear or dislike him and become emotionally detached from him. As they grow older, they may avoid contact with him or refuse to see him altogether.

Breaking the Anger Habit

Becoming aware of anger: To break the anger habit, you must develop an awareness of the events, circumstances, and behaviors of others that "trigger" your anger. This awareness also involves understanding the negative consequences that result from anger. For example, you may be in line at the supermarket and become impatient because the lines are too long. You could become angry, then boisterously demand that the checkout clerk call for more help. As your anger escalates, you may become involved in a heated exchange with the clerk or another customer.

The store manager may respond by having a security officer remove you from the store. The negative consequences that result from this event are not getting the groceries that you wanted and the embarrassment and humiliation you suffer from being removed from the store.

Strategies for controlling anger: In addition to becoming aware of anger, you need to develop strategies to effectively manage it. These strategies can be used to stop the escalation of anger before you lose control and experience negative consequences. An effective set of strategies for controlling anger should include both immediate and preventive strategies. Immediate strategies include taking a timeout, deep-breathing exercises, and thought stopping. Preventive strategies include developing an exercise program and changing your irrational beliefs.

One example of an immediate anger management strategy worth exploring at this point is the timeout. The timeout can be used formally or informally. For now, we will only describe the informal use of a timeout. This use involves leaving a situation if you feel your anger is escalating out of control. For example, you may be a passenger on a crowded bus and become angry because you perceive that people are deliberately bumping into you. In this situation, you can simply get off the bus and wait for a less crowded bus.

The informal use of a timeout may also involve stopping yourself from engaging in a discussion or argument if you feel that you are becoming too angry. In these situations, it may be helpful to actually call a timeout or to give the timeout sign with your hands. This lets the other person know that you wish to immediately stop talking about the topic and are becoming frustrated, upset, or angry.

Cognitive-Behavioral Therapy

Cognitive behavioral therapy (CBT) treatments have been found to be effective, time-limited treatments for anger problems. Four types of CBT interventions, theoretically unified by principles of social learning theory, are most often used when treating anger disorders:

- relaxation interventions, which target emotional and physiological components of anger;
- cognitive interventions, which target cognitive processes such as hostile appraisals and attributions, irrational beliefs, and inflammatory thinking;
- communication skills interventions, which target deficits in assertiveness and conflict resolution skills; and
- combined interventions, which integrate two or more CBT interventions and target multiple response domains.

Meta-analysis studies conclude that there are moderate anger reduction effects for CBT interventions, with average effect sizes ranging from 0.7 to 1.2. From these studies, it can be inferred that the average participant under CBT conditions fared better than 76 percent of control participants. These results are consistent with other meta-analysis studies examining the effectiveness of CBT interventions in the treatment of depression and anxiety.

Some treatment models use a combined CBT approach that employs relaxation, cognitive, and communication skills interventions. This combined approach presents the participants with options that draw on these different interventions and then encourages them to develop individualized anger control plans using as many of the techniques as possible. Not all the participants use all the techniques and interventions presented in the treatment (e.g., cognitive restructuring), but almost all finish the treatment with more than one technique or intervention on their anger control plans.

Theoretically, the more techniques and interventions an individual has on his or her anger control plan, the better equipped he or she will be to manage anger in response to anger-provoking events.

Chapter 63

What to Do When Depression Enters a Relationship

The pressure of being in a relationship can feel overwhelming to someone living with depression. When you're struggling with an illness that makes you tired, sad, and generally uninterested in life, often the last thing on your mind are the needs of others. Equally frustrating and emotionally draining is trying to maintain a relationship with someone who's depressed. It's hurtful and confusing when loved ones increasingly isolate themselves, pull away, and reject others' efforts to help. All of these feelings and reactions can damage relationships, whether they're with spouses, partners, children, or friends.

Each year, depression affects an estimated 19 million Americans and countless numbers of loved ones. It can test even the most secure of relationships. The good news is that depression is very treatable and by taking the appropriate steps to combat the illness, your relationship can survive.

Steps to Overcome Depression and Keep Your Relationship Healthy

- The most important step toward successful recovery is to seek treatment. With the appropriate combination of "talk" therapy

---

and medication, people with depression can achieve remission (virtual elimination) of symptoms and reconnect with life and with relationships.

If you're experiencing symptoms of depression:

- Share your feelings with others as much as possible. Your reluctance to talk about how you feel only creates distance between you and your loved ones. It's especially important to keep the lines of communication open during trying times.
- Let your partner know that you still find him or her attractive. An affectionate touch and a few reassuring words can mean a lot, even if you don't feel inclined toward more intimate relations.
- Consider couples or family counseling. Your willingness to talk about your relationship and how it may be affected by depression speaks volumes to family members and loved ones about their importance in your life.
- Keep working toward recovery. Today's treatment options make that more realistic than ever.
- To resolve all your symptoms, a combination of medication and "talk" therapy may be recommended. Your physician will help you determine the right levels of medication and how long you should stay on them.

If you're in a relationship with someone experiencing depression:

- Remember, your role is to offer support and encourage your loved one to seek professional help. Encourage your partner not to settle for partial improvement and explain that with the right treatment, people with depression can regain their lives.
- Although you may be prepared to do anything and everything to help, don't try to take over the life of someone who is depressed. Your loved one may seem overwhelmed, incapable, or frustrated, but you can't reconstruct his or her life.
- Give advice in the form of options. For example, recommend a physician for your partner to see or suggest support groups you think may be a step toward alleviating his or her symptoms.

- Remember that depression is a real illness that should be taken seriously. Don't belittle the person by saying things such as "Snap out of it," "Get over it," or "Everyone feels down now and then." Try your best to understand the illness.
- Recognize that depression is not rational. It is painful to be rejected, scorned, or ignored, but this may be how your loved one responds to your efforts to help.
- Care for yourself. Carve out time to pursue your own interests and to socialize even when your partner can't join you. You might also want to consider seeking individual counseling.

Chapter 64

Rights, Protection, and Advocacy: Information for People with Mental Health Disorders

Where can I obtain free mental health advocacy and/or technical or legal assistance?

Each State, the District of Columbia, and the six Territories (American Indian Consortium, American Samoa, Guam, the Northern Mariana Islands, Puerto Rico, and the Virgin Islands) have a Protection and Advocacy for Individuals with Mental Illness (PAIMI) program. PAIMI programs safeguard the rights of people with significant mental illnesses who are at risk for abuse, neglect, or civil rights violations while receiving care or treatment in a public or private residential facility. If a violation is found, PAIMI programs may pursue various remedies such as mediation, administrative hearings, and litigation (the remedy of last resort) to ensure protection of the rights of PAIMI-eligible clients. People with mental illnesses who are not eligible for PAIMI services may be eligible for services from other programs within their State Protection and Advocacy (P&A) system, such as the Protection and Advocacy for Individual Rights (PAIR) Program, Client Assistance Program (CAP), Protection and Advocacy for Beneficiaries of Social Security (PABSS) Program, Protection and Advocacy for Developmental Disabilities (PADD) Program, Protection and

---

From "Rights and Protection and Advocacy," by the Substance Abuse and Mental Health Services Administration (SAMHSA, mentalhealth.samhsa.gov), part of the U.S. Department of Health and Human Services, May 2003. Despite the older date of this document, the information it provides is still relevant.

Advocacy for Assistive Technology (PAAT) Program, Protection and Advocacy for Voters Rights (PAVR) Program, and Protection and Advocacy for Traumatic Brain Injury (PATBI) Program.

What are the eligibility requirements for the PAIMI Program?

Individuals eligible for PAIMI:

- Are diagnosed with a significant mental illness or emotional impairment, as determined by a mental health professional qualified under the laws and regulations of the State; and
- Are inpatients or residents in public or private residential facilities that provide care or treatment to individuals with mental illnesses; and
- Were abused, neglected, or had their rights violated, or were in danger of abuse, neglect, or rights violations, while receiving care or treatment in a public or private residential facility.

In addition, the services requested must be within the State P&A system's PAIMI program priorities and objectives for the current Federal fiscal year. To see if your request is within your State protection and advocacy agency's annual service priorities, contact your State system.

What can I do if I feel my employer, or a potential employer, has discriminated against me because of my mental disability?

The Americans with Disabilities Act (ADA) is a legal tool to fight discrimination. Any person who believes he or she has experienced employment discrimination based on a psychiatric disability has a right to file an administrative "charge" or "complaint" with the U.S. Equal Employment Opportunity Commission (EEOC) or with a State or local anti-discrimination agency. Such individuals also may file a lawsuit in court, but only after filing an administrative charge. For information on how to file a discrimination charge, the publication Filing an ADA Employment Discrimination Charge: Making It Work for You [http://mentalhealth.samhsa.gov/publications/allpubs/SMA00-3471/default.asp] may be helpful.

You also may find it useful to contact the:

U.S. Equal Employment Opportunity Commission
1801 L Street, NW
Washington, DC 20507
Phone: 202-663-4900
Website: www.eeoc.gov

U.S. Department of Justice
950 Pennsylvania Avenue, NW
Civil Rights Division
Disability Rights Section–NYAVE
Washington, DC. 20530
ADA Information Line: 800-514-0301
TDD: 800-514-0383
Website: www.usdoj.gov

National Disability Rights Network
900 Second Street, NE, Suite 211
Washington, DC 20002
Phone: 202-408-9514
Website: www.ndrn.org

What can I do if I was discriminated against in a private or commercial facility or could not get into a government program because the building lacked access?

The U.S. Department of Justice provides information on how to file complaints against private facilities, government programs, and public transportation services. Complaints against private or commercial facilities are covered under Title III of the Americans with Disabilities Act (ADA) According to the Department of Justice, facilities included under Title III are "places of lodging, establishments serving food and drink, places of exhibition or entertainment, places of public gathering, sales or rental establishments, service establishments, stations used for specified public transportation, places of public display or collection, places of recreation, places of education, social service center establishments, and places of exercise or recreation. Title III also covers commercial facilities (such as warehouses, factories, and office buildings), private transportation services, and licensing and testing practices." Title II of the ADA covers access to government programs and public transportation. To find out how to file a formal complaint under either Title III or Title II, you can access these documents from the Department of Justice: Title III Complaints [http://www.ada.gov/t3compfm.htm] or Title II Complaints [http://www.ada.gov/t2cmpfrm.htm]. The Department of Justice also offers an informal method for resolving some Title III and Title II complaints. Through the Department of Justice ADA Mediation Program, professional mediators will handle complaints that are appropriate for mediation at no expense to the persons involved in the complaint. To request help from the mediation program, you will need to submit either a Title II or Title III complaint form and note on the form that you wish to resolve the dispute by mediation.

What can I do if I have a complaint about the mental health treatment that someone is receiving?

You may want to start by contacting the facility or program administrators to make them aware of your complaint. If you cannot reach a resolution in this way, you may want to contact your State Mental Health Agency to determine if your State has a commission that reviews quality of care. If not, each State, the District of Columbia, and the six Territories have a Protection and Advocacy for Individuals with Mental Illness (PAIMI) program. PAIMI programs investigate reports of abuse, neglect, and civil rights violations in facilities providing mental health care or treatment. Other programs within your State Protection and Advocacy (P&A) system are listed in the answer to the first question.

Chapter 65

Employment and Housing Concerns for People with Mental Health Disorders

Chapter Contents

Section 65.1

Getting and Keeping a Job

Excerpted from "Mental Illness Is Not a Full-Time Job," by the Substance Abuse and Mental Health Services Administration (SAMHSA, www.mentalhealth.samhsa.gov), part of the U.S. Department of Health and Human Services, 1996. Reviewed by David A. Cooke, M.D., January 10, 2009.

Like all workers, people with severe mental illnesses can benefit greatly from the security and self-sufficiency that come with stable and fulfilling employment.

In addition to providing a living, work gives people a sense of belonging and community. It also creates a network of friends and colleagues.

Mental health problems can occur at any age. Young people with mental health problems may be looking for entry-level jobs. Adults with mental illness may need to learn new skills, pursue different employment paths, or develop ways to stay on their current job. At any point in a person's life, severe mental illness will present challenges which, with the right support, people can overcome.

Getting and Keeping a Job

Many communities have resources to help people with mental illness acquire the skills needed to find and keep a job.

Supported employment—which can include vocational training or retraining and job coaching—is one way that people with mental illness can make their way into the work world. Models of supported employment include individual placement and support (IPS) and clubhouses. The Employment Intervention Demonstration Program, an initiative funded by the Center for Mental Health Services in the Substance Abuse and Mental Health Services Administration, is studying ways to help consumers keep competitive jobs—real work for real wages in the real world.

Taking the First Steps

For people with severe mental illness who are just entering the workforce, there are a few ways to start their job search. They may ask their therapist, social worker, case manager, or psychiatrist to recommend a supported employment agency. They can ask friends to recommend helpful programs. Consumer advocacy organizations often offer employment guidance or can refer people to agencies in their community.

State and local governments have local employment service agencies. Most also have vocational rehabilitation agencies that can help people with mental illness acquire new skills and be successful in the job market.

Equal Protection Under the Law: The Americans with Disabilities Act (ADA)

The ADA mandates that all people have a fair chance to pursue their dreams. The Act prohibits businesses that employ 15 or more people from discriminating against a qualified candidate on the basis of his or her disability—including mental illness. Businesses must make reasonable accommodations—such as adapting training materials and providing flexible work schedules or routines—for qualified people with disabilities.

Adapted with permission from *Working on the Dream: A Guide to Career Planning and Job Success*, by Don Lavin and Andrea Everett. Rise, Inc., 1996.

Section 65.2

Supported Employment

From "Supported Employment: For Consumers," by the Substance Abuse and Mental Health Services Administration (SAMHSA, mentalhealth.samhsa.gov), part of the U.S. Department of Health and Human Services, 2003. Reviewed by David A. Cooke, M.D., January 23, 2009.

For many people, work is an important part of the recovery process. But sometimes our talents and abilities are overlooked. Some people believe that because we have a mental illness, we are unable to work a job in the community. However, experience and research have shown that mental health consumers want to work and can work. We are capable of surprising those who doubt our ability to have a meaningful job. With the right type of work support, work can become a reality for many of us.

It can feel that all vocational programs are the same because they try to get people to work in workshops or places that only have jobs for people with disabilities. Fortunately, this is not always the case.

This text provides information about supported employment—a service that helps consumers find and maintain meaningful jobs in the community. The jobs are competitive (paying at least minimum wage) and are based on a person's preferences and abilities.

Work can have many benefits.

For most of us, work is part of our identity. When we feel good about having a job, we often see ourselves in a more positive way. Work provides structure and routines. Job income gives us more choices about what to buy, where to live, and gives us a chance to build savings.

When researchers have asked consumers if they want to work, nearly 7 out of every 10 consumers said they would like to have a job. Research shows 6 out of every 10 consumers can work at a job in the community if they are provided with the right types of services and supports.

Supported employment has helped many consumers already.

Researchers have studied different types of programs that help consumers find and keep employment. These studies compare supported employment to many other vocational approaches and they consistently find that supported employment assists more consumers with getting and keeping their jobs than any other approach.

Supported employment is based on six principles.

- Eligibility is based on consumer choice. No one is excluded who wants to participate.
- Supported employment is integrated with treatment. Employment specialists coordinate plans with your treatment team: your case manager, therapist, psychiatrist, etc.
- Competitive employment is the goal. The focus is community jobs anyone can apply for that pay at least minimum wage, including part-time and full-time jobs.
- Job search starts soon after a consumer expresses interest in working. There are no requirements for completing extensive pre-employment assessment and training, or intermediate work experiences (like prevocational work units, transitional employment, or sheltered workshops).
- Follow-along supports are continuous. Individualized supports to maintain employment continue as long as consumers want the assistance.
- Consumer preferences are important. Choices and decisions about work and support are individualized based on the person's preferences, strengths, and experiences.

Supported employment starts with you.

This program does not force you to work. With supported employment, you let employment specialists (people who work for a supported employment team) or other members of your treatment team (case manager, therapist, psychiatrist, etc.) know that you are interested in having a job. If you want to work, you will be given the supports and services to help you make your career goals a possibility.

Working part-time is also your choice. Employment specialists are trained to understand that you will be happier with a career that fits your needs rather than a job that you have to fit into.

Your job choices are important.

You may know of some careers that interest you, or have a work history. Employment specialists will listen to your preferences. The type of job that you will get through supported employment depends on your choices. If you are unsure about what specific career you want, your employment specialist can help you with questions and ideas about employment.

Taking tests, filling out forms and waiting for referrals are not required before starting in supported employment. Your employment specialist will start meeting with you soon after you identify work as a goal.

Employment specialists help you obtain information on how your benefits, such as Social Security or Medicaid, are affected by working.

Many consumers worry about starting work and how their benefits may be affected. Employment specialists assist you in obtaining accurate information. There are benefit programs that can help you continue to receive benefits, or partial benefits even when you are earning an income from work.

Supported employment is an ongoing service.

Employment specialists are available to help you plan your career, manage surprises that may come up at work, and develop ways to help you succeed after you have obtained a job. Working is sometimes stressful. When you are hired, an employment specialist will continue to provide supports and services.

It is not uncommon for people to change jobs a few times before finding a job they want to keep. Your employment specialist can talk with you about ending an unsatisfying job and looking for a better job match.

For More Information

Supported employment services are provided by numerous agencies across the country. If you are interested in knowing more about supported employment, or want to receive these services, contact staff at your local mental health or vocational agency.

Section 65.3

Housing Options for People with Mental Health Disorders

"Housing Options For People With Mental Illness," by the Substance Abuse and Mental Health Services Administration (SAMHSA, mental health.samhsa.gov), part of the U.S. Department of Health and Human Services, April 2003. Despite the older date of this document, the information it provides is still relevant.

Why are housing choices so important?

For people with severe mental illness, home can be a space to live in dignity and move toward recovery.

What factors should be considered as part of a housing decision?

- How much can you afford to pay?
- Is the neighborhood pleasant? Is it safe?
- If you share your living space, will your housemates be compatible?
- Is the house, apartment, or room in good condition?
- Is transportation to shopping and your treatment center nearby?
- How much support will you need to carry out everyday activities?
- Does your prospective landlord have a reputation for responding promptly and courteously to tenants' requests?

Also, have the lease reviewed before you sign on the dotted line. If you need help with finding a place, filling out forms, or reviewing a lease, your caseworker is a valuable resource. If you do not have a caseworker, contact the advocacy group or the housing specialist at the public mental health agency nearest you.

What are the different types of housing programs that are available?

Public housing: Although the kinds of housing vary from state to state, public housing programs basically operate as follows:

- **Section 8:** The tenant-based rental assistance program provides vouchers or certificates to subsidize rent. Under this program, a person pays either 30 percent of his or her adjusted income, 10 percent of gross income, or the welfare assistance amount designated for housing. The certificate or voucher pays the remainder of the rent to the landlord.
- **Chapter 9:** The project-based rental assistance program offers landlords an incentive to provide housing for people with disabilities by tying the subsidy to the rental building. The demand for this housing also outstrips the number of available units.

Other housing: States and localities also fund housing programs. In addition, some for-profit organizations offer housing for people with disabilities. Contact your local or state mental health authority to find out about licensing and required services. In general, many localities offer several of the following options:

- private residential housing,
- commercial boarding homes,
- supported independent living,
- personal care group homes,
- community residential rehabilitation centers,
- structured residential programs, and
- 24-hour care homes and nursing facilities.

Who can I contact for more information?

To find the best housing option for you, work closely with your mental health caseworker. In addition, your local affiliates of the National Alliance on Mental Illness (NAMI) and Mental Health America should have information on housing options in your area. Check your telephone directory, or call the national offices for a referral to your local affiliate.

Section 65.4

Mental Health Disorders and Homelessness

"Mental Illness and Homelessness," © 2006 National Coalition for the Homeless. Reprinted with permission.

An average of 16% of the single adult homeless population suffers from some form of severe and persistent mental illness (National Resource and Training Center on Homelessness and Mental Illness, 2003). While 22% of the American population suffers from a mental illness, a small percentage of the 44 million people who have a serious mental illness are homeless at any given point in time (National Institute of Mental Health, 2005). In a 2007 survey performed by the U.S. Conference of Mayors, of the 23 cities surveyed, 7.9% of the homeless population of individuals in a family suffer from some type of mental illness. Additionally, 22.4% of the homeless individuals in this survey have a mental illness.

Despite the disproportionate number of mentally ill people among the homeless population, the growth in homelessness is not attributable to the release of seriously mentally ill people from institutions. Most patients were released from mental hospitals in the 1950s and 1960s, yet vast increases in homelessness did not occur until the 1980s when incomes and housing options for those living on the margins began to diminish rapidly. The mass deinstitutionalization from mental health facilities occurred over forty years ago, yet the promise of community-based programs and outpatient services has not been kept especially towards the homeless and others living in poverty (Mental Illness, *Chronic Homelessness: An American Disgrace*, 2000). A new wave of deinstitutionalization and the denial of services or premature and unplanned discharge brought about by managed care arrangements may be contributing to the continued presence of seriously mentally ill persons within the homeless population.

Mental disorders prevent people from carrying out essential aspects of daily life, such as self-care, household management, and interpersonal relationships. Homeless people with mental disorders remain homeless for longer periods of time and have less contact with family and friends. Many of the mentally ill (especially those with severe disorders such as schizophrenia, bipolar disorder, and major depression), both the homeless and others, often misinterpret the guidance of others and react irrationally because of their condition(s). This pushes away friends and family and other caregivers occasionally leading to homelessness or a longer a period of homelessness (Mental Illness, *Chronic Homelessness: An American Disgrace*, 2000).

The mentally ill homeless population encounters more barriers to employment, tend to be in poorer physical health, and have more contact with the legal system than homeless people who do not suffer from mental disorder. All people with mental disorders, including those who are homeless, require ongoing access to a full range of treatment and rehabilitation services to lessen the impairment and disruption produced by their condition. However, most people with mental disorder do not need hospitalization, and even fewer require long-term institutional care.

According to the 2003 U.S. Department of Health and Human Services Report, most homeless persons with mental illness do not need to be institutionalized, but can live in the community with the appropriate supportive housing options (U.S. Department of Health and Human Services, 2003). Unfortunately, there are not enough community-based treatment services, nor enough appropriate, affordable housing, to accommodate the number of people disabled by mental disorders in the United States. However, studies have found that a supported housing treatment program would most likely be more effective than other methods of treatment for homeless mentally ill individuals, and though the cost may be slightly be more, the increased benefits make supported housing the most effective method (Rosenheck, et al., 2003).

Federal demonstration programs have produced a large body of knowledge on the service and treatment needs of homeless individuals with serious mental illnesses. The research exists to make effective programs, yet the political support and finances to support these programs has been minimal (Mental Illness, *Chronic Homelessness: An American Disgrace*, 2000). Many homeless people who have mental illnesses need independent housing with supports (National Resource and Training Center on Homelessness and Mental Illness, 2003). Findings also reveal that persons with mental disorder and persons with addictive disorders share many of the same treatment needs, including carefully designed client engagement and case management, housing options, and long-term follow-up and support services. Studies also emphasize the importance of service integration, outreach, and engagement; the use of case management to negotiate care systems; the need for a range of supportive housing and treatment options that are responsive to consumer preferences; and the importance of meaningful daily activity. When combined with supportive services, meaningful daily activity in the community (including work), access to therapy, and appropriate housing can provide the framework necessary to end homelessness for many individuals.

Policy Issues

Low-income people with mental disorders are at increased risk of homelessness. A variety of approaches must be employed to help them obtain and retain stable housing to prevent homelessness.

In addition, programs that assure access to mainstream and targeted community-based services for homeless people with serious mental illness, such as the Projects for Assistance in Transition from Homelessness (PATH) program, should be expanded. It was founded in FY [fiscal year] 2006 at only $54 million making it unable to meet the needs of many people with serious mental illness who are homeless or at risk of becoming homeless (National Health Care for the Homeless Council, 2007).

Supplemental Security Income (SSI) benefit levels must be increased so that disabled Americans are not forced to live in poverty. Individual recipients of SSI receive $603 a month, and for many this is their sole source of income. This allows an individual to afford only $180 for rent, making any kind of housing unaffordable (NLIHC, 2004). In most states, even if the SSI grant does cover the rent, only a few dollars remain for other expenses. Benefit levels have not kept up with increases in the cost of rent and therefore do not provide disabled individuals with adequate allowances for housing.

Finally, the commitment to making deinstitutionalization work as it was intended must be renewed. People with mental illness must be able to live as independently as possible with the help of expanded comprehensive, community-based mental health services and other supports. It is crucial that policies be proactive rather than reactive. Services such as crisis intervention, landlord-tenant intervention, continuous treatment teams, and appropriate discharge planning in jails and inpatient facilities must be made available in all communities.

References

Federal Task Force on Homelessness and Severe Mental Illness. *Outcasts on Main Street: A Report of the Federal Task Force on Homelessness and Severe Mental Illness*, 1992. Available, free, from the National Resource Center on Homelessness and Mental Illness, 262 Delaware Ave., Delmar, NY, 12054-1123; 800-444-7415.

Kaufman, Tracy L. *Out of Reach: Rental Housing At What Cost?* 1997. Available for $25.00 from the National Low Income Housing Coalition, 1012 14th St., NW, #610, Washington, DC 20005-3410, 202-662-1530.

Koegel, Paul, et al. "The Causes of Homelessness," in *Homelessness in America*, 1996, Oryx Press. National Coalition for the Homeless, 2201 P St., NW, Washington, DC, 20037; 202-462-4822.

Lezak, Anne and Elizabeth Edgar. *Preventing Homelessness Among People with Serious Mental Illness: A Guide for States*, 1998. Available, free, from the National Resource Center on Homelessness and Mental Illness, 262 Delaware Ave., Delmar, NY, 12054-1123; 800-444-7415.

National Institute of Mental Health. "The Numbers Count," 2005. Available at www.nimh.nih.gov.

"Mental Illness, Chronic Homelessness: An American Disgrace." *Healing Hands*, October 2000. Available from http://www.nhchc.org/healinghands.html.

National Low Income Housing Coalition. "Out of Reach 2004." Available at www.nlihc.org.

National Resource and Training Center on Homelessness and Mental Illness, "Get the Facts," 2003. Available at www.nrchmi.samhsa.gov.

Oakley, Deirdre and Deborah L. Dennis, "Responding to the Needs of Homeless People with Alcohol, Drug, and/or Mental Disorders," in *Homelessness in America*, Oryx Press, 1996. National Coalition for the Homeless, 2201 P St., NW, Washington, DC, 20037; 202-462-4822.

Wells, Susan Milstrey. *Projects for Assistance in Transition from Homelessness: A Summary of Fiscal Year 1994 State Implementation Reports*, 1996. Available, free, from National Coalition for the Homeless, 1012 14th Street, NW, Suite 600, Washington, DC 20005; 202-737-6444.

Rosenheck, R., Kasprow, W., Frisman, L., and Liu-Mares, W. "Cost-effectiveness of Supported Housing for Homeless Persons with Mental Illnesses." *Archive of General Psychiatry*, September 2003. Available from www.archgenpsychiatry.com.

Chapter 66

Psychiatric Advance Directives: Frequently Asked Questions

What are the advantages of a psychiatric advance directive?

If you expect to need mental health treatment in the future and believe that you might be found incompetent to make your decisions at that time:

- An advance directive empowers you to make your treatment preferences known.
- An advance directive will improve communication between you and your physician. It can prevent clashes with professionals over treatment and may prevent forced treatment.
- Having an advance directive may shorten your hospital stay.

Will my psychiatric advance directive be legally binding?

While advance directives for health care have been around a long time, their use for psychiatric care is a very new area of law. We do not yet know how courts will deal with them, especially when safety issues arise. State laws vary and it is possible that part or all of this document will not be effective in your state. However, many mental health consumers who are now using these documents find that an

---

advance directive increases the likelihood that doctors, hospitals, and judges honor their choices.

Please note that template forms at http://www.bazelon.org do not constitute legal advice. Before you assume that the advance directive you create using these forms will be legally valid in your state, you should consult a lawyer.

Where can I get legal advice about advance directives in my state?

Your state Protection and Advocacy System (P&A) may be able to tell you about your state's requirements or refer you to a lawyer who can. For the name and number of the system in your state, visit the website of the National Disability Rights Network or call NDRN at 202-408-9514. The Bazelon Center is not able to respond to individual inquiries.

Additional information is available from the following:

- For an analysis of state statutes relating to advance directives for mental health care, see Robert Fleishner's article [http://www.napas.org].
- A bibliography of cases and materials on advance directives for people with mental illness [http://www.napas.org].
- Two articles on Advance Directives are available on the National Empowerment Center website: "Making Advance Directives Work for You," [http://www.power2u.org/articles/selfhelp/directives_work.html] by Daniel Fisher, M.D., Ph.D. and "Advance Directives Are What You Make Them," [http://www.power2u.org/articles/selfhelp/directives.html] by Xenia Williams.
- California Protection and Advocacy, Inc. has "Advance Health Care Directives" [http://www.pai-ca.org/pubs/508801.pdf] on its website (also available en español) [http://www.pai-ca.org/pubs/508802.pdf].
- In New York, the Resource Center [http://www.peer-resource.org] provides training, educational materials, and technical assistance to consumers, survivors, and providers in New York. The center's Advance Directive Training Project is designed to provide training to recipients of mental health services (in particular, those who might be impacted by involuntary outpatient commitment under New York's Assisted Outpatient Treatment Law)

in developing and implementing advance directive documents for use when they are unable to make their own health care decisions. The Resource Center website includes information about the use of psychiatric advance directives in New York, along with sample forms.

- The New York State Commission on Quality Care [http://www.cqc.state.ny.us/hottopics/advdi.htm] also has information about mental health care advance directives on its website.
- In New York, the Office of Mental Health Bureau of Children and Families has been working with consumers to develop the "Prime Directive Initiative," the goal of which is to give young people a voice in their treatment and service planning. They are developing two documents, "My Prime Directive Journal" and "My Prime Directive." The Journal is designed to inform youth of some of the choices they might want to think about for their self-care and the Prime Directive is a place to record what they need from others. It was announced in June 2001 that the documents, which are designed for use by consumers who will decide whether to share them with others, will be available soon. More information is in *OMH Quarterly* [http://www.omh.state.ny.us/], June 2001, Vol. 7, No. 1.
- North Carolina has a law governing "Advance Instructions for Mental Health Treatment" (AIMHT), in addition to its laws on living wills and general health care power of attorney documents. Many have found this separate statutory scheme problematic. Some attorneys in the state advise clients to incorporate mental health treatment powers in a general health care power of attorney to minimize potential problems with, for example, automatic expiration, revocation rules, witnessing requirements and ambiguities in a provider's obligation to comply with advance instructions. An analysis of the law and sample forms are available in Schwab, Carol, "A Critical Analysis of North Carolina's Advance Instruction for Mental Health Treatment," [http://www.ncsu.edu/ffci/index.php] The Forum for Family and Consumer Issues 3.1 (1998) (March 7, 1998).
- Ohio Legal Rights Service (the protection and advocacy system) [http://olrs.ohio.gov/ASP/olrs_AdvanceDirect.asp] has on its website information about "Advance Directives for Health Care" and a form for a "Durable Power of Attorney for Health Care and Declaration of Treatment Instructions."

- The Oregon Advocacy Center (the state's protection and advocacy system) [http://www.oradvocacy.org] has produced a guide for consumers and families on the state's mental health law, which includes information on a "Mental Health Declaration," which can include decisions on medications, ECT and hospitalization, under certain circumstances.
- Advocacy Inc., the Texas P&A, has information on its website [http://www.advocacyinc.org] about how to make a Declaration for Mental Health Treatment under Texas law, including sample forms.
- The West Virginia Mental Health Consumers Association has a Toolkit on Advance Directives for consumers, family members, and providers. [http://www.contac.org]

Have any courts upheld the validity of psychiatric advance directives?

Permitting people who are not mentally ill to engage in advance planning through advance directive instruments on a wider basis than people with mental illnesses raises significant issues. To date one federal court has addressed such an issue. A Vermont law allows doctors to go to court to nullify mental health provisions in a durable power of attorney/advance directive if the treatment choices made by the agent do not result in improvement of the declarant's condition. In October 2001, a federal Magistrate Judge ruled that this provision is discriminatory and violates the Americans with Disabilities Act. The decision is *Hargrave v. State of Vermont*, No. 2:99-CV-128 (D. Vt. Oct. 11, 2001). Also available is a brief of 18 former state mental health commissioners, the National Mental Health Association, and other as *amici curiae* in support of the appellees in *Hargrave v. State of Vermont*.

The plaintiff, Nancy Hargrave, had been diagnosed with a serious mental illness. She was involuntarily medicated, in direct contravention of her wishes expressly stated in her Durable Power of Attorney for Health Care. At issue in the case was whether the State of Vermont had the right to override a durable power of attorney with involuntary psychiatric medication in a non-emergency situation, thereby depriving individuals with mental illnesses from executing a durable power of attorney for health care that is afforded the same recognition and enforcement as the advance directives instruments executed by people who do not have mental illnesses.

Do I have to appoint an agent?

That depends on the law in your state. In some states, you may set up an advance directive without appointing a person to act for you. In most states, however, an advance directive for psychiatric care is only valid if you have named an agent. The Bazelon Center's study of advance directives suggests that these tools are much more likely to be honored when an agent has been appointed. We strongly urge consumers to name an agent whenever possible.

If you appoint an agent, it should be someone you trust. You can direct your agent to present the choices you have expressed in your advance directive. You can also authorize him or her to make other decisions about your care that are not in your directive. Or you can appoint an agent without giving any written instructions, but if you do this, you should clearly explain what your wishes are so he or she can advocate effectively on your behalf.

The template includes a provision (item 5 in Section II) that your agent's decisions about mental health treatment would prevail even if a court appoints a guardian or conservator for you.

Does the document cover health care, too?

No. The document you produce with these template forms will be an advance directive for mental health decision-making only; it will not cover decisions about other medical or surgical treatment. It is a good idea to have an advance directive for health care as well, stating your preferences about emergency medical treatment. Forms to create one are available from most hospitals and health agencies. A form for New York State can be downloaded at http://www.cqc.state.ny.us.

Part Eight

Mental Health Concerns in Children and Adolescents

Chapter 67

What Every Child Needs for Good Mental Health

It is easy for parents to identify their child's physical needs: nutritious food, warm clothes when it's cold, bedtime at a reasonable hour. However, a child's mental and emotional needs may not be as obvious. Good mental health allows children to think clearly, develop socially, and learn new skills. Additionally, good friends and encouraging words from adults are all important for helping children develop self-confidence, high self-esteem, and a healthy emotional outlook on life.

A child's physical and mental health are both important.

Basics for a child's good physical health:

- Nutritious food
- Adequate shelter and sleep
- Exercise
- Immunizations
- Healthy living environment

Basics for a child's good mental health:

- Unconditional love from family
- Self-confidence and high self-esteem

- The opportunity to play with other children
- Encouraging teachers and supportive caretakers
- Safe and secure surroundings
- Appropriate guidance and discipline

Give Children Unconditional Love

Love, security, and acceptance should be at the heart of family life. Children need to know that your love does not depend on his or her accomplishments.

Mistakes and/or defeats should be expected and accepted. Confidence grows in a home that is full of unconditional love and affection.

Nurture Children's Confidence and Self-Esteem

- **Praise them:** Encouraging children's first steps or their ability to learn a new game helps them develop a desire to explore and learn about their surroundings. Allow children to explore and play in a safe area where they cannot get hurt. Assure them by smiling and talking to them often. Be an active participant in their activities. Your attention helps build their self-confidence and self-esteem.
- **Set realistic goals:** Young children need realistic goals that match their ambitions with their abilities. With your help, older children can choose activities that test their abilities and increase their self-confidence.
- **Be honest:** Do not hide your failures from your children. It is important for them to know that we all make mistakes. It can be very reassuring to know that adults are not perfect.
- **Avoid sarcastic remarks:** If a child loses a game or fails a test, find out how he or she feels about the situation. Children may get discouraged and need a pep talk. Later, when they are ready, talk and offer assurance.
- **Encourage children:** To not only strive to do their best, but also to enjoy the process. Trying new activities teaches children about teamwork, self-esteem, and new skills.

Make Time for Play!

- **Encourage children to play.** To children, play is just fun. However, playtime is as important to their development as food and good care. Playtime helps children be creative, learn problem-solving skills and learn self-control. Good, hardy play, which includes running and yelling, is not only fun, but helps children to be physically and mentally healthy.

- **Children need playmates.** Sometimes it is important for children to have time with their peers. By playing with others, children discover their strengths and weaknesses, develop a sense of belonging, and learn how to get along with others. Consider finding a good children's program through neighbors, local community centers, schools, or your local park and recreation department.

- **Parents can be great playmates.** Join the fun! Playing Monopoly or coloring with a child gives you a great opportunity to share ideas and spend time together in a relaxed setting.

- **Play for fun.** Winning is not as important as being involved and enjoying the activity. One of the most important questions to ask children is "Did you have fun?" not "Did you win?" In our goal-oriented society, we often acknowledge only success and winning. This attitude can be discouraging and frustrating to children who are learning and experimenting with new activities. It's more important for children to participate and enjoy themselves.

TV use should be monitored.

Try not to use TV as a "baby-sitter" on a regular basis. Be selective in choosing television shows for children. Some shows can be educational as well as entertaining.

School Should Be Fun!

Starting school is a big event for children. "Playing school" can be a positive way to give them a glimpse of school life.

Try to enroll them in a pre-school, Head Start, or similar community program which provides an opportunity to be with other kids and make new friends. Children can also learn academic basics as well as how to make decisions and cope with problems.

Provide Appropriate Guidance and Instructive Discipline

Children need the opportunity to explore and develop new skills and independence. At the same time, children need to learn that certain behaviors are unacceptable and that they are responsible for the consequences of their actions.

As members of a family, children need to learn the rules of the family unit. Offer guidance and discipline that is fair and consistent. They will take these social skills and rules of conduct to school and eventually to the workplace.

Suggestions on Guidance and Discipline

- Be firm, but kind and realistic with your expectations. Children's development depends on your love and encouragement.
- Set a good example. You cannot expect self-control and self-discipline from a child if you do not practice this behavior.
- Criticize the behavior, not the child. It is best to say, "That was a bad thing you did," rather than "You are a bad boy or girl."
- Avoid nagging, threats, and bribery. Children will learn to ignore nagging, and threats and bribes are seldom effective.
- Give children the reasons "why" you are disciplining them and what the potential consequences of their actions might be.
- Talk about your feelings. We all lose our temper from time to time. If you do "blow your top," it is important to talk about what happened and why you are angry. Apologize if you were wrong! Remember, the goal is not to control the child, but for him or her to learn self-control.

Provide a Safe and Secure Home

It's okay for children to feel afraid sometimes. Everyone is afraid of something at some point in their life. Fear and anxiety grow out of experiences that we do not understand.

If your children have fears that will not go away and affect his or her behavior, the first step is to find out what is frightening them. Be loving, patient, and reassuring, not critical. Remember: the fear may be very real to the child.

Signs of Fear

Nervous mannerisms, shyness, withdrawal, and aggressive behavior may be signs of childhood fears. A change in normal eating and sleeping patterns may also signal an unhealthy fear. Children who "play sick" or feel anxious regularly may have some problems that need attention. Fear of school can occur following a stressful event such as moving to a new neighborhood, changing schools, or after a bad incident at school.

Children may not want to go to school after a period of being at home because of an illness.

When to seek help

Parents and family members are usually the first to notice if a child has problems with emotions or behavior. Your observations with those of teachers and other caregivers may lead you to seek help for your child. If you suspect a problem or have questions, consult your pediatrician or contact a mental health professional.

Warning signs

The following signs may indicate the need for professional assistance or evaluation:

- Decline in school performance
- Poor grades despite strong efforts
- Regular worry or anxiety
- Repeated refusal to go to school or take part in normal children's activities
- Hyperactivity or fidgeting
- Persistent nightmares
- Persistent disobedience or aggression
- Frequent temper tantrums
- Depression, sadness, or irritability

Where to seek help

Information and referrals regarding the types of services that are available for children may be obtained from:

- Mental health organizations, hotlines, and libraries
- Other professionals such as the child's pediatrician or school counselor
- Other families in the community
- Family network organizations
- Community-based psychiatric care
- Crisis outreach teams
- Education or special education services
- Family resource centers and support groups
- Health services
- Protection and advocacy groups and organizations
- Self-help and support groups

Chapter 68

Children and Adolescents Can Have Serious Mental Health Problems

Mental health is how people think, feel, and act as they face life's situations. It affects how people handle stress, relate to one another, and make decisions. Mental health influences the ways individuals look at themselves, their lives, and others in their lives. Like physical health, mental health is important at every stage of life.

All aspects of our lives are affected by our mental health. Caring for and protecting our children is an obligation and is critical to their daily lives and their independence.

Children and adolescents can have serious mental health problems

Like adults, children and adolescents can have mental health disorders that interfere with the way they think, feel, and act. When untreated, mental health disorders can lead to school failure, family conflicts, drug abuse, violence, and even suicide. Untreated mental health disorders can be very costly to families, communities, and the health care system.

From "Child and Adolescent Mental Health," a fact sheet by the Substance Abuse and Mental Health Services Administration (SAMHSA, mentalhealth .samhsa.gov), U.S. Department of Health or Human Services, November 2003. Reviewed by David A. Cooke, M.D., January 10, 2009.

Mental health disorders are more common in young people than many realize

Studies show that at least one in five children and adolescents have a mental health disorder. At least one in 10, or about 6 million people, have a serious emotional disturbance.

The causes are complicated

Mental health disorders in children and adolescents are caused mostly by biology and environment. Examples of biological causes are genetics, chemical imbalances in the body, or damage to the central nervous system, such as a head injury. Many environmental factors also put young people at risk for developing mental health disorders. Examples include:

- exposure to environmental toxins, such as high levels of lead;
- exposure to violence, such as witnessing or being the victim of physical or sexual abuse, drive-by shootings, muggings, or other disasters;
- stress related to chronic poverty, discrimination, or other serious hardships; and
- the loss of important people through death, divorce, or broken relationships.

Signs of mental health disorders can signal a need for help

Children and adolescents with mental health issues need to get help as soon as possible. A variety of signs may point to mental health disorders or serious emotional disturbances in children or adolescents. Pay attention if a child or adolescent you know has any of these warning signs:

A child or adolescent is troubled by feeling:

- sad and hopeless for no reason, and these feelings do not go away;
- very angry most of the time and crying a lot or overreacting to things;
- worthless or guilty often;
- anxious or worried often;
- unable to get over a loss or death of someone important;

- extremely fearful or having unexplained fears;
- constantly concerned about physical problems or physical appearance; and/or
- frightened that his or her mind either is controlled or is out of control.

A child or adolescent experiences big changes, such as:

- showing declining performance in school;
- losing interest in things once enjoyed;
- experiencing unexplained changes in sleeping or eating patterns;
- avoiding friends or family and wanting to be alone all the time;
- daydreaming too much and not completing tasks;
- feeling life is too hard to handle;
- hearing voices that cannot be explained; and/or
- experiencing suicidal thoughts.

A child or adolescent experiences:

- poor concentration and is unable to think straight or make up his or her mind;
- an inability to sit still or focus attention;
- worry about being harmed, hurting others, or doing something "bad";
- a need to wash, clean things, or perform certain routines hundreds of times a day, in order to avoid an unsubstantiated danger;
- racing thoughts that are almost too fast to follow; and/or
- persistent nightmares.

A child or adolescent behaves in ways that cause problems, such as:

- using alcohol or other drugs;
- eating large amounts of food and then purging, or abusing laxatives, to avoid weight gain;

- dieting and/or exercising obsessively;
- violating the rights of others or constantly breaking the law without regard for other people;
- setting fires;
- doing things that can be life threatening; and/or
- killing animals.

Comprehensive services through systems of care can help

Some children diagnosed with severe mental health disorders may be eligible for comprehensive and community-based services through systems of care. Systems of care help children with serious emotional disturbances and their families cope with the challenges of difficult mental, emotional, or behavioral problems. To learn more about systems of care, call the National Mental Health Information Center at 800-789-2647, and request fact sheets on systems of care and serious emotional disturbances, or visit the Center's web site at http://mentalhealth.samhsa.gov.

Finding the right services is critical

To find the right services for their children, families can do the following:

- Get accurate information from hotlines, libraries, or other sources.
- Seek referrals from professionals.
- Ask questions about treatments and services.
- Talk to other families in their communities.
- Find family network organizations.

It is critical that people who are not satisfied with the mental health care they receive discuss their concerns with providers, ask for information, and seek help from other sources.

Chapter 69

Depression in Children and Adolescents

Chapter Contents

Section 69.1

Depression in Children

Depression is more than just "feeling blue" or having a bad day. And it's different from feelings of grief or sorrow that follow a major loss, such as a death in the family. It's not a personal weakness or a character flaw. Children and teens with clinical depression cannot simply "snap out of it."

Depression is a serious health problem that affects feelings, thoughts and actions, and can appear as a physical illness. As many as one in eight teens and one in 33 children have clinical depression. Fortunately, depression in youth is treatable.

Signs of Depression

- Persistent sadness
- Withdrawal from family, friends, and activities that were once enjoyed
- Increased irritability or agitation
- Changes in eating and sleeping habits (e.g., significant weight loss, insomnia, excessive sleep)
- Frequent physical complaints, such as headaches and stomachaches
- Lack of enthusiasm or motivation
- Decreased energy level and chronic fatigue
- Play that involves excessive aggression toward self or others, or that involves persistently sad themes
- Indecision, lack of concentration, or forgetfulness
- Feelings of worthlessness or excessive guilt
- Recurring thoughts of death or suicide

What Can Parents and Other Adults Do If They Suspect a Child May Have Depression?

- Know the warning signs for depression, and note the duration, frequency, and severity of troubling behavior.
- Get accurate information from libraries, hotlines, the internet, and other sources.
- Take the child to see a mental health professional or doctor for evaluation and diagnosis if he or she is exhibiting several of the warning signs. The evaluation may include psychological testing, laboratory tests, and consultation with other specialists.
- Ask questions about treatments and services. A comprehensive treatment plan may include psychotherapy, ongoing evaluation and, in some cases, medication. Optimally, the treatment plan is developed with the family, and whenever possible, the child.
- Talk to other families in your community or find a family network organization.

Section 69.2

Understanding Depression in Adolescents

"Depression," October 2007, reprinted with permission from www.kidshealth.org. Copyright ©2007 The Nemours Foundation. This information was provided by KidsHealth, one of the largest resources online for medically reviewed health information written for parents, kids, and teens. For more articles like this one, visit www.KidsHealth.org, or www.TeensHealth.org.

Lately Lindsay hasn't felt like herself. Her friends have noticed it, too. Kia was surprised when Lindsay turned down her invitation to go to the mall last Saturday (Lindsay could always be counted on to shop!). There was really no reason not to go, but Lindsay just didn't feel like it. Instead, she spent most of Saturday sleeping.

Staying in more than usual isn't the only change in Lindsay. She's always been a really good student. But over the past couple of months her grades have fallen and she has trouble concentrating. She forgot to turn in a paper that was due and is having a hard time getting motivated to study for her finals.

Lindsay feels tired all the time but has difficulty falling asleep. She's gained weight too. When her mother asks her what's wrong, Lindsay just feels like crying. But she doesn't know why. Nothing particularly bad has happened. Yet Lindsay feels sad all the time and can't shake it.

Lindsay may not realize it yet, but she is depressed.

Depression is very common and affects as many as 1 in 8 people in their teen years. Depression affects people of every color, race, economic status, or age; however, it does seem to affect more girls than guys.

How Do People Respond to Someone Who's Depressed?

Sometimes friends or family members recognize that someone is depressed. They may respond with love, kindness, or support, hoping that the sadness will soon pass. They may offer to listen if the person wants to talk. If the depressed feeling doesn't pass with a little time, friends or loved ones may encourage the person to get help from a doctor, therapist, or counselor.

But not everyone recognizes depression when it happens to someone they know.

Some people don't really understand about depression. For example, they may react to a depressed person's low energy with criticism, yelling at the person for acting lazy or not trying harder. Some people mistakenly believe that depression is just an attitude or a mood that a person can shake off. It's not that easy.

Sometimes even people who are depressed don't take their condition seriously enough. Some people feel that they are weak in some way because they are depressed. This is wrong—and it can even be harmful if it causes people to hide their depression and avoid getting help.

Occasionally, when depression causes physical symptoms (things like headaches or other stress-related problems), a person may see a doctor. Once in a while, even a well-meaning doctor may not realize a person is depressed, and just treat the physical symptoms.

Why Do People Get Depressed?

There is no single cause for depression. Many factors play a role including genetics, environment, life events, medical conditions, and the way people react to things that happen in their lives.

Genetics

Research shows that depression runs in families and that some people inherit genes that make it more likely for them to get depressed. Not everyone who has the genetic makeup for depression gets depressed, though. And many people who have no family history of depression have the condition. So although genes are one factor, they aren't the single cause of depression.

Life Events

The death of a family member, friend, or pet can go beyond normal grief and sometimes lead to depression. Other difficult life events, such as when parents divorce, separate, or remarry, can trigger depression. Even events like moving or changing schools can be emotionally challenging enough that a person becomes depressed.

Family and Social Environment

For some teens, a negative, stressful, or unhappy family atmosphere can affect their self-esteem and lead to depression. This can also include high-stress living situations such as poverty; homelessness; and violence in the family, relationships, or community.

Substance use and abuse also can cause chemical changes in the brain that affect mood—alcohol and some drugs are known to have depressant effects. The negative social and personal consequences of substance abuse also can lead to severe unhappiness and depression.

Medical Conditions

Certain medical conditions can affect hormone balance and therefore have an effect on mood. Some conditions, such as hypothyroidism, are known to cause a depressed mood in some people. When these medical conditions are diagnosed and treated by a doctor, the depression usually disappears.

For some teens, undiagnosed learning disabilities might block school success, hormonal changes might affect mood, or physical illness might present challenges or setbacks.

What Happens in the Brain When Someone Is Depressed?

Depression involves the brain's delicate chemistry—specifically, it involves chemicals called neurotransmitters. These chemicals help send messages between nerve cells in the brain. Certain neurotransmitters regulate mood, and if they run low, people can become depressed, anxious, and stressed. Stress also can affect the balance of neurotransmitters and lead to depression.

Sometimes, a person may experience depression without being able to point to any particular sad or stressful event. People who have a genetic predisposition to depression may be more prone to the imbalance of neurotransmitter activity that is part of depression.

Medications that doctors use to treat depression work by helping to restore the proper balance of neurotransmitters.

Types of Depression

For some people, depression can be intense and occur in bouts that last for weeks at a time. For others, depression can be less severe but can linger at a low level for years.

Doctors who treat depression distinguish between these two types of depression. They call the more severe, short-lasting type major depression, and the longer-lasting but less severe form dysthymia (pronounced: diss-thy-me-uh).

A third form of depression that doctors may diagnose is called adjustment disorder with depressed mood. This diagnosis refers to a depressive reaction to a specific life event (such as a death, divorce, or other loss), when adjusting to the loss takes longer than the normally expected timeframe or is more severe than expected and interferes with the person's daily activities.

Bipolar disorder (also sometimes called manic depressive illness) is another depressive condition that involves periods of major depression mixed with periods of mania. Mania is the term for abnormally high mood and extreme bursts of unusual activity or energy.

What Are the Symptoms of Depression?

Symptoms that people have when they're depressed can include:

- depressed mood or sadness most of the time (for what may seem like no reason)
- lack of energy and feeling tired all the time
- inability to enjoy things that used to bring pleasure
- withdrawal from friends and family
- irritability, anger, or anxiety

- inability to concentrate
- significant weight loss or gain
- significant change in sleep patterns (inability to fall asleep, stay asleep, or get up in the morning)
- feelings of guilt or worthlessness
- aches and pains (with no known medical cause)
- pessimism and indifference (not caring about anything in the present or future)
- thoughts of death or suicide

When someone has five or more of these symptoms most of the time for 2 weeks or longer, that person is probably depressed.

Teens who are depressed may show other warning signs or symptoms, such as lack of interest or motivation, poor concentration, and low mental energy caused by depression. They also might have increased problems at school because of skipped classes.

Some teens with depression have other problems, too, and these can intensify feelings of worthlessness or inner pain. For example, people who cut themselves or who have eating disorders may have unrecognized depression that needs attention.

How Is Depression Different from Regular Sadness?

Everyone has some ups and downs, and sadness is a natural emotion. The normal stresses of life can lead anyone to feel sad every once in a while. Things like an argument with a friend, a breakup, doing poorly on a test, not being chosen for a team, or a best friend moving out of town can lead to feelings of sadness, hurt, disappointment, or grief. These reactions are usually brief and go away with a little time and care.

Depression is more than occasionally feeling blue, sad, or down in the dumps, though. Depression is a strong mood involving sadness, discouragement, despair, or hopelessness that lasts for weeks, months, or even longer. It interferes with a person's ability to participate in normal activities.

Depression affects a person's thoughts, outlook, and behavior as well as mood. In addition to a depressed mood, a person with depression can also feel tired, irritable, and notice changes in appetite.

When someone has depression, it can cloud everything. The world looks bleak and the person's thoughts reflect that hopelessness and helplessness. People with depression tend to have negative and self-critical thoughts. Sometimes, despite their true value, people with depression can feel worthless and unlovable.

Because of feelings of sadness and low energy, people with depression may pull away from those around them or from activities they once enjoyed. This usually makes them feel more lonely and isolated, making the depression and negative thinking worse.

Depression can be mild or severe. At its worst, depression can create such feelings of despair that a person thinks about suicide.

Depression can cause physical symptoms, too. Some people have an upset stomach, loss of appetite, weight gain or loss, headaches, and sleeping problems when they're depressed.

Getting Help

Depression is one of the most common emotional problems in the United States and around the world. The good news is that it's also one of the most treatable conditions. Therapists and other professionals can help. In fact, about 80% of people who get help for their depression have a better quality of life—they feel better and enjoy themselves in a way that they weren't able to before.

Treatment for depression can include talk therapy, medication, or a combination of both.

Talk therapy with a mental health professional is very effective in treating depression. Therapy sessions can help people understand more about why they feel depressed, and ways to combat it.

Sometimes, doctors prescribe medicine for a person who has depression. When prescribing medicine, a doctor will carefully monitor patients to make sure they get the right dose. The doctor will adjust the dose as necessary. It can take a few weeks before the person feels the medicine working. Because every person's brain is different, what works well for one person might not be good for another.

Everyone can benefit from mood-boosting activities like exercise, yoga, dance, journaling, or art. It can also help to keep busy no matter how tired you feel.

People who are depressed shouldn't wait and hope it will go away on its own because depression can be effectively treated. Friends or others need to step in if someone seems severely depressed and isn't getting help.

Many people find that it helps to open up to parents or other adults they trust. Simply saying, "I've been feeling really down lately and I think I'm depressed," can be a good way to begin the discussion. Ask your parent to arrange an appointment with a therapist. If a parent or family member can't help, turn to your school counselor, best friend, or a helpline to get help.

When Depression Is Severe

People who are extremely depressed and who may be thinking about hurting themselves or about suicide need help as soon as possible. When depression is this severe, it is a very real medical emergency, and an adult must be notified. Most communities have suicide hotlines where people can get guidance and support in an emergency.

Although it's important to be supportive, trying to cheer up a friend or reasoning with him or her probably won't work to help depression or suicidal feelings go away. Depression can be so strong that it outweighs a person's ability to respond to reason. Even if your friend has asked you to promise not to tell, severe depression is a situation where telling can save a life. The most important thing a depressed person can do is to get help. If you or a friend feels unsafe or out of control, get help now. Tell a trusted adult, call 911, or go to the emergency room.

Depression doesn't mean a person is "crazy." Depression (and the suffering that goes with it) is a real and recognized medical problem. Just as things can go wrong in all other organs of the body, things can go wrong in the most important organ of all: the brain. Luckily, most teens who get help for their depression go on to enjoy life and feel better about themselves.

Section 69.3

Antidepressant Medications for Children and Adolescents: Information for Parents and Caregivers

From the National Institute of Mental Health (NIMH, www.nimh.nih.gov), part of the National Institutes of Health, June 26, 2008.

Depression is a serious disorder that can cause significant problems in mood, thinking, and behavior at home, in school, and with peers. It is estimated that major depressive disorder (MDD) affects about 5 percent of adolescents.

Research has shown that, as in adults, depression in children and adolescents is treatable. Certain antidepressant medications, called selective serotonin reuptake inhibitors (SSRIs), can be beneficial to children and adolescents with MDD. Certain types of psychological therapies also have been shown to be effective. However, our knowledge of antidepressant treatments in youth, though growing substantially, is limited compared to what we know about treating depression in adults.

Recently, there has been some concern that the use of antidepressant medications themselves may induce suicidal behavior in youths. Following a thorough and comprehensive review of all the available published and unpublished controlled clinical trials of antidepressants in children and adolescents, the U.S. Food and Drug Administration (FDA) issued a public warning in October 2004 about an increased risk of suicidal thoughts or behavior (suicidality) in children and adolescents treated with SSRI antidepressant medications. In 2006, an advisory committee to the FDA recommended that the agency extend the warning to include young adults up to age 25.

More recently, results of a comprehensive review of pediatric trials conducted between 1988 and 2006 suggested that the benefits of antidepressant medications likely outweigh their risks to children and adolescents with major depression and anxiety disorders. The study, partially funded by NIMH, was published in the April 18, 2007, issue of *the Journal of the American Medical Association*.

What Did the FDA Review Find?

In the FDA review, no completed suicides occurred among nearly 2,200 children treated with SSRI medications. However, about 4 percent of those taking SSRI medications experienced suicidal thinking or behavior, including actual suicide attempts—twice the rate of those taking placebo, or sugar pills.

In response, the FDA adopted a "black box" label warning indicating that antidepressants may increase the risk of suicidal thinking and behavior in some children and adolescents with MDD. A black-box warning is the most serious type of warning in prescription drug labeling.

The warning also notes that children and adolescents taking SSRI medications should be closely monitored for any worsening in depression, emergence of suicidal thinking or behavior, or unusual changes in behavior, such as sleeplessness, agitation, or withdrawal from normal social situations. Close monitoring is especially important during the first 4 weeks of treatment. SSRI medications usually have few side effects in children and adolescents, but for unknown reasons, they may trigger agitation and abnormal behavior in certain individuals.

What Do We Know about Antidepressant Medications?

The SSRIs include:

- fluoxetine (Prozac);
- sertraline (Zoloft);
- paroxetine (Paxil);
- citalopram (Celexa);
- escitalopram (Lexapro); and
- fluvoxamine (Luvox).

Another antidepressant medication, venlafaxine (Effexor), is not an SSRI but is closely related.

SSRI medications are considered an improvement over older antidepressant medications because they have fewer side effects and are less likely to be harmful if taken in an overdose, which is an issue for patients with depression already at risk for suicide. They have been shown to be safe and effective for adults.

However, use of SSRI medications among children and adolescents ages 10 to 19 has risen dramatically in the past several years.

Fluoxetine (Prozac) is the only medication approved by the FDA for use in treating depression in children ages 8 and older. The other SSRI medications and the SSRI-related antidepressant venlafaxine have not been approved for treatment of depression in children or adolescents, but doctors still sometimes prescribe them to children on an "off-label" basis. In June 2003, however, the FDA recommended that paroxetine not be used in children and adolescents for treating MDD.

Fluoxetine can be helpful in treating childhood depression, and can lead to significant improvement of depression overall. However, it may increase the risk for suicidal behaviors in a small subset of adolescents. As with all medical decisions, doctors and families should weigh the risks and benefits of treatment for each individual patient.

What Should You Do for a Child with Depression?

A child or adolescent with MDD should be carefully and thoroughly evaluated by a doctor to determine if medication is appropriate. Psychotherapy often is tried as an initial treatment for mild depression. Psychotherapy may help to determine the severity and persistence of the depression and whether antidepressant medications may be warranted. Types of psychotherapies include "cognitive behavioral therapy," which helps people learn new ways of thinking and behaving, and "interpersonal therapy," which helps people understand and work through troubled personal relationships.

Those who are prescribed an SSRI medication should receive ongoing medical monitoring. Children already taking an SSRI medication should remain on the medication if it has been helpful, but should be carefully monitored by a doctor for side effects. Parents should promptly seek medical advice and evaluation if their child or adolescent experiences suicidal thinking or behavior, nervousness, agitation, irritability, mood instability, or sleeplessness that either emerges or worsens during treatment with SSRI medications.

Once started, treatment with these medications should not be abruptly stopped. Although they are not habit-forming or addictive, abruptly ending an antidepressant can cause withdrawal symptoms or lead to a relapse. Families should not discontinue treatment without consulting their doctor.

All treatments can be associated with side effects. Families and doctors should carefully weigh the risks and benefits, and maintain appropriate follow-up and monitoring to help control for the risks.

Section 69.4

Medication Considerations for Teens with Depression

From "Medication-Only Therapy and Combination Therapy Both Cost Effective for Treating Teens with Depression," by the National Institute of Mental Health (NIMH, www.nimh.nih.gov), part of the National Institutes of Health, May 12, 2008.

Treating depressed teenagers with either the antidepressant fluoxetine (Prozac) or a combination of fluoxetine and psychotherapy can be cost effective, according to a recent economic analysis of the NIMH-funded Treatment for Adolescents with Depression Study (TADS). The study was published online ahead of print April 15, 2008, in the *American Journal of Psychiatry.*

Marisa Elena Domino, Ph.D., of the University of North Carolina at Chapel Hill, and colleagues compared costs associated with each of the trial's three active treatment groups—fluoxetine only, cognitive behavioral therapy (CBT) only, and a combination of fluoxetine and CBT—to costs associated with a placebo (sugar pill) group during the first 12 weeks of the trial. The researchers studied direct costs of medication and CBT sessions, and other costs outside the trial, such as visits to primary care providers, school-based services, and lost wages associated with caregivers transporting the adolescent to and from services.

Overall, cost was highest for participants in the combination group—a median of $2,832 per participant. Median cost per participant was $2,287 in the CBT-only group, $942 in the fluoxetine-only group, and $841 in the placebo group.

Combination therapy was associated with the highest time and travel costs at $762, but medication costs were lower than those associated with the fluoxetine-only group because those in combination treatment tended to take lower doses of the medication. CBT costs for participants in the CBT-only group and participants receiving it as part of combination treatment did not differ.

Combination treatment cost more, but it also was shown to be more effective than the fluoxetine-only treatment in the first 12 weeks, as reported in August 2004. By assigning a monetary value to clinical improvement, the researchers deduced that both the fluoxetine-only treatment and combination treatment were cost-effective choices.

Finally, CBT was not found to be as effective or as cost effective as the other treatment groups in the first 12 weeks of the trial. However, by the end of the 36-week study, response rates in the CBT-only group had essentially caught up with the other two groups. Therefore, the researchers predicted that if long-term costs remain stable, CBT-only may become a cost-effective treatment choice as well.

Reference

Domino ME, Burns BJ, Silva SG, Kratochvil CJ, Vitiello B, Reinecke MA, Mario J, March JS. Cost-effectiveness of treatments for adolescent depression: results from TADS. *American Journal of Psychiatry.* Published online ahead of print April 15, 2008.

Section 69.5

Maintenance Treatment Crucial for Teens' Recovery from Depression

From the National Institute of Mental Health (NIMH, www.nimh.nih.gov), part of the National Institutes of Health, April 8, 2008.

Long-term maintenance treatment is likely to sustain improvement and prevent recurrence among adolescents with major depression, according to an NIMH-funded study published in the April 2008 issue of the *Archives of General Psychiatry.*

The study, led by Paul Rohde, Ph.D., of Oregon Research Institute, analyzed data from the Treatment of Adolescents with Depression Study (TADS), a large, NIMH-funded trial in which depressed teens were randomized to one of three treatments for 36 weeks—fluoxetine (Prozac), cognitive behavior therapy (CBT), or a combination of both.

Teens with depression, even if they show a good initial response to treatment, are at high risk for relapse and recurrence. However, guidelines for depression maintenance treatment are based on adult needs. Rohde and colleagues aimed to identify whether the available guidelines are appropriate for depressed adolescents.

Among the 242 TADS participants analyzed for this study, 61 percent significantly improved by week 12. The combination group achieved the highest rate of sustained response (71 percent) compared to the fluoxetine-only group (68 percent) and CBT-only group (42 percent).

The majority (82 percent) of teens who reached a sustained positive response by week 12 maintained this level of recovery through week 36. Among those in combination treatment, about 89 percent maintained improvement for the full 36 weeks. Among those in the fluoxetine-only group, 74 percent maintained improvement, but among those in CBT-only treatment, 97 percent maintained their improvement.

The high long-term success rate of CBT suggests that for teens who initially respond to it, CBT may have a preventive effect that helps to sustain positive improvement and potentially avoid relapse or recurrence, even if treatment visits become infrequent, as was the case after the first 12 weeks in the TADS study. Additionally, the relatively lower sustained success rate for fluoxetine suggests that the effectiveness of fluoxetine therapy may plateau at a certain point for some responders, triggering a need for the addition of psychosocial treatment.

"For those teens who respond to fluoxetine only, adding CBT to their treatment regimen early on would likely increase their chances for continued improvement," suggested Rohde.

The findings help guide clinicians in deciding on the best maintenance course after a teen responds to an initial treatment. They also emphasize the value of ongoing, long-term treatment, even if treatment visits are infrequent, Rohde and colleagues concluded.

Reference

Rohde P, Silva SG, Tonev ST, Kennard BD, Vitiello B, Kratochvil CJ, Reinecke MA, Curry JF, Simons AD, March JS. Achievement and maintenance of sustained improvement during TADS continuation and maintenance therapy. *Archives of General Psychiatry.* 2008 Apr; 65(4): 447-455.

Chapter 70

Bipolar Disorder in Youth

Children's Mental Health Facts: Bipolar Disorder

This text provides basic information on bipolar disorder in children and describes an approach to getting services and supports, called "systems of care," that helps children, youth, and families thrive at home, in school, in the community, and throughout life.

What is bipolar disorder?

Bipolar disorder is a brain disorder that causes persistent, overwhelming, and uncontrollable changes in moods, activities, thoughts, and behaviors. A child has a much greater chance of having bipolar disorder if there is a family history of the disorder or depression. This means that parents cannot choose whether or not their children will have bipolar disorder.

Although bipolar disorder affects at least 750,000 children in the United States, it is often difficult to recognize and diagnose in children. If left untreated, the disorder puts a child at risk for school failure, drug abuse, and suicide. That is why it is important that you seek the advice of a qualified professional when trying to find out if your child has bipolar disorder.

This chapter contains text from "Children's Mental Health Facts: Bipolar Disorder," by the Substance Abuse and Mental Health Services Administration (SAMHSA, mentalhealth.samhsa.gov), November 2005, and "Rates of Bipolar Diagnosis in Youth Rapidly Climbing, Treatment Patterns Similar to Adults," from the National Institute of Mental Health (NIMH, www.nimh.nih.gov), part of the National Institutes of Health, September 3, 2007.

Symptoms of bipolar disorder can be mistaken for other medical/mental health conditions, and children with bipolar disorder can have other mental health needs at the same time. Other disorders that can occur at the same time as bipolar disorder include, but are not limited to, attention-deficit/hyperactivity disorder, conduct disorder, oppositional defiant disorder, anxiety disorders, autistic spectrum disorders, and drug abuse disorders. The roles that a family's culture and language play in how causes and symptoms are perceived and then described to a mental health care provider are important, too. Misperceptions and misunderstandings can lead to delayed diagnoses, misdiagnoses, or no diagnoses—which are serious problems when a child needs help. That is why it is important that supports be in place to bridge differences in language and culture. Once bipolar disorder is properly diagnosed, treatment can begin to help children and adolescents with bipolar disorder live productive and fulfilling lives.

What are the signs of bipolar disorder?

Unlike some health problems where different people experience the same symptoms, children experience bipolar disorder differently. Often, children with the illness experience mood swings that alternate, or cycle, between periods of "highs" and "lows," called "mania" and "depression," with varying moods in between. These cycles can happen much more rapidly than in adults, sometimes occurring many times within a day. Mental health experts differ in their interpretation of what symptoms children experience. The following are commonly reported signs of bipolar disorder:

- excessively elevated moods alternating with periods of depressed or irritable moods;
- periods of high, goal-directed activity, and/or physical agitation;
- racing thoughts and speaking very fast;
- unusual/erratic sleep patterns and/or a decreased need for sleep;
- difficulty settling as babies;
- severe temper tantrums, sometimes called "rages";
- excessive involvement in pleasurable activities, daredevil behavior, and/or grandiose, "super-confident" thinking and behaviors;
- impulsivity and/or distractibility;
- inappropriate sexual activity, even at very young ages;
- hallucinations and/or delusions;

- suicidal thoughts and/or talks of killing self; and
- inflexible, oppositional/defiant, and extremely irritable behavior.

What happens after a bipolar disorder diagnosis?

If a qualified mental health provider has diagnosed your child with bipolar disorder, the provider may suggest several different treatment options, including strategies for managing behaviors, medications, and/or talk therapy. Your child's mental health care provider may also suggest enrolling in a system of care, if one is available.

What is a system of care?

A system of care is a coordinated network of community-based services and supports that are organized to meet the challenges of children and youth with serious mental health needs and their families. Families, children, and youth work in partnership with public and private organizations so services and supports are effective, build on the strengths of individuals, and address each person's cultural and linguistic needs.

Specifically, a system of care can help by tailoring services to the unique needs of your child and family, making services and supports available in your language and connecting you with professionals who respect your values and beliefs, encouraging you and your child to play as much of a role in the design of a treatment plan as you want, and providing services from within your community, whenever possible.

How can I find a system of care for my child with bipolar disorder?

Visit mentalhealth.samhsa.gov/cmhs and click "Child, Adolescent & Family" and then "Systems of Care" to locate a system of care close to you. If you prefer to speak to someone in person to locate a system of care, or if there is not a system of care in your area, contact the National Mental Health Information Center by calling toll-free 800-789-2647 or visiting mentalhealth.samhsa.gov.

Rates of Bipolar Diagnosis in Youth Rapidly Climbing, Treatment Patterns Similar to Adults

The number of visits to a doctor's office that resulted in a diagnosis of bipolar disorder in children and adolescents has increased by

40 times over the last decade, reported researchers funded in part by the National Institutes of Health (NIH). Over the same time period, the number of visits by adults resulting in a bipolar disorder diagnosis almost doubled. The cause of these increases is unclear. Medication prescription patterns for the two groups were similar. The study was published in the September 2007 issue of the *Archives of General Psychiatry*.

Mark Olfson, M.D., M.P.H., of New York State Psychiatric Institute of Columbia University, along with National Institute of Mental Health (NIMH) researcher Gonzalo Laje, M.D., and their colleagues examined 10 years of data from the National Ambulatory Medical Care Survey (NAMCS), an annual, nationwide survey of visits to doctors' offices over a one-week period, conducted by the National Center for Health Statistics. The researchers estimated that in the United States from 1994–1995, the number of office visits resulting in a diagnosis of bipolar disorder (http://www.nimh.nih.gov/healthinformation/bipolar menu.cfm) for youths ages 19 and younger was 25 out of every 100,000 people. By 2002–2003, the number had jumped to 1,003 office visits resulting in bipolar diagnoses per 100,000 people. In contrast, for adults ages 20 and older, 905 office visits per 100,000 people resulted in a bipolar disorder diagnosis in 1994–1995; a decade later the number had risen to 1,679 per 100,000 people.

While the increase in bipolar diagnoses in youth far outpaces the increase in diagnosis among adults, the researchers are cautious about interpreting these data as an actual rise in the number of people who have the illness (prevalence) or the number of new cases each year (incidence).

"It is likely that this impressive increase reflects a recent tendency to overdiagnose bipolar disorder in young people, a correction of historical under recognition, or a combination of these trends. Clearly, we need to learn more about what criteria physicians in the community are actually using to diagnose bipolar disorder in children and adolescents and how physicians are arriving at decisions concerning clinical management," said Dr. Olfson.

The fourth edition of the *Diagnostic and Statistical Manual of Mental Disorders* (*DSM-IV*) provides general guidelines that can help doctors identify bipolar disorder in young patients. However, some studies show that youths with symptoms of mania (over-excited, elated mood)—one of the classic signs of bipolar disorder—often do not meet the full criteria for a diagnosis of bipolar disorder.

Other disorders, such as attention-deficit hyperactivity disorder (ADHD) (http://www.nimh.nih.gov/healthinformation/adhdmenu.cfm), may have symptoms that overlap, so some of these conditions may be mistaken for bipolar disorder as well. For example, in a study conducted in 2001, nearly one-half of bipolar diagnoses in adolescent inpatients made by community clinicians were later re-classified as other mental disorders.

Doctors also face tough questions when deciding on proper treatment for young people. Guidelines for treating adults with bipolar disorder are well-documented by research, but few studies have looked at the safety and effectiveness of psychiatric medications for treating children and adolescents with the disorder. Despite this limited evidence, the researchers found similar treatment patterns for both age groups in terms of use of psychotherapy and prescription medications.

Of the medications studied, mood stabilizers, including lithium—which was the only medication approved at the time of the study by the U.S. Food and Drug Administration for treating bipolar disorder in children—were prescribed in two thirds of the visits by youth and adults. Anticonvulsant medications, such as valproate (Depakote) and carbamazepine (Tegretol), were the most frequently prescribed type of mood stabilizers in both groups.

Doctors prescribed antidepressant medications in slightly over one third of visits by youth and adults. Antidepressant medications include the older classes of antidepressant medications, such as tricyclics, tetracyclics, and monoamine oxidase inhibitors (MAOIs); selective serotonin reuptake inhibitors, such as fluoxetine (Prozac) and paroxetine (Paxil); and also newer types of antidepressants, including venlafaxine (Effexor). In both age groups, about one third of the visits where antidepressant medications were prescribed did not include prescription of a mood stabilizer. This trend raises concerns, considering an earlier NIMH-funded study (Thase & Sachs, 2000) which reported that treating adults who have bipolar disorder with an antidepressant in the absence of a mood stabilizer may put them at risk of switching to mania. Also, a recent NIMH study showed that for depressed adults with bipolar disorder who are taking a mood stabilizer, adding an antidepressant medication was no more effective in managing bipolar symptoms (http://www.nimh.nih.gov/press/stepbd-medication.cfm) than a placebo (sugar pill).

Roughly the same percentage of youth and adult bipolar visits included a prescription for an antipsychotic medication, although young patients were more likely to be prescribed one of the newer, atypical antipsychotic medications, such as aripiprazole (Abilify) or olanzapine (Zyprexa), than other types of antipsychotics. This finding suggests that doctors may be basing their treatment choices for bipolar youth on prescribing practices for adults with the disorder.

However, one main difference between youth and adult treatment was that children and teens were more likely than adults to be prescribed a stimulant medication—usually prescribed for treating ADHD—and adults were more likely than youth to be prescribed benzodiazepines, a type of medication used to treat anxiety disorders (http://www.nimh.nih.gov/healthinformation/anxietymenu.cfm). More than half of all diagnosed youths and adults were prescribed a combination of medications. Given the relative lack of studies on appropriate treatments for youth with bipolar disorder, the researchers noted the urgent need for more research on the safety and effectiveness of medication treatments that are commonly prescribed to this age group.

The study had several important limitations. For example, the survey relied on the judgment of the treating physicians, rather than an independent assessment. As a result, the researchers' findings reveal more about patterns in diagnosis among office-based doctors than about definitive numbers of people affected by the illness.

Another limitation is that the survey recorded the number of office visits instead of the number of individual patients, so some people may have been counted more than once.

"A forty-fold increase in the diagnosis of bipolar disorder in children and adolescents is worrisome," said NIMH Director Thomas R. Insel, M.D. "We do not know how much of this increase reflects earlier underdiagnosis, current overdiagnosis, possibly a true increase in prevalence of this illness, or some combination of these factors. However, these new results confirm what we are hearing increasingly from families who tell us about disabling, sometimes dangerous psychiatric symptoms in their children. This report reminds us of the need for research that validates the diagnosis of bipolar disorder and other disorders in children and the importance of developing treatments that are safe, effective, and feasible for use in primary care."

"This research, performed at a National Center on Minority Health and Health Disparities (NCMHD) Center of Excellence, underscores the need to fully engage the community with their health care providers to better understand the actual prevalence of bipolar disease in children and adolescents," said John Ruffin, Ph.D., Director of NCMHD.

Moreno C, Laje G, Blanco C, Jiang H, Schmidt AB, Olfson M. National trends in the outpatient diagnosis and treatment of bipolar disorder in youth. *Arch Gen Psychiatry.* 2007 Sep;64(9).

Chapter 71

Anxiety Disorders in Children and Adolescents

What are anxiety disorders?

Children and adolescents with anxiety disorders typically experience intense fear, worry, or uneasiness that can last for long periods of time and significantly affect their lives. If not treated early, anxiety disorders can lead to:

- repeated school absences or an inability to finish school;
- impaired relations with peers;
- low self-esteem;
- alcohol or other drug use;
- problems adjusting to work situations; and
- anxiety disorder in adulthood.

What are the types and signs of anxiety disorders?

Many different anxiety disorders affect children and adolescents. Several disorders and their signs are described below:

From "Children's Mental Health Facts: Children and Adolescents with Anxiety Disorders," from the Substance Abuse and Mental Health Services Administration (SAMHSA, mentalhealth.samhsa.gov), part of the U.S. Department of Health and Human Services, April 2003. Reviewed by David A. Cooke, M.D., January 23, 2009.

Generalized anxiety disorder: Children and adolescents with generalized anxiety disorder engage in extreme, unrealistic worry about everyday life activities. They worry unduly about their academic performance, sporting activities, or even about being on time. Typically, these young people are very self-conscious, feel tense, and have a strong need for reassurance. They may complain about stomachaches or other discomforts that do not appear to have any physical cause.

Separation anxiety disorder: Children with separation anxiety disorder often have difficulty leaving their parents to attend school or camp, stay at a friend's house, or be alone. Often, they "cling" to parents and have trouble falling asleep. Separation anxiety disorder may be accompanied by depression, sadness, withdrawal, or fear that a family member might die. About one in every 25 children experiences separation anxiety disorder.

Phobias: Children and adolescents with phobias have unrealistic and excessive fears of certain situations or objects. Many phobias have specific names, and the disorder usually centers on animals, storms, water, heights, or situations, such as being in an enclosed space. Children and adolescents with social phobias are terrified of being criticized or judged harshly by others. Young people with phobias will try to avoid the objects and situations they fear, so the disorder can greatly restrict their lives.

Panic disorder: Repeated "panic attacks" in children and adolescents without an apparent cause are signs of a panic disorder. Panic attacks are periods of intense fear accompanied by a pounding heartbeat, sweating, dizziness, nausea, or a feeling of imminent death. The experience is so scary that young people live in dread of another attack. Children and adolescents with the disorder may go to great lengths to avoid situations that may bring on a panic attack. They also may not want to go to school or to be separated from their parents.

Obsessive-compulsive disorder: Children and adolescents with obsessive-compulsive disorder, sometimes called OCD, become trapped in a pattern of repetitive thoughts and behaviors. Even though they may recognize that the thoughts or behaviors appear senseless and distressing, the pattern is very hard to stop. Compulsive behaviors may include repeated hand washing, counting, or arranging and rearranging objects. About two in every 100 adolescents experience obsessive-compulsive disorder (U.S. Department of Health and Human Services, 1999).

Posttraumatic stress disorder: Children and adolescents can develop posttraumatic stress disorder after they experience a very stressful event. Such events may include experiencing physical or sexual abuse; being a victim of or witnessing violence; or living through a disaster, such as a bombing or hurricane. Young people with posttraumatic stress disorder experience the event over and over through strong memories, flashbacks, or other kinds of troublesome thoughts. As a result, they may try to avoid anything associated with the trauma. They also may overreact when startled or have difficulty sleeping.

How common are anxiety disorders?

Anxiety disorders are among the most common mental, emotional, and behavioral problems to occur during childhood and adolescence. About 13 of every 100 children and adolescents ages 9 to 17 experience some kind of anxiety disorder; girls are affected more than boys. About half of children and adolescents with anxiety disorders have a second anxiety disorder or other mental or behavioral disorder, such as depression. In addition, anxiety disorders may coexist with physical health conditions requiring treatment.

Who is at risk?

Researchers have found that the basic temperament of young people may play a role in some childhood and adolescent anxiety disorders. For example, some children tend to be very shy and restrained in unfamiliar situations, a possible sign that they are at risk for developing an anxiety disorder. Research in this area is very complex, because children's fears often change as they age.

Researchers also suggest watching for signs of anxiety disorders when children are between the ages of 6 and 8. During this time, children generally grow less afraid of the dark and imaginary creatures and become more anxious about school performance and social relationships.

An excessive amount of anxiety in children this age may be a warning sign for the development of anxiety disorders later in life.

Studies suggest that children or adolescents are more likely to have an anxiety disorder if they have a parent with anxiety disorders. However, the studies do not prove whether the disorders are caused by biology, environment, or both. More data are needed to clarify whether anxiety disorders can be inherited.

What help is available for young people with anxiety disorders?

Children and adolescents with anxiety disorders can benefit from a variety of treatments and services. Following an accurate diagnosis, possible treatments include: cognitive-behavioral treatment, in which young people learn to deal with fears by modifying the ways they think and behave; relaxation techniques; biofeedback (to control stress and muscle tension); family therapy; parent training; and medication.

While cognitive-behavioral approaches are effective in treating some anxiety disorders, medications work well with others. Some people with anxiety disorders benefit from a combination of these treatments. More research is needed to determine what treatments work best for the various types of anxiety disorders.

What can parents do?

If parents or other caregivers notice repeated symptoms of an anxiety disorder in their child or adolescent, they should:

- Talk with the child's health care provider. He or she can help to determine whether the symptoms are caused by an anxiety disorder or by some other condition and can also provide a referral to a mental health professional.
- Look for a mental health professional trained in working with children and adolescents, who has used cognitive-behavioral or behavior therapy and has prescribed medications for this disorder, or has cooperated with a physician who does.
- Get accurate information from libraries, hotlines, or other sources.
- Ask questions about treatments and services.
- Talk with other families in their communities.
- Find family network organizations.

People who are not satisfied with the mental health care they receive should discuss their concerns with the provider, ask for information, and/or seek help from other sources.

Chapter 72

Obsessive-Compulsive Disorder in Children and Adolescents

All kids have worries and doubts. But kids with obsessive-compulsive disorder (OCD) can't stop worrying, no matter how much they try to. And those worries compel them to behave in certain ways over and over again.

About OCD

OCD is a type of anxiety disorder. Kids with OCD become preoccupied with whether something could be harmful, dangerous, wrong, or dirty—or with thoughts about bad stuff that might happen. With OCD, upsetting or scary thoughts or images, called obsessions, pop into a person's mind and are hard to shake.

Someone with OCD feels strong urges to do certain things repeatedly—called rituals or compulsions—in order to banish the scary thoughts, ward off something dreaded, or make extra sure that things are safe or clean or right. By doing a ritual, someone with OCD is trying to feel absolutely certain that something bad won't happen.

Think of OCD as an "overactive alarm system." The rise in anxiety or worry is so strong that a child feels like he or she must perform the task or dwell on the thought, over and over again, to the point

---

where it interferes with everyday life. Most kids with OCD realize that they really don't have to repeat the behaviors over and over again, but the anxiety can be so great that they feel that repetition is "required" to neutralize the uncomfortable feeling.

An estimated 2% of children in the United States experience OCD, which is characterized as a pattern of rituals and obsessive thinking that generally lasts more than an hour each day, causes a child distress, and interferes with daily activities. It's more prevalent than many other childhood disorders or illnesses, but kids often keep the symptoms hidden from their families because they're embarrassed about them.

OCD in kids is usually diagnosed between the ages of 7 and 12. Since these are the years when kids naturally feel concerned about fitting in with their friends, the discomfort and stress brought on by OCD can make them feel scared, out of control, and alone.

It's important to understand that the obsessive-compulsive behavior is not something that a child can stop by trying harder. OCD is a disorder, just like any physical disorder and is not something a child can control.

Common OCD Behaviors in Kids

OCD can make daily life difficult for the kids that it affects and their families. The behaviors often take up a great deal of time and energy, making it more difficult to complete tasks, such as homework or chores, or to enjoy life. In addition to feeling frustrated or guilty for not being able to control their own thoughts or actions, kids with OCD also may suffer from low self-esteem from shame or embarrassment about what they're thinking or feeling.

They also may feel pressured because they don't have enough time to do everything. A child might become irritable because he or she feels compelled to stay awake late into the night or miss an activity or outing to complete the compulsive rituals. Kids might have difficulties with attention or concentration because of the intrusive thoughts.

Among kids and teens with OCD, the most common obsessions include:

- fear of dirt or germs
- fear of contamination
- a need for symmetry, order, and precision
- religious obsessions

- preoccupation with body wastes
- lucky and unlucky numbers
- sexual or aggressive thoughts
- fear of illness or harm coming to oneself or relatives
- preoccupation with household items
- intrusive sounds or words

These compulsions are the most common among kids and teens:

- grooming rituals, including hand washing, showering, and teeth brushing
- repeating rituals, including going in and out of doorways, needing to move through spaces in a special way, checking to make sure that an appliance is off or a door is locked, and checking homework
- rituals to undo contact with a "contaminated" person or object
- touching rituals
- rituals to prevent harming self or others
- ordering or arranging objects
- counting rituals
- hoarding and collecting things
- cleaning rituals related to the house or other items

Signs and Symptoms of OCD

Recognizing OCD is often difficult because kids can become adept at hiding the behaviors. It's not uncommon for a child to engage in ritualistic behavior for months, or even years, before parents know about it. Also, a child may not engage in the ritual at school, so parents might think that it's just a phase.

When a child with OCD tries to contain these thoughts or behaviors, this creates anxiety. Kids who feel embarrassed or as if they're "going crazy" may try to blend the OCD into the normal daily routine until they can't control it anymore.

It's common for kids to ask a parent to join in the ritualistic behavior: First the child has to do something and then the parent has to do something else. If a child says, "I didn't touch something with germs, did I?" the parent might have to respond, "No, you're OK," and the ritual will begin again for a certain number of times. Initially, the parent might not notice what is happening. Tantrums, overt signs of worry, and difficult behaviors are common when parents fail to participate in their child's rituals. It is often this behavior, as much as the OCD itself, that brings families into treatment.

Parents can look for the following possible signs of OCD:

- raw, chapped hands from constant washing
- unusually high rate of soap or paper towel usage
- high, unexplained utility bills
- a sudden drop in test grades
- unproductive hours spent doing homework
- holes erased through test papers and homework
- requests for family members to repeat strange phrases or keep answering the same question
- a persistent fear of illness
- a dramatic increase in laundry
- an exceptionally long amount of time spent getting ready for bed
- a continual fear that something terrible will happen to someone
- constant checks of the health of family members
- reluctance to leave the house at the same time as other family members

Environmental and stress factors can signal the onset of OCD. These can include ordinary developmental transitions (such as starting school) as well as significant losses or changes (such as the death of a loved one or moving).

Diagnosing OCD

If your child shows signs of OCD, talk to your doctor. In screening for OCD, a doctor or mental health professional will ask about your child's obsessions and compulsions in language that kids will understand, such as:

- Do you have worries, thoughts, images, feelings, or ideas that bother you?
- Do you have to check things over and over again?
- Do you have to wash your hands a lot, more than most kids?
- Do you count to a certain number or do things a certain number of times?
- Do you collect things that others might throw away (like hair or fingernail clippings)?
- Do things have to be "just so"?
- Are there things you have to do before you go to bed?

Because it might be normal for a child who doesn't have OCD to answer yes to any of these questions, the doctor also will ask about your family's history of OCD, Tourette syndrome, and other motor or vocal tic disorders. OCD has a genetic component, which means that children whose family members have had any of these disorders may be more prone to it.

Tic disorders often resemble OCD symptoms: up to half of people with Tourette syndrome also have OCD (but only a small percentage of kids with OCD also have Tourette syndrome).

Disorders that frequently occur with OCD include other anxiety disorders, depression, disruptive behavior disorders such as attention deficit hyperactivity disorder, learning disorders, trichotillomania (compulsive hair pulling), and habit disorders such as nail biting or skin picking.

In rare cases, OCD symptoms or tics that come on very suddenly may be associated with a recent group A streptococcus infection (strep throat or, less commonly, scarlet fever). This phenomenon is known as PANDAS (Pediatric Autoimmune Neuropsychiatric Disorders Associated with Streptococcal Infections). No one knows for sure why PANDAS occurs. One theory is that strep infections trigger an antibody response in some kids that causes changes in the basal ganglia, a part of the brain that has been implicated in OCD.

Of course, just because a child has had strep throat doesn't mean he or she will also have PANDAS. Almost all school-age kids have strep throat at some point, and the vast majority recover with no complications. Similarly, most kids who have OCD or tics do not have PANDAS. The condition may be considered only if a child's OCD symptoms or tics are directly preceded by, or significantly worsen after, a strep infection.

Treating OCD

The most successful treatments for kids with OCD are behavioral therapy and medication. Behavioral therapy, also known as cognitive-behavioral psychotherapy (CBT), helps kids learn to change thoughts and feelings by first changing behavior. It involves exposing a child to his or her fears to decrease the surrounding anxiety. For example, kids who are afraid of dirt might be exposed to something they consider dirty until they no longer fear it.

For exposure to be successful, it is often combined with response prevention, in which the child's rituals or avoidance behaviors are blocked. For example, a child who fears dirt must not only stay in contact with the dirty object, but also must not be allowed to wash repeatedly. Some treatment plans involve having the child "bossing back" the OCD, giving it a nasty nickname, and visualizing it as something the child can control.

OCD can sometimes worsen if it's not treated in a consistent, logical, and supportive manner. So it's important to find a therapist who has training and experience in treating OCD. Family support and cooperation also go a long way toward helping a child cope.

Many kids can do well with behavioral therapy alone while others will need a combination of behavioral therapy and medication. Therapy can help your child and family learn strategies to manage the ebb and flow of OCD symptoms, while medication, such as selective serotonin reuptake inhibitors (SSRIs), often can reduce the impulse to engage in the ritualistic behavior.

Help Kids with OCD

It's important to understand that OCD is never a child's fault. Once a child is in treatment, it's important for parents to participate, to learn more about OCD, and to modify expectations and be supportive.

Kids with OCD get better at different rates so try to avoid any day-to-day comparisons, and recognize and praise any small improvements. Keep in mind that it's the OCD that is causing the problem, not the child. The more that personal criticism can be avoided, the better.

It can be helpful to keep family routines as normal as possible, and for all family members to learn strategies to help the child with OCD.

Chapter 73

Conduct Disorder

What is conduct disorder?

Children with conduct disorder repeatedly violate the personal or property rights of others and the basic expectations of society. A diagnosis of conduct disorder is likely when symptoms continue for 6 months or longer. Conduct disorder is known as a "disruptive behavior disorder" because of its impact on children and their families, neighbors, and schools.

Another disruptive behavior disorder, called oppositional defiant disorder, may be a precursor of conduct disorder. A child is diagnosed with oppositional defiant disorder when he or she shows signs of being hostile and defiant for at least 6 months. Oppositional defiant disorder may start as early as the preschool years, while conduct disorder generally appears when children are older. Oppositional defiant disorder and conduct disorder are not co-occurring conditions.

What are the signs of conduct disorder?

Symptoms of conduct disorder include:

From "Children's Mental Health Facts: Children and Adolescents with Conduct Disorder," by the Substance Abuse and Mental Health Services Administration (SAMHSA, mentalhealth.samhsa.gov), part of the U.S. Department of Health and Human Services, April 2003. Reviewed by David A. Cooke, M.D., January 23, 2009.

- aggressive behavior that harms or threatens other people or animals;
- destructive behavior that damages or destroys property;
- lying or theft;
- truancy or other serious violations of rules;
- early tobacco, alcohol, and substance use and abuse; and
- precocious sexual activity.

Children with conduct disorder or oppositional defiant disorder also may experience:

- higher rates of depression, suicidal thoughts, suicide attempts, and suicide;
- academic difficulties;
- poor relationships with peers or adults;
- sexually transmitted diseases;
- difficulty staying in adoptive, foster, or group homes; and
- higher rates of injuries, school expulsions, and problems with the law.

How common is conduct disorder?

Conduct disorder affects 1 to 4 percent of 9- to 17-year-olds, depending on exactly how the disorder is defined. The disorder appears to be more common in boys than in girls and more common in cities than in rural areas.

Who is at risk for conduct disorder?

Research shows that some cases of conduct disorder begin in early childhood, often by the preschool years. In fact, some infants who are especially "fussy" appear to be at risk for developing conduct disorder.

Other factors that may make a child more likely to develop conduct disorder include:

- early maternal rejection;
- separation from parents, without an adequate alternative caregiver;

- early institutionalization;
- family neglect;
- abuse or violence;
- parental mental illness;
- parental marital discord;
- large family size;
- crowding; and
- poverty.

What help is available for families?

Although conduct disorder is one of the most difficult behavior disorders to treat, young people often benefit from a range of services that include:

- training for parents on how to handle child or adolescent behavior;
- family therapy;
- training in problem solving skills for children or adolescents; and
- community-based services that focus on the young person within the context of family and community influences.

What can parents do?

Some child and adolescent behaviors are hard to change after they have become ingrained. Therefore, the earlier the conduct disorder is identified and treated, the better the chance for success. Most children or adolescents with conduct disorder are probably reacting to events and situations in their lives. Some recent studies have focused on promising ways to prevent conduct disorder among at-risk children and adolescents. In addition, more research is needed to determine if biology is a factor in conduct disorder.

Parents or other caregivers who notice signs of conduct disorder or oppositional defiant disorder in a child or adolescent should:

- pay careful attention to the signs, try to understand the underlying reasons, and then try to improve the situation;

- if necessary, talk with a mental health or social services professional, such as a teacher, counselor, psychiatrist, or psychologist specializing in childhood and adolescent disorders;
- get accurate information from libraries, hotlines, or other sources;
- talk to other families in their communities; and
- find family network organizations.

People who are not satisfied with the mental health services they receive should discuss their concerns with their provider, ask for more information, and/or seek help from other sources.

Chapter 74

Oppositional Defiant Disorder

Oppositional defiant disorder (ODD) is a diagnosis given to children who display a pattern of negative and defiant behavior to parents, teachers, and others who have authority over them.

Many children disobey their parents or teachers from time to time. In fact, oppositional behavior is very common in pre-school children and teenagers. It's important that we don't mislabel these normal "phases" of childhood as signs of a behavioral disorder. Children with ODD have frequent run-ins with authority figures and are oppositional far more often than other children their age.

Boys are more likely to be diagnosed with ODD than girls, especially before puberty. Children typically begin to show signs of ODD before age 8 and no later than 13-15. While mental health professionals are very cautious with diagnosing ODD before the school-aged years, many children with ODD had "difficult" temperaments as toddlers. They were often fussy, argumentative, and likely to throw temper tantrums even as very young children.

The following is a list of signs that may suggest that a child has ODD (APA, 1994). Be careful; as mentioned earlier, many children are oppositional from time to time. Children with ODD really stand out from other kids due to their poor behavior. Also, this pattern of behavior must have been going on for at least 6 months before the diagnosis of ODD can be considered.

"Oppositional Defiant Disorder (ODD)" by Garret D. Evans, Psy.D., © 1999 University of Florida Institute of Food and Agricultural Sciences. Reviewed February 2007. Reprinted with permission.

Signs of Oppositional Defiant Disorder

- Temper tantrums, even over small disagreements, very upset when they don't get their own way.
- Argues with adults, especially with those in authority.
- Defies or deliberately refuses to follow rules or directions given by adults.
- Deliberately annoys people, continues a behavior after being asked to stop several times (e.g., touching things, saying something, making sounds, etc.).
- Blames others for his or her mistakes or misbehavior.
- Seems touchy or easily annoyed by others.
- Seems angry and resentful much of the time, walks around with a "sour-puss" much of the time.
- Often wants to "even the score" with others, is spiteful toward others.

These children often need special attention while growing up to overcome their behavior problems. Unfortunately, the "special attention" they receive often comes in the form of almost non-stop punishment, teasing by siblings and peers, and being singled-out as the "problem child" at home and school.

Like other children with behavior problems, they often have low self-esteem and don't get along with brothers, sisters, and kids their own age. They also may have school problems related to their poor classroom behavior and problems with classmates.

If the condition is not successfully treated in childhood and the early teens, the child is likely to have greater problems in their teenage and early adult years. For example, children with ODD are vulnerable to having problems with drugs, alcohol, tobacco, and early sexual activity. As teenagers, their parents often complain that they are "running around with the wrong crowd" and that they can't seem to control them anymore.

While this report gives specific information for identifying signs and symptoms of ODD in children, parents and others should not try to diagnose any type of behavioral or emotional disorder in their children or themselves. A diagnosis of ODD can only be made with confidence by a mental health professional who has been specifically trained in the assessment and treatment of this disorder.

Reference

American Psychiatric Association. (2000). *Diagnostic and statistical manual of mental disorders (text revision).* Washington, DC: Author.

Footnotes

1. This document is FCS 2135, one of a series of the Family Youth and Community Sciences Department, Florida Cooperative Extension Service, Institute of Food and Agricultural Sciences, University of Florida. Original publication date July 1, 1999. Reviewed February 27, 2007 by Heidi Radunovich, Assistant Professor, Department of Family, Youth and Community Sciences. Visit the EDIS Web Site at http://edis.ifas.ufl.edu.

2. Garret D. Evans, Psy.D., associate professor, Clinical Psychology, Department of Family, Youth and Community Sciences, Cooperative Extension Service, Institute of Food and Agricultural Sciences, University of Florida, Gainesville, 32611.

Chapter 75

Substance Abuse in Youth

Substance use has fluctuated nationally since the mid-1970s when the government and other independent sources began collecting data on this behavior. Over the past 5–10 years, the level of substance use has remained relatively stable; however, research indicates changes in the types of drugs used. Each year, a number of national surveys are conducted to determine the prevalence of substance use in this country, the number of new users (or incidence of the behavior), and the attitudes of users and non-users.

Overview

The National Survey on Drug Use and Health (NSDUH) is a household survey conducted by the federal government's Substance Abuse and Mental Health Services Administration (SAMHSA). In the past, this survey was referred to as The National Household Survey on Drug Abuse (NHSDA). The most recent data report:

- An estimated 19.9 million Americans currently use illicit drugs, representing 8% of the population 12 and older.
- Marijuana is the most common illicit drug, used by 73% of people reporting illicit substance use.

Excerpted from "Substance Abuse," by the National Youth Violence Prevention Resource Center (www.safeyouth.org), sponsored by the Centers for Disease Control and Prevention, 2001. Reviewed and revised by David A. Cooke, M.D., January 22, 2009.

- Approximately 3.7% of the population (an estimated 9.3 million Americans) use other illicit drugs, such as cocaine, heroin, crack, hallucinogens, and other psychotherapeutic medications taken non-medically or without prescription.

Tobacco and alcohol misuse are other aspects of substance use that are tracked by national surveys.

- Over 28% of the population surveyed in the 2007 NSDUH reported current use of tobacco, with the vast majority smoking cigarettes.
- About 58 million Americans (an estimated 23.3%) reported engaging in binge drinking episodes, defined as having 5 or more drinks on one occasion during the 30 days prior to the survey.
- Over 17 million Americans (an estimated 6.9%) were identified as heavy drinkers, having 5 or more drinks on one occasion 5 or more times during the 30 days prior to the survey.
- Although consumption of alcohol is illegal for those under 21, 10.7 million drinkers were ages 12–20 in 2007. In this group, 7.2 million (approximately 67%) engaged in binge drinking.

Variation by Age

Rates and patterns of drug use tend to vary by age. For example, 3.3% of 12-year-olds surveyed in the NSDUH reported current (use within the past month) illicit drug use. Among this age group, the primary illicit drugs of choice were inhalants and psychotherapeutics (1.1% and 1.4%, respectively). Only 0.9% of the 12-year-olds used marijuana. However, by age 14, marijuana was the dominant drug, with a prevalence of 5.7%. Overall, the rate of current illicit drug use among 14-year-olds was 8.9%.

Among youth 12 to 17 years of age, 9.5% had used an illicit drug within the 30 days prior to survey. Of this group, 6.7% had used marijuana, and 3.7% had used some illicit drug other than marijuana. Nearly 10% of youth in this age group report current cigarette smoking, compared to 36.2% of young adults aged 18–25 and 24% of adults 26 and older. More than 10.7 million youth under age 20, report current alcohol use, with 67% of these individuals reporting binge drinking.

Risk and Protective Factors

All young people are exposed to both risk and protective factors for substance abuse. Risk factors place individuals at greater than average risk for substance use, whereas protective factors buffer youth from initiating or continuing use. Typically, the greater the number of risk factors, the higher a youth's susceptibility. In contrast, the accumulation of protective factors appears to reduce risk.

It is important to note that the importance of a given risk or protective factor can vary with the type of substance, a youth's stage of development, and a youth's gender or ethnic/racial group. For example:

- parental communication of norms has been found to be a protective factor for alcohol use, but not for marijuana use;
- repeating a grade in school increases a youth's risk for cigarette use in grades 7–8, but not in grades 9–12; and
- aggressive behavior in early childhood is predictive of later substance abuse for boys, but not for girls.

Also, it is important to keep in mind that factors significant for earlier stages of use and initiation (such as "trying" marijuana) may differ from those related to the transition to dependence (for example, heroin addiction or alcoholism). Social, situational, and environmental factors are likely to be more influential in initial or low-level substance use, while individuals who progress from use to abuse or addiction are influenced to a greater extent by biological, psychological, and psychiatric factors.

Risk and protective factors exist in six different domains: the individual environment, family environment, peer association, school-related, society-related, and community environment.

Individual Risk and Protective Factors

Numerous individual factors have been identified that increase an individual's risk for substance use and abuse. Boys are typically at much greater risk for early initiation and later substance abuse than girls.

The age at which one first drinks alcohol or tries other substances is also an important factor. Age at initiation is predictive of later problems with a substance, with earlier use placing individuals at greater risk for later abuse. About 40% of those who start drinking at age 14 years or under develop alcohol dependence at some point in their lives; for those who start drinking at age 21 years or older, only 10% develop alcohol dependence.

Age at onset of alcohol and marijuana use is also a strong predictor of progression to other drugs. In one study, researchers found that if a child smoked tobacco or drank alcohol, he/she was 65 times more likely to use marijuana than a child who never smoked or drank. Children who used marijuana were 104 times as likely to use cocaine compared with their peers who never used marijuana.

Youth with emotional and psychological problems are at greater risk for substance use and abuse. Boys with a history of aggressive behavior early in childhood are more likely to use drugs, as are youth with persistent antisocial behavior in early adolescence, such as misbehaving in school, skipping school, and getting into fights with other children. A history of sensation-seeking, low harm-avoidance, and lack of impulse control also puts boys at risk.

Finally, antisocial beliefs and values and specific positive beliefs about a substance can increase the likelihood of substance use.

Identified individual-level protective factors that promote resistance to drug use include: positive self-esteem, self-control, assertiveness, social competence, a spiritual or religious identity, and academic achievement.

Family Environment Risk and Protective Factors

If children are raised in a family with a history of addiction to alcohol or other drugs, the risk of their having substance abuse problems themselves increases. Access to alcohol and drugs in their homes also increases youth's likelihood of substance use.

Parental family management and discipline practices can also put youth at risk, including a lack of clear expectations for behavior, failure of parents to monitor their children (knowing where they are and who they are with), and use of excessively severe or inconsistent punishment. A low level of parent/child attachment and nurturing can also increase a youth's risk for substance use, as can a chaotic home environment. Finally, abuse in the home has also been implicated as a significant risk factor for later substance abuse.

In contrast, factors such as parent/family connectedness, warmth and attachment, parent/ adolescent shared activities, parent supervision, high parental school expectations, and parental communication of norms against a substance, can promote resistance to drug use.

Chapter 76

Treating Youth with Mental Health Disorders

There has been public concern over reports that very young children are being prescribed psychotropic medications. The studies to date are incomplete, and much more needs to be learned about young children who are treated with medications for all kinds of illnesses. In the field of mental health, new studies are needed to tell us what the best treatments are for children with emotional and behavioral disturbances.

Children are in a state of rapid change and growth during their developmental years. Diagnosis and treatment of mental disorders must be viewed with these changes in mind. While some problems are short-lived and don't need treatment, others are persistent and very serious, and parents should seek professional help for their children.

Not long ago, it was thought that many brain disorders such as anxiety disorders, depression, and bipolar disorder began only after childhood. We now know they can begin in early childhood. An estimated 1 in 10 children and adolescents in the United States suffers from mental illness severe enough to cause some level of impairment. Fewer than one in five of these ill children receives treatment. Perhaps the most studied, diagnosed, and treated childhood-onset mental disorder is attention deficit hyperactivity disorder (ADHD), but even with this disorder there is a need for further research in very young children.

From "Treatment of Children with Mental Disorders," a booklet by the National Institute of Mental Health (NIMH, www.nimh.nih.gov), part of the National Institutes of Health, 2004.

Questions and Answers

What should I do if I am concerned about mental, behavioral, or emotional symptoms in my young child?

Talk to your child's doctor. Ask questions and find out everything you can about the behavior or symptoms that worry you. Every child is different and even normal development varies from child to child. Sensory processing, language, and motor skills are developing during early childhood, as well as the ability to relate to parents and to socialize with caregivers and other children. If your child is in daycare or preschool, ask the caretaker or teacher if your child has been showing any worrisome changes in behavior, and discuss this with your child's doctor.

How do I know if my child's problems are serious?

Many everyday stresses cause changes in behavior. The birth of a sibling may cause a child to temporarily act much younger. It is important to recognize such behavior changes, but also to differentiate them from signs of more serious problems. Problems deserve attention when they are severe, persistent, and impact on daily activities. Seek help for your child if you observe problems such as changes in appetite or sleep, social withdrawal, or fearfulness; behavior that seems to slip back to an earlier phase such as bed-wetting; signs of distress such as sadness or tearfulness; self-destructive behavior such as head banging; or a tendency to have frequent injuries. In addition, it is essential to review the development of your child, any important medical problem he/she might have had, family history of mental disorders, as well as physical and psychological traumas or situations that may cause stress.

Whom should I consult to help my child?

First, consult your child's doctor. Ask for a complete health examination of your child. Describe the behaviors that worry you. Ask whether your child needs further evaluation by a specialist in child behavioral problems. Such specialists may include psychiatrists, psychologists, social workers, and behavioral therapists. Educators may also be needed to help your child.

How are mental disorders diagnosed in young children?

Similar to adults, disorders are diagnosed by observing signs and symptoms. A skilled professional will consider these signs and symptoms in the context of the child's developmental level, social and physical environment, and reports from parents and other caretakers or teachers, and an assessment will be made according to criteria established by experts. Very young children often cannot express their thoughts and feelings, which makes diagnosis a challenging task. The signs of a mental disorder in a young child may be quite different from those of an older child or an adult.

Stimulant medications: There are four stimulant medications that are approved for use in the treatment of attention deficit hyperactivity disorder (ADHD), the most common behavioral disorder of childhood. These medications have all been extensively studied and are specifically labeled for pediatric use. Children with ADHD exhibit such symptoms as short attention span, excessive activity, and impulsivity that cause substantial impairment in functioning. Stimulant medication should be prescribed only after a careful evaluation to establish the diagnosis of ADHD and to rule out other disorders or conditions. Medication treatment should be administered and monitored in the context of the overall needs of the child and family, and consideration should be given to combining it with behavioral therapy. If the child is of school age, collaboration with teachers is essential.

Antidepressant and antianxiety medications: These medications follow the stimulant medications in prevalence among children and adolescents. They are used for depression, a disorder recognized only in the last 20 years as a problem for children, and for anxiety disorders, including obsessive-compulsive disorder (OCD). The medications most widely prescribed for these disorders are the selective serotonin reuptake inhibitors (the SSRIs).

In the human brain, there are many "neurotransmitters" that affect the way we think, feel, and act. Three of these neurotransmitters that antidepressants influence are serotonin, dopamine, and norepinephrine. SSRIs affect mainly serotonin and have been found to be effective in treating depression and anxiety without as many side effects as some older antidepressants.

Antipsychotic medications: These medications are used to treat children with schizophrenia, bipolar disorder, autism, Tourette syndrome, and severe conduct disorders. Some of the older antipsychotic medications have specific indications and dose guidelines for children. Some of the newer "atypical" antipsychotics, which have fewer side effects, are also being used for children. Such use requires close monitoring for side effects.

Mood stabilizing medications: These medications are used to treat bipolar disorder (manic-depressive illness). However, because there is very limited data on the safety and efficacy of most mood stabilizers in youth, treatment of children and adolescents is based mainly on experience with adults. The most typically used mood stabilizers are lithium and valproate (Depakote®), which are often very effective for controlling mania and preventing recurrences of manic and depressive episodes in adults. Research on the effectiveness of these and other medications in children and adolescents with bipolar disorder is ongoing. In addition, studies are investigating various forms of psychotherapy, including cognitive-behavioral therapy, to complement medication treatment for this illness in young people.

Effective treatment depends on appropriate diagnosis of bipolar disorder in children and adolescents. There is some evidence that using antidepressant medication to treat depression in a person who has bipolar disorder may induce manic symptoms if it is taken without a mood stabilizer. In addition, using stimulant medications to treat co-occurring ADHD or ADHD-like symptoms in a child with bipolar disorder may worsen manic symptoms. While it can be hard to determine which young patients will become manic, there is a greater likelihood among children and adolescents who have a family history of bipolar disorder. If manic symptoms develop or markedly worsen during antidepressant or stimulant use, a physician should be consulted immediately, and diagnosis and treatment for bipolar disorder should be considered.

What difference does it make if a medication is specifically approved for use in children or not?

Approval of a medication by the FDA [U.S. Food and Drug Administration] means that adequate data have been provided to the FDA by the drug manufacturer to show safety and efficacy for a particular therapy in a particular population. Based on the data, a label indication for the drug is established that includes proper dosage, potential side effects, and approved age. Doctors prescribe medications as they feel appropriate even if those uses are not included in the labeling. Although in some cases there is extensive clinical experience in using medications for children or adolescents, in many cases there is not. Everyone agrees that more studies in children are needed if we are to know the appropriate dosages, how a drug works in children, and what effects there are on learning and development.

What does "off-label" use of a medication mean?

Many medications that are on the market have not been officially approved by the FDA for use in children. Treatment of children with

Table 76.1. Medications Used to Treat Mental Health Disorders in Children

Type of Medication	Brand Name	Generic Name	Approved Age
Stimulant Medications	Adderall	amphetamines	3 and older
	Concerta	methylphenidate	6 and older
	Cylert	pemoline	6 and older[1]
	Dexedrine	dextroamphetamine	3 and older
	Dextrostat	dextroamphetamine	3 and older
	Ritalin	methylphenidate	6 and older
Antidepressant and Antianxiety Medications	Anafranil	clomipramine	10 and older (for OCD)
	BuSpar	buspirone	18 and older
	Effexor	venlafaxine	18 and older
	Luvox (SSRI)	fluvoxamine	8 and older (for OCD)
	Paxil (SSRI)	paroxetine	18 and older
	Prozac (SSRI)	fluoxetine	18 and older
	Serzone (SSRI)	nefazodone	18 and older
	Sinequan	doxepin	12 and older
	Tofranil	imipramine	6 and older (for bed-wetting)
	Wellbutrin	bupropion	18 and older
	Zoloft (SSRI)	sertraline	6 and older (for OCD)
Antipsychotic Medications	Clozaril(atypical)	clozapine	18 and older
	Haldol	haloperidol	3 and older
	Risperdal (atypical)	risperidone	5 to 16 years[2] ; 18 and older[3]
	Seroquel (atypical)	quetiapine	18 and older
	(Generic Only)	thioridazine	2 and older
	Zyprexa (atypical)	olanzapine	18 and older
	Orap	pimozide	12 and older[4]
Mood Stabilizing Medications	Cibalith-S	lithium citrate	12 and older
	Depakote	divalproex sodium	2 and older (for seizures)
	Eskalith	lithium carbonate	12 and older
	Lithobid	lithium carbonate	12 and older
	Tegretol	carbamazepine	any age (for seizures)

Notes:

1. Because of its potential for serious side effects affecting the liver, Cylert should not ordinarily be considered as first line drug therapy for ADHD.
2. For irritability associated with autistic disorder.
3. For schizophrenia and bipolar mania.
4. For Tourette syndrome. Data for age 2 and older indicate similar safety profile.

these medications is called "off-label" use. For some medications, the off-label use is supported by data from well-conducted studies in children. For instance, some antidepressant medications have been shown to be effective in children and adolescents with depression. For other medications, there are no controlled studies in children, but only isolated clinical reports. In particular, the use of psychotropic medications in preschoolers has not been adequately studied and must be considered very carefully by balancing severity of symptoms, degree of impairment, and potential benefits and risks of treatment.

Why haven't many medications been tested in children?

In the past, medications were not studied in children because of ethical concerns about involving children in clinical trials. However, this created a new problem: lack of knowledge about the best treatments for children. In clinical settings where children are suffering from mental or behavioral disorders, medications are being prescribed at increasingly early ages. The FDA has been urging that products be appropriately studied in children and has offered incentives to drug manufacturers to carry out such testing. The NIH [National Institutes of Health] and the FDA are examining the issue of medication research in children and are developing new research approaches.

Does the FDA approve medications for different age groups among children?

Yes. However, this is based on the data provided to the FDA by the drug manufacturer and the policies in effect at the time of approval. For example, Ritalin® is approved for children age 6 and older, whereas Dexedrine® is approved for children as young as 3. When Ritalin® was tested for efficacy by its manufacturer, only children age 6 and above were involved; therefore, age 6 was approved as the lower age limit for Ritalin®.

Can events such as a death in the family, illness in a parent, onset of poverty, or divorce cause symptoms?

Yes. When a tragedy occurs or some extreme stress hits, every member of a family is affected, even the youngest ones. This should also be considered when evaluating mental, emotional, or behavioral symptoms in a child.

Chapter 77

Taking Your Child to a Therapist

Sometimes kids, like adults, can benefit from therapy. Therapy can help kids develop problem-solving skills and also teach them the value of seeking help. Therapists can help kids and families cope with stress and a variety of emotional and behavioral issues.

Many kids need help dealing with school stress, such as homework, test anxiety, bullying, or peer pressure. Others need help to discuss their feelings about family issues, particularly if there's a major transition, such as a divorce, move, or serious illness.

Should My Child See a Therapist?

Significant life events—such as the death of a family member, friend, or pet; divorce or a move; abuse; trauma; a parent leaving on military deployment; or a major illness in the family—can cause stress that might lead to problems with behavior, mood, sleep, appetite, and academic or social functioning.

In some cases, it's not as clear what's caused a child to suddenly seem withdrawn, worried, stress, sulky, or tearful. But if you feel your

---

"Taking Your Child to a Therapist," August 2007, reprinted with permission from www.kidshealth.org. This information was provided by KidsHealth, one of the largest resources online for medically reviewed health information written for parents, kids, and teens. For more articles like this one, visit www.KidsHealth.org, or www.TeensHealth.org.

child might have an emotional or behavioral problem or needs help coping with a difficult life event, trust your instincts.

Signs that your child may benefit from seeing a psychologist or licensed therapist include:

- developmental delay in speech, language, or toilet training
- learning or attention problems (such as ADHD)
- behavioral problems (such as excessive anger, acting out, bedwetting or eating disorders)
- a significant drop in grades, particularly if your child normally maintains high grades
- episodes of sadness, tearfulness, or depression
- social withdrawal or isolation
- being the victim of bullying or bullying other children
- decreased interest in previously enjoyed activities
- overly aggressive behavior (such as biting, kicking, or hitting)
- sudden changes in appetite (particularly in adolescents)
- insomnia or increased sleepiness
- excessive school absenteeism or tardiness
- mood swings (e.g., happy one minute, upset the next)
- development of or an increase in physical complaints (such as headache, stomachache, or not feeling well) despite a normal physical exam by your doctor
- management of a serious, acute, or chronic illness
- signs of alcohol, drug, or other substance use (such as solvents or prescription drug abuse)
- problems in transitions (following separation, divorce, or relocation)
- bereavement issues
- custody evaluations
- therapy following sexual, physical, or emotional abuse or
- other traumatic events

Kids who aren't yet school-age could benefit from seeing a developmental or clinical psychologist if there's a significant delay in achieving developmental milestones such as walking, talking, and potty training, and if there are concerns regarding autism or other developmental disorders.

It's also helpful to speak to caregivers and teachers who interact regularly with your child. Is your child paying attention in class and turning in assignments on time? What's his or her behavior like at recess and with peers? Gather as much information as possible to determine the best course of action.

Discuss your concerns with your child's doctor, who can offer perspective and evaluate your child to rule out any medical conditions that could be having an effect. The doctor also may be able to refer you to a qualified therapist for the help your child needs.

Finding the Right Therapist

How do you find a qualified clinician who has experience working with kids and teens? While experience and education are important, it's also important to find a counselor your child feels comfortable talking to. Look for one who not only has the right experience, but also the best approach to help your child in the current circumstances.

Your doctor can be a good source of a referral. Most doctors have working relationships with mental health specialists such as child psychologists or clinical social workers. Friends, colleagues, or family members might also be able to recommend someone.

Consider a number of factors when searching for the right therapist for your child. A good first step is to ask if the therapist is willing to meet with you for a brief consultation or to talk with you during a phone interview before you commit to regular visits. Not all therapists are able to do this, given their busy schedules. Most therapists charge a fee for this type of service; others consider it a complimentary visit.

Consider the following factors when evaluating a potential therapist:

- Is the therapist licensed to practice in your state? (You can check with the state board for that profession or check to see if the license is displayed in the office.)
- Is the therapist covered by your health insurance plan's mental health benefits? If so, how many sessions are covered by your plan? What will your co-pay be?
- What are his or her credentials?

- What type of experience does the therapist have?
- How long has the therapist worked with children and adolescents?
- Would your child find the therapist friendly?
- What is the cancellation policy if you're unable to keep an appointment?
- Is the therapist available by phone during an emergency?
- Who will be available to your child during the therapist's vacation or illness or during off-hours?
- What types of therapy does the therapist specialize in?
- Is the therapist willing to meet with you in addition to working with your child?

The right therapist-client match is critical, so you might need to meet with a few before you find one who clicks with both you and your child.

As with other medical professionals, therapists may have a variety of credentials and specific degrees. As a general rule, your child's therapist should hold a professional degree in the field of mental health (psychology, social work, or psychiatry) and be licensed by your state. Psychologists, social workers, and psychiatrists all diagnose and treat mental health disorders.

It's also a good idea to know what those letters that follow a therapist's name mean:

Psychiatrists

Psychiatrists (MDs or DOs) are medical doctors who have advanced training and experience in psychotherapy and pharmacology. They can also prescribe medications.

Clinical Psychologists

Clinical psychologists (PhDs, PsyDs, or EdDs) are therapists who have a doctorate degree that includes advanced training in the practice of psychology, and many specialize in treating children and teens and their families. Psychologists may help clients manage medications but do not prescribe medication.

Clinical Social Workers

A licensed clinical social worker (LCSW) has a master's degree, specializes in clinical social work, and is licensed in the state in which he or she practices. An LICSW is also a licensed clinical social worker. A CSW is a certified social worker. Many social workers are trained in psychotherapy, but the credentials vary from state to state. Likewise, the designations (i.e., LCSW, LICSW, CSW) can vary from state to state.

Different Types of Therapy

There are many types of therapy. Therapists choose the strategies that are most appropriate for a particular problem and for the individual child and family. Therapists will often spend a portion of each session with the parents alone, with the child alone, and with the family together.

Any one therapist may use a variety of strategies, including:

Cognitive Behavioral Therapy (CBT)

This type of therapy is often helpful with kids and teens who are depressed, anxious, or having problems coping with stress.

Cognitive behavioral therapy restructures negative thoughts into more positive, effective ways of thinking. It can include work on stress management strategies, relaxation training, practicing coping skills, and other forms of treatment.

Psychoanalytic therapy is less commonly used with children but can be used with older kids and teens who may benefit from more in-depth analysis of their problems. This is the quintessential "talk therapy" and does not focus on short-term problem-solving in the same way as CBT and behavioral therapies.

In some cases, kids benefit from individual therapy, one-on-one work with the therapist on issues they need guidance on, such as depression, social difficulties, or worry. In other cases, the right option is group therapy, where kids meet in groups of 6 to 12 to solve problems and learn new skills (such as social skills or anger management).

Family therapy can be helpful in many cases, such as when family members aren't getting along; disagree or argue often; or when a child or teen is having behavior problems. Family therapy involves counseling sessions with some, or all, family members, helping to improve communication skills among them. Treatment focuses on problem-solving techniques and can help parents re-establish their role as authority figures.

Preparing for the First Visit

You may be concerned that your child will become upset when told of an upcoming visit with a therapist. Although this is sometimes the case, it's essential to be honest about the session and why your child (or family) will be going. The issue will come up during the session, but it's important for you to prepare your child for it.

Explain to young kids that this type of visit to the doctor doesn't involve a physical exam or shots. You may also want to stress that this type of doctor talks and plays with kids and families to help them solve problems and feel better. Kids might feel reassured to learn that the therapist will be helping the parents and other family members too.

Older kids and teens may be reassured to hear that anything they say to the therapist is confidential and cannot be shared with anyone else, including parents or other doctors, without their permission—the exception is if they indicate that they're having thoughts of suicide or otherwise hurting themselves or others.

Giving kids this kind of information before the first appointment can help set the tone, prevent your child from feeling singled out or isolated, and provide reassurance that the family will be working together on the problem.

Providing Additional Support

While your child copes with emotional issues, be there to listen and care, and offer support without judgment. Patience is critical, too, as many young children are unable to verbalize their fears and emotions.

Try to set aside some time to discuss your child's worries or concerns. To minimize distractions, turn off the TV and let voice mail answer your phone calls. This will let your child know that he or she is your first priority.

Other ways to communicate openly and problem-solve include:

- Talk openly and as frequently with your child as you can.
- Show love and affection to your child, especially during troubled times.
- Set a good example by taking care of your own physical and emotional needs.
- Enlist the support of your partner, immediate family members, your child's doctor, and teachers.

- Improve communication at home by having family meetings that end with a fun activity (e.g., playing a game, making ice-cream sundaes).
- No matter how hard it is, set limits on inappropriate or problematic behaviors. Ask the therapist for some strategies to encourage your child's cooperation.
- Communicate frequently with the therapist.
- Be open to all types of feedback from your child and from the therapist.
- Respect the relationship between your child and the therapist. If you feel threatened by it, discuss this with the therapist (it's nothing to be embarrassed about).
- Enjoy favorite activities or hobbies with your child.

By recognizing problems and seeking help early on, you can help your child—and your entire family—move through the tough times toward happier, healthier times ahead.

Chapter 78

Helping Children and Adolescents Exposed to Violence and Disasters

Violence or disasters can cause trauma in young people. Trauma is hurt or harm. It can be hurt to a person's body. It can be harm to a person's mind.

Parents and family members play important roles. They help children who experience violence or disaster. They help children cope with trauma. They help protect children from further trauma. They help children get medical care and counseling. They also help young people avoid or overcome emotional problems. These problems can result from trauma.

Coping with Trauma after Violence and Disasters

Disasters cause major damage. Hurricanes Katrina and Rita were examples. They occurred in 2005. Many homes were destroyed. Whole communities were damaged. Many survivors were displaced. There were also many deaths.

Trauma is also caused by major acts of violence. The September 11, 2001 terrorist attacks were examples. Another example was the 1999 shootings at Columbine High School in Colorado. The Oklahoma City bombing in 1995 was also an example. These acts claim lives. They also threaten our sense of security.

From "Helping Children and Adolescents Cope with Violence and Disasters: What Parents Can Do," by the National Institute of Mental Health (NIMH, www.nimh.nih.gov), part of the National Institutes of Health, June 26, 2008.

Beyond these events, children face many other traumas. Each year, they are injured. They see others harmed by violence. They suffer sexual abuse. They lose loved ones. Or, they witness other tragic events.

Children are very sensitive. They struggle to make sense of trauma. They also respond differently to traumas. They may have emotional reactions. They may hurt deeply. They may find it hard to recover from frightening experiences. They need support. Adult helpers can provide this support. This may help children resolve emotional problems.

What Is Trauma?

There are two types of trauma—physical and mental. Physical trauma includes the body's response to serious injury and threat. Mental trauma includes frightening thoughts and painful feelings. They are the mind's response to serious injury. Mental trauma can produce strong feelings. It can also produce extreme behavior; such as intense fear or helplessness, withdrawal or detachment, lack of concentration, irritability, sleep disturbance, aggression, hypervigilance (intensely watching for more distressing events), or flashbacks (sense that event is reoccurring).

A response could be fear. It could be fear that a loved one will be hurt or killed. It is believed that more direct exposures to traumatic events causes greater harm. For instance, in a school shooting, an injured student will probably be more severely affected emotionally than a student who was in another part of the building. However, secondhand exposure to violence can also be traumatic. This includes witnessing violence such as seeing or hearing about death and destruction after a building is bombed or a plane crashes.

Helping Young Trauma Survivors

Helping children begins at the scene of the event. It may need to continue for weeks or months. Most children recover within a few weeks. Some need help longer. Grief (a deep emotional response to loss) may take months to resolve. It could be for a loved one or a teacher. It could be for a friend or pet. Grief may be re-experienced or worsened by news reports or the event's anniversary.

Some children may need help from a mental health professional. Some people may seek other kinds of help. They may turn to religious leaders. They may turn to community leaders.

Identify children who need the most support. Help them obtain it. Monitor their healing.

Identify children who refuse to go places that remind them of the event; seem numb emotionally; show little reaction to the event; or behave dangerously. These children may need extra help.

In general adult helpers should:

- Attend to children:
    - Listen to them.
    - Accept/do not argue about their feelings.
    - Help them cope with the reality of their experiences.
- Reduce effects of other sources of stress including:
    - frequent moving or changes in place of residence;
    - long periods away from family and friends;
    - pressures at school;
    - transportation problems;
    - fighting within the family; and
    - being hungry.
- Monitor healing:
    - It takes time.
    - Do not ignore severe reactions.
    - Attend to sudden changes in behaviors, speech, language use, or in emotional/feeling states.
- Remind children that adults:
    - love them;
    - support them; and
    - will be with them when possible.

How Parents Can Help

After violence or a disaster parents and family should:

- identify and address their own feelings—this will allow them to help others;
- explain to children what happened; and
- let children know:
    - you love them;
    - the event was not their fault;

- you will take care of them, but only if you can; be honest; and
- it's okay for them to feel upset.

Do:

- allow children to cry;
- allow sadness;
- let children talk about feelings;
- let them write about feelings; and
- let them draw pictures.

Don't:

- expect children to be brave or tough;
- make children discuss the event before they are ready;
- get angry if children show strong emotions; or
- get upset if they begin:
  - bed-wetting;
  - acting out; or
  - thumb-sucking.

If children have trouble sleeping:

- give them extra attention;
- let them sleep with a light on;
- let them sleep in your room (for a short time); and
- try to keep normal routines (such routines may not be normal for some children):
  - bedtime stories
  - eating dinner together;
  - watching TV together; and
  - reading books, exercising, and playing games.
- If you can't keep normal routines, make new ones together.
- Help children feel in control:
  - let them choose meals, if possible;

- let them pick out clothes, if possible; and
- let them make some decisions for themselves, when possible.

Help for All People in the First Days and Weeks

Key steps after a disaster can help adults cope. Adults can then provide better care for children. Create an environment of safety. Be calm. Be hopeful. Be friendly, even if people are difficult. Connect to others. Listen to their stories. But, listen only if they want to share. Encourage respect for adult decision-making.

In general help people:

- get food;
- get a safe place to live;
- get help from a doctor or nurse if hurt;
- contact loved ones or friends;
- keep children with parents or relatives;
- become aware of available help;
- become aware of where to get help;
- understand what happened;
- understand what is being done; and
- move toward meeting their own needs.

Avoid certain things:

- Don't force people to tell their stories.
- Don't probe for personal details.
- Do not say:
    - "Everything will be OK";
    - "At least you survived";
    - what you think people should feel;
    - how people should have acted;
    - people suffered for personal behaviors or beliefs; or
    - negative things about available help.
- Don't make promises that you can't keep (Ex: "You will go home soon.")

How Children React to Trauma

Children's reactions to trauma can be immediate. Reactions may also appear much later. Reactions differ in severity. They also cover a range of behaviors. People from different cultures may have their own ways of reacting. Other reactions vary according to age.

One common response is loss of trust. Another is fear of the event reoccurring. Some children are more vulnerable to trauma's effects. Children with existing mental health problems may be more affected. Children who have experienced other traumatic events may be more affected.

Children Age 5 and Under

Children under 5 can react in a number of ways:

- facial expressions of fear;
- clinging to parent or caregiver;
- crying or screaming;
- whimpering or trembling;
- moving aimlessly;
- becoming immobile;
- returning to behaviors common to being younger;
- thumb sucking;
- bedwetting; and
- being afraid of the dark.

Young children's reactions are strongly influenced by parent reactions to the event.

Children Age 6 to 11

Children between 6 and 11 have a range of reactions. They may:

- isolate themselves;
- become quiet around friends, family, and teachers;
- have nightmares or other sleep problems;
- become irritable or disruptive;
- have outbursts of anger;
- start fights;
- be unable to concentrate;

- refuse to go to school;
- complain of unfounded physical problems;
- develop unfounded fears;
- become depressed;
- become filled with guilt;
- feel numb emotionally; or
- do poorly with school and homework.

Adolescents Age 12 to 17

Children between 12 and 17 have various reactions:

- flashbacks to the traumatic event (flashbacks are the mind reliving the event);
- avoiding reminders of the event;
- drug, alcohol, tobacco use and abuse;
- antisocial behavior i.e. disruptive, disrespectful, or destructive behavior;
- physical complaints;
- nightmares or other sleep problems;
- isolation or confusion;
- depression; or
- suicidal thoughts.

Adolescents may feel guilty about the event. They may feel guilt for not preventing injury or deaths. They may also have thoughts of revenge.

More about Trauma and Stress

Some children will have prolonged problems after a traumatic event. These may include grief, depression, anxiety, and post-traumatic stress disorder (PTSD). Children may show a range of symptoms:

- Re-experiencing the event:
    - through play;
    - through trauma-specific nightmares/dreams;
    - in flashbacks and unwanted memories; or
    - by distress over events that remind them of the trauma
- avoidance of reminders of the event;

- lack of responsiveness;
- lack of interest in things that used to interest them;
- a sense of having "no future";
- increased sleep disturbances;
- irritability;
- poor concentration;
- be easily startled; or
- behavior from earlier life stages.

Children experience trauma differently. It is difficult to tell how many will develop mental health problems. Some trauma survivors get better with only good support. Others need counseling by a mental health professional.

If, after a month in a safe environment children are not able to perform normal routines or new symptoms develop, then, contact a health professional.

Some people are more sensitive to trauma. Factors that may influence how someone may respond include:

- being directly involved in the trauma, especially as a victim;
- severe and/or prolonged exposure to the event;
- personal history of prior trauma;
- family or personal history of mental illness and severe behavioral problems;
- lack of social support;
- lack of caring family and friends; and
- on-going life stressors such as moving to a new home, or new school, divorce, job change, or financial troubles.

Some symptoms may require immediate attention. Contact a mental health professional if these symptoms occur:

- flashbacks;
- racing heart and sweating;
- being easily startled;
- being emotionally numb;
- being very sad or depressed; and
- thoughts or actions to end life.

Chapter 79

Helping Kids Deal with Bullies

Each day, 10-year-old Seth asked his mom for more and more lunch money. Yet he seemed skinnier than ever and came home from school hungry. It turned out that Seth was handing his lunch money to a fifth-grader, who was threatening to beat him up if he didn't pay.

Kayla, 13, thought things were going well at her new school, since all the popular girls were being so nice to her. But then she found out that one of them had posted mean rumors about her on a website. Kayla cried herself to sleep that night and started going to the nurse's office complaining of a stomachache to avoid the girls in study hall.

Unfortunately, the kind of bullying that Seth and Kayla experienced is widespread. In national surveys, most kids and teens say that bullying happens at school.

A bully can turn something like going to the bus stop or recess into a nightmare for kids. Bullying can leave deep emotional scars that last for life. And in extreme situations, it can culminate in violent threats, property damage, or someone getting seriously hurt.

If your child is being bullied, there are ways to help him or her cope with it on a day-to-day basis and lessen its lasting impact. And even if bullying isn't an issue right in your house right now, it's important to discuss it so your kids will be prepared if it does happen.

What Is Bullying?

Most kids have been teased by a sibling or a friend at some point. And it's not usually harmful when done in a playful, friendly, and mutual way, and both kids find it funny. But when teasing becomes hurtful, unkind, and constant, it crosses the line into bullying and needs to stop.

Bullying is intentional tormenting in physical, verbal, or psychological ways. It can range from hitting, shoving, name-calling, threats, and mocking to extorting money and treasured possessions. Some kids bully by shunning others and spreading rumors about them. Others use e-mail, chat rooms, instant messages, social networking websites, and text messages to taunt others or hurt their feelings.

It's important to take bullying seriously and not just brush it off as something that kids have to "tough out." The effects can be serious and affect kids' sense of self-worth and future relationships. In severe cases, bullying has contributed to tragedies, such as school shootings.

Why Do Kids Bully?

Kids bully for a variety of reasons. Sometimes they pick on kids because they need a victim—someone who seems emotionally or physically weaker, or just acts or appears different in some way—to feel more important, popular, or in control. Although some bullies are bigger or stronger than their victims, that's not always the case.

Sometimes kids torment others because that's the way they've been treated. They may think their behavior is normal because they come from families or other settings where everyone regularly gets angry, shouts, or calls names. Some popular TV shows even seem to promote meanness—people are "voted off," shunned, or ridiculed for their appearance or lack of talent.

Signs of Bullying

Unless your child tells you about bullying—or has visible bruises or injuries—it can be difficult to figure out if it's happening.

But there are some warning signs. You might notice your child acting differently or seeming anxious, or not eating, sleeping well, or doing the things that he or she usually enjoys. When kids seem moodier or more easily upset than usual, or when they start avoiding certain situations, like taking the bus to school, it may be because of a bully.

If you suspect bullying but your child is reluctant to open up, find opportunities to bring up the issue in a more roundabout way. For instance, you might see a situation on a TV show and use it as a conversation starter, asking "What do you think of this?" or "What do you think that person should have done?" This might lead to questions like: "Have you ever seen this happen?" or "Have you ever experienced this?" You might want to talk about any experiences you or another family member had at that age.

Let your child know that if he or she is being bullied—or sees it happening to someone else—it's important to talk to someone about it, whether it's you, another adult (a teacher, school counselor, or family friend), or a sibling.

Helping Kids

If your child tells you about a bully, focus on offering comfort and support, no matter how upset you are. Kids are often reluctant to tell adults about bullying. They feel embarrassed and ashamed that it's happening. They worry that their parents will be disappointed.

Sometimes kids feel like it's their own fault, that if they looked or acted differently it wouldn't be happening. Sometimes they're scared that if the bully finds out that they told, it will get worse. Others are worried that their parents won't believe them or do anything about it. Or kids worry that their parents will urge them to fight back when they're scared to.

Praise your child for being brave enough to talk about it. Remind your child that he or she isn't alone—a lot of people get bullied at some point. Emphasize that it's the bully who is behaving badly—not your child. Reassure your child that you will figure out what to do about it together.

Sometimes an older sibling or friend can help deal with the situation. It may help your daughter to hear how the older sister she idolizes was teased about her braces and how she dealt with it. An older sibling or friend may also be able to give you some perspective on what's happening at school, or wherever the bullying is happening, and help you figure out the best solution.

Take it seriously if you hear that the bullying will get worse if the bully finds out that your child told. Sometimes it's useful to approach the bully's parents. In other cases, teachers or counselors are the best ones to contact first. If you've tried those methods and still want to speak to the bullying child's parents, it's best to do so in a context where a school official, such as a counselor, can mediate.

Many states have bullying laws and policies. Find out about the laws in your community. In certain cases, if you have serious concerns about your child's safety, you may need to contact legal authorities.

Advice for Kids

The key to helping kids is providing strategies that deal with bullying on an everyday basis and also help restore their self-esteem and regain a sense of dignity.

It may be tempting to tell a kid to fight back. After all, you're angry that your child is suffering and maybe you were told to "stand up for yourself" when you were young. And you may worry that your child will continue to suffer at the hands of the bully.

But it's important to advise kids not to respond to bullying by fighting or bullying back. It can quickly escalate into violence, trouble, and someone getting injured. Instead, it's best to walk away from the situation, hang out with others, and tell an adult.

Here are some other strategies to discuss with kids that can help improve the situation and make them feel better:

- **Avoid the bully and use the buddy system.** Use a different bathroom if a bully is nearby and don't go to your locker when there is nobody around. Make sure you have someone with you so that you're not alone with the bully. Buddy up with a friend on the bus, in the hallways, or at recess—wherever the bully is. Offer to do the same for a friend.

- **Hold the anger.** It's natural to get upset by the bully, but that's what bullies thrive on. It makes them feel more powerful. Practice not reacting by crying or looking red or upset. It takes a lot of practice, but it's a useful skill for keeping off of a bully's radar. Sometimes kids find it useful to practice "cool down" strategies such as counting to 10, writing down their angry words, taking deep breaths or walking away. Sometimes the best thing to do is to teach kids to wear a "poker face" until they are clear of any danger (smiling or laughing may provoke the bully).

- **Act brave, walk away, and ignore the bully.** Firmly and clearly tell the bully to stop, then walk away. Practice ways to ignore the hurtful remarks, like acting uninterested or texting someone on your cell phone. By ignoring the bully, you're showing that you don't care. Eventually, the bully will probably get bored with trying to bother you.

- **Tell an adult.** Teachers, principals, parents, and lunchroom personnel at school can all help stop bullying.
- **Talk about it.** Talk to someone you trust, such as a guidance counselor, teacher, sibling, or friend. They may offer some helpful suggestions, and even if they can't fix the situation, it may help you feel a little less alone.
- **Remove the incentives.** If the bully is demanding your lunch money, start bringing your lunch. If he's trying to get your music player, don't bring it to school.

Reaching Out

At home you can lessen the impact of the bullying. Encourage your kids to get together with friends that help build their confidence. Help them meet other kids by joining clubs or sports programs. And find activities that can help a child feel confident and strong. Maybe it's a self-defense class like karate or a movement or other gym class.

And just remember: as upsetting as bullying can be for you and your family, lots of people and resources are available to help.

Part Nine

Additional Help and Information

Chapter 80

Glossary of Terms Related to Mental Health Disorders

agoraphobia: Severe and pervasive anxiety about being in situations from which escape might be difficult or avoidance of situations such as being alone outside of the home, traveling in a car, bus, or airplane, or being in a crowded area.

anorexia nervosa: An eating disorder characterized by unusual eating habits such as avoiding food and meals, picking out a few foods and eating them in small amounts, weighing food, and counting the calories of all foods. Individuals with anorexia nervosa may also exercise excessively.

anxiety disorders: Disorders range from feelings of uneasiness to immobilizing bouts of terror. If a person cannot shake unwarranted worries, or if the feelings are jarring to the point of avoiding everyday activities, he or she most likely has an anxiety disorder.

assertive community treatment: A multidisciplinary clinical team approach of providing 24-hour, intensive community services in the individual's natural setting that help individuals with serious mental illness live in the community.

behavioral therapy: Therapy focused on behavior-changing unwanted behaviors through rewards, reinforcements, and desensitization.

This glossary contains terms excerpted from glossaries and documents produced by the following government agencies: Office of Women's Health and the Substance Abuse and Mental Health Services Administration (SAMHSA).

Desensitization, or exposure therapy, is a process of confronting something that arouses anxiety, discomfort, or fear and overcoming the unwanted responses. Behavioral therapy often involves the cooperation of others, especially family and close friends, to reinforce a desired behavior.

binge eating disorder: An eating disorder characterized by frequent episodes of compulsive overeating, but unlike bulimia, the eating is not followed by purging. During food binges, individuals with this disorder often eat alone and very quickly, regardless of whether they feel hungry or full.

biofeedback: Learning to control muscle tension and "involuntary" body functioning, such as heart rate and skin temperature; it can be a path to mastering one's fears. It is used in combination with, or as an alternative to, medication to treat disorders such as anxiety, panic, and phobias.

bipolar disorder: Extreme mood swings punctuated by periods of generally even-keeled behavior characterize this disorder. Bipolar disorder tends to run in families. This disorder typically begins in the mid-twenties and continues throughout life. Without treatment, people who have bipolar disorder often go through devastating life events such as marital breakups, job loss, substance abuse, and suicide.

body dysmorphic disorder: A condition in which the compulsive and obsessive behavior centers around a preoccupation with one's appearance.

borderline personality disorder: Pervasive instability in moods, interpersonal relationships, self-image, and behavior. The instability can affect family and work life, long-term planning, and the individual's sense of self-identity.

bulimia nervosa: Bulimia nervosa is an eating disorder characterized by excessive eating. People who have bulimia will eat an excessive amount of food in a single episode and almost immediately make themselves vomit or use laxatives or diuretics (water pills) to get rid of the food in their bodies. This behavior often is referred to as the "binge/purge" cycle. Like people with anorexia, people with bulimia have an intense fear of gaining weight.

caregiver: A person who has special training to help people with mental health problems. Examples include social workers, teachers, psychologists, psychiatrists, and mentors.

clinical psychologist: A professional with a doctoral degree in psychology who specializes in therapy.

cognitive therapy: Therapy aims to identify and correct distorted thinking patterns that can lead to feelings and behaviors that may be troublesome, self-defeating, or even self-destructive. The goal is to replace such thinking with a more balanced view that, in turn, leads to more fulfilling and productive behavior.

cognitive/behavioral therapy: A combination of cognitive and behavioral therapies, this approach helps people change negative thought patterns, beliefs, and behaviors so they can manage symptoms and enjoy more productive, less stressful lives.

conduct disorders: Children with conduct disorder repeatedly violate the personal or property rights of others and the basic expectations of society. A diagnosis of conduct disorder is likely when these symptoms continue for 6 months or longer. Conduct disorder is known as a "disruptive behavior disorder" because of its impact on children and their families, neighbors, and schools.

***DSM-IV-TR (Diagnostic and Statistical Manual of Mental Disorders, Fourth Edition, Text Revision)*:** An official manual of mental health problems developed by the American Psychiatric Association. Psychiatrists, psychologists, social workers, and other health and mental health care providers use this reference book to understand and diagnose mental health problems. Insurance companies and health care providers also use the terms and explanations in this book when discussing mental health problems.

depression: A mood disorder characterized by intense feelings of sadness that persist beyond a few weeks. Two neurotransmitters—natural substances that allow brain cells to communicate with one another—are implicated in depression: serotonin and norepinephrine.

dually diagnosed: A person who has both an alcohol or drug problem and an emotional/psychiatric problem is said to have a dual diagnosis.

electroconvulsive therapy: Also known as ECT, this highly controversial technique uses low voltage electrical stimulation of the brain to treat some forms of major depression, acute mania, and some forms of schizophrenia. This potentially life-saving technique is considered only when other therapies have failed, when a person is seriously medically ill and/or unable to take medication, or when a person is very likely to commit suicide. Substantial improvements in the equipment, dosing guidelines, and anesthesia have significantly reduced the possibility of side effects.

group therapy: This form of therapy involves groups of usually four to 12 people who have similar problems and who meet regularly with a therapist. The therapist uses the emotional interactions of the group's members to help them get relief from distress and possibly modify their behavior.

hallucinations: Experiences of sensations that have no source. Some examples of hallucinations include hearing nonexistent voices, seeing nonexistent things, and experiencing burning or pain sensations with no physical cause.

individual therapy: Therapy tailored for a patient/client that is administered one-on-one.

inpatient hospitalization: Mental health treatment provided in a hospital setting 24 hours a day. Inpatient hospitalization provides: (1) short-term treatment in cases where a person is in crisis and possibly a danger to his/herself or others, and (2) diagnosis and treatment when the patient cannot be evaluated or treated appropriately in an outpatient setting.

intake screening: Services designed to briefly assess the type and degree of a client's/patient's mental health condition to determine whether services are needed and to link him/her to the most appropriate and available service. Services may include interviews, psychological testing, physical examinations including speech/hearing, and laboratory studies.

kleptomania: Compulsive stealing.

mental health: How a person thinks, feels, and acts when faced with life's situations. Mental health is how people look at themselves, their lives, and the other people in their lives; evaluate their challenges and problems; and explore choices. This includes handling stress, relating to other people, and making decisions.

obsessive-compulsive disorder: A chronic, relapsing illness. People who have it suffer from recurrent and unwanted thoughts or rituals. The obsessions and the need to perform rituals (compulsions) can take over a person's life if left untreated. They feel they cannot control these thoughts or rituals.

panic disorder: Heart-pounding terror that strikes suddenly and without warning. Since they cannot predict when a panic attack will seize them, many people live in persistent worry that another one could overcome them at any moment.

paranoia and paranoid disorders: Symptoms of paranoia include feelings of persecution and an exaggerated sense of self-importance. The disorder is present in many mental disorders and it is rare as an isolated mental illness.

phobias: Irrational fears that lead people to altogether avoid specific things or situations that trigger intense anxiety.

postpartum depression: Depression after childbirth.

posttraumatic stress disorder (PTSD): An anxiety disorder that develops as a result of witnessing or experiencing a traumatic occurrence, especially life-threatening events.

psychiatrist: A professional who completed both medical school and training in psychiatry and is a specialist in diagnosing and treating mental illness.

psychoanalysis: Psychoanalysis focuses on past conflicts as the underpinnings to current emotional and behavioral problems. In this long-term and intensive therapy, an individual meets with a psychoanalyst three to five times a week, using "free association" to explore unconscious motivations and earlier, unproductive patterns of resolving issues.

pyromania: Compulsive fire setting.

schizophrenia: A mental disorder with symptoms including delusions, hallucinations, and disordered thinking (apparent from a person's fragmented, disconnected and sometimes nonsensical speech), social withdrawal, extreme apathy, diminished motivation, and blunted emotional expression.

seasonal affective disorder (SAD): A form of depression that appears related to fluctuations in the exposure to natural light. It usually strikes during autumn and often continues through the winter when natural light is reduced.

suicide: Taking or attempting to take one's own life.

supported employment: Supportive services that include assisting individuals in finding work; assessing individuals' skills, attitudes, behaviors, and interest relevant to work; providing vocational rehabilitation and/or other training; and providing work opportunities. Includes transitional and supported employment services.

trichotillomania: Compulsive hair pulling.

Chapter 81

Directory of Agencies That Provide Information about Mental Health Disorders

Government Agencies That Provide Information about Mental Health

Administration on Aging
Washington, DC 20201
Toll-Free: 800-677-1116
(Eldercare Locator)
Phone: 202-619-0724
Website: www.aoa.gov
E-mail: aoainfo@aoa.hhs.gov

Agency for Healthcare Research and Quality
Office of Communications and Knowledge Transfer
540 Gaither Road, Second Floor
Rockville, MD 20850
Phone: 301-427-1364
Fax: 301-427-1873
Website: www.ahrq.gov

Center for Mental Health Services
Substance Abuse and Mental Health Services Administration
P.O. Box 2345
Rockville, MD 20847
Toll-Free: 800-789-2647
Fax: 240-221-4295
Website: mentalhealth.samhsa.gov
Mental Health Services Locator: mentalhealth.samhsa.gov/databases

---

Resources in this chapter were compiled from several sources deemed reliable; all contact information was verified and updated in January 2009.

Centers for Disease Control and Prevention
1600 Clifton Road
Atlanta, GA 30333
Toll-Free: 800-CDC-INFO (232-4636)
Phone: 404-639-3311
Website: www.cdc.gov
E-mail: cdcinfo@cdc.gov

Centers for Medicare and Medicaid Services
7500 Security Boulevard
Baltimore, MD 21244-1850
Toll-Free: 800-633-4227
Website: www.medicare.gov

Healthfinder®
National Health Information Center
P.O. Box 1133
Washington, DC 20013-1133
Toll-Free: 800-336-4797
Phone: 301-565-4167
Fax: 301-984-4256
Website: www.healthfinder.gov
E-mail: healthfinder@nhic.org

National Cancer Institute
Cancer Information Service
6116 Executive Boulevard
Room 3036A
Bethesda, MD 20892-8322
Toll-Free: 800-4-CANCER (422-6237)
TTY Toll-Free: 800-332-8615
Website: www.cancer.gov
E-mail: cancergovstaff@mail.nih.gov

National Center for Complementary and Alternative Medicine
National Institutes of Health
9000 Rockville Pike
Bethesda, MD 20892
Toll-Free: 888-644-6226
TTY: 866-464-3615
Fax: 866-464-3616
Website: nccam.nih.gov
E-mail: info@nccam.nih.gov

National Center for Post-traumatic Stress Disorder
Website: www.ncptsd.va.gov

National Institute of Child Health and Human Development
P.O. Box 3006
Rockville, MD 20847
Toll-Free: 800-370-2943
Phone: 800-370-2943
TTY: 888-320-6942
Fax: 301-984-1473
Website: www.nichd.nih.gov
E-mail: NICHDInformationResourceCenter@mail.nih.gov

National Institute of Mental Health
National Institutes of Health, DHHS
6001 Executive Boulevard
Room 8184, MSC 9663
Bethesda, MD 20892-9663
Toll-Free: 866-615-NIMH (615-6464)
Phone: 301-443-4513
TTY: 301-443-8431
Toll-Free TTY: 866-415-8051
Fax: 301-443-4279
Website: www.nimh.nih.gov
E-mail: nimhinfo@nih.gov

National Institute of Neurological Disorders and Stroke
NIH Neurological Institute
P.O. Box 5801
Bethesda, MD 20824
Toll-Free: 800-352-9424
Phone: 301-496-5751
TTY: 301-468-5981
Website: www.ninds.nih.gov
E-mail: braininfo@ninds.nih.gov

National Institute on Aging
Building 31, Room 5C27
31 Center Drive, MSC 2292
Bethesda, MD 20892
Publications Toll-Free: 800-222-2225
Phone: 301-496-1752
TTY: 800-222-4225
Fax: 301-496-1072
Websites: www.nia.nih.gov
Publications Website: www.niapublications.org
E-mail: niainfo@nia.nih.gov

National Institute on Drug Abuse
6001 Executive Boulevard, Room 5213
Bethesda, MD 20892-9561
Phone: 301-443-1124
Website: www.nida.nih.gov
E-mail: information@nida.nih.gov

National Institutes of Health
9000 Rockville Pike
Bethesda, MD 20892
Phone: 301-496-4000
TTY: 301-402-9612
Website: www.nih.gov
E-mail: NIHinfo@od.nih.gov

National Women's Health Information Center
8270 Willow Oaks Corporate Drive
Fairfax, VA 22031
Toll-Free: 800-994-9662
TDD: 888-220-5446
Website: www.4women.gov

Office of Minority Health
P.O. Box 37337
Washington, DC 20013-7337
Toll-Free: 800-444-6472
Fax: 301-251-2160
Website: www.omhrc.gov
E-mail: info@omhrc.gov

U.S. Department of Health and Human Services
200 Independent Avenue, SW
Washington, DC 20201
Toll-Free: 877-696-6775
Phone: 202-619-0257
Website: www.hhs.gov

U.S. Food and Drug Administration
10903 New Hampshire Avenue
Silver Spring, MD 20903
Toll-Free: 888-463-6332
Website: www.fda.gov

U.S. National Library of Medicine
8600 Rockville Pike
Bethesda, MD 20894
Toll-Free: 888-346-3656
Phone: 301-594-5983
TDD: 800-735-2258
Website: www.nlm.nih.gov
E-mail: custserv@nlm.nih.gov

Private Agencies That Provide Information about Mental Health

AIDS InfoNet
P.O. Box 810
Arroyo Seco, NM 87514
Website: www.aidsinfonet.org
E-mail:
AIDSInfoNet@taosnet.com

Alzheimer's Association
225 N. Michigan Avenue
Floor 17
Chicago, IL 60601-7633
Toll-Free: 800-272-3900
Phone: 312-335-8700
TDD: 312-335-5886
Fax: 866-699-1246
Website: www.alz.org
E-mail: info@alz.org

American Academy of Child and Adolescent Psychiatry
3615 Wisconsin Avenue, NW
Washington, DC 20016-3007
Phone: 202-966-7300
Fax: 202-966-2891
Website: www.aacap.org
E-mail:
communications@aacap.org

American Academy of Pediatrics
141 Northwest Point Boulevard
Elk Grove Village, IL 60007
Phone: 847-434-4000
Fax: 847-434-8000
Website: www.aap.org
E-mail: kidsdocs@aap.org

American Art Therapy Association
11160-C1 South Lakes Drive, Suite 813
Reston, VA 20191
Toll-Free: 888-290-0878
Phone: 571-252-7573
Website: www.arttherapy.org
E-mail: info@arttherapy.org

American Association for Geriatric Psychiatry
7910 Woodmont Avenue
Suite 1050
Bethesda, MD 20814-3004
Phone: 301-654-7850
Fax: 301-654-4137
Website: www.aagpgpa.org
E-mail: main@aagponline.org

American Association for Marriage and Family Therapy
112 South Alfred Street
Alexandria, VA 22314
Phone: 703-838-9808
Fax: 703-838-9805
Website: www.aamft.org
E-mail: central@aamft.org

American Association of Suicidology
5221 Wisconsin Avenue, NW
Washington, DC 20015
Phone: 202-237-2280
Fax: 202-237-2282
Website: www.suicidology.org
E-mail: info@suicidology.org

American Counseling Association
5999 Stevenson Avenue
Alexandria, VA 22304
Toll-Free: 800-347-6647
TDD: 703-823-6862
Fax: 703-823-0252
Website: www.counseling.org
E-mail:
webmaster@counseling.org

American Foundation for Suicide Prevention
120 Wall Street, 22nd Floor
New York, NY 10005
Toll-free: 888-333-AFSP (333-2377)
Phone: 212-363-3500
Fax: 212-363-6237
Website: www.afsp.org
E-mail: inquiry@afsp.org

American Medical Association/Medem
100 Pine Street, 3rd Floor
San Francisco, CA 94111
Toll-Free: 877-926-3336
Phone: 415-644-3800
Fax: 415-644-3950
Website: www.medem.com
E-mail: info@medem.com

American Psychiatric Association
1000 Wilson Boulevard
Suite 1825
Arlington, VA 22209-3901
Phone: 703-907-7300
E-mail: apa@psych.org
Website: www.psych.org

American Psychiatric Nurses Association
1555 Wilson Boulevard
Suite 530
Arlington, VA 22209
Toll-Free: 866-243-2443
Phone: 703-243-2443
Fax: 703-243-3390
Website: www.apna.org

American Psychological Association
750 First Street, NE
Washington, DC 20002-4242
Toll-Free: 800-374-2721
Phone: 202-336-5500
Website: www.apa.org

American Psychotherapy Association
2750 E. Sunshine Street
Springfield, MO 65804
Toll-Free: 800-205-9165
Fax: 417-823-9959
Website:
www.americanpsychotherapy.com

American Public Health Association
800 I Street, NW
Washington, DC 20001-3710
Phone: 202-777-APHA (777-2742)
Fax: 202-777-2532
Website: www.apha.org
E-mail: comments@apha.org

American School Health Association
7263 State Route 43
P.O. Box 708
Kent, OH 44240
Phone: 330-678-1601
Fax: 330-678-4526
Website: www.ashaweb.org
E-mail: asha@ashaweb.org

American Therapeutic Recreation Association
207 3rd Avenue
Hattiesburg, MS 39401
Phone: 601-450-2872
Fax: 601-582-3354
Website: atra-online.com/cms
E-mail: national@atra-online.com

Anxiety Disorders Association of America
8730 Georgia Avenue, Suite 600
Silver Spring, MD 20910
Phone: 240-485-1001
Fax: 240-485-1035
Website: www.adaa.org
E-mail: information@adaa.org

Association for Applied Psychophysiology and Biofeedback
10200 West 44th Avenue
Suite 304
Wheat Ridge, CO 80033
Toll-Free: 800-477-8892
Phone: 303-422-8436
Website: www.aapb.org
E-mail: aapb@resourcenter.com

Association for Death Education and Counseling
111 Deer Lake Road, Suite 100
Deerfield, IL 60015
Phone: 847-509-0403
Fax: 847-480-9282
Website: www.adec.org

Association of Maternal and Child Health Programs
2030 M Street, NW, Suite 350
Washington, DC 20036
Phone: 202-775-0436
Fax: 202-775-0061
Website: www.amchp.org

Child and Adolescent Bipolar Foundation
1000 Skokie Boulevard
Suite 570
Wilmette, IL 60091
Phone: 847-256-8525
Website: www.bpkids.org
E-mail: cabf@bpkids.org

Children of Alcoholics Foundation
Website: www.coaf.org
E-mail: coaf@phoenixhouse.org

Cleveland Clinic
9500 Euclid Avenue
Cleveland, OH 44195
Toll-Free: 800-223-2273
Phone: 216-444-2200
TTY: 216-444-0261
Website:
www.clevelandclinic.org

Depressed Anonymous
P.O. Box 17414
Louisville, KY 40217
Phone: 502-569-1989
Website:
www.depressedanon.com
E-mail: info@depressedanon.com

Depression and Bipolar Support Alliance
730 N. Franklin Street
Suite 501
Chicago, IL 60654-7225
Toll-Free: 800-826-3632
Fax: 312-642-7243
Website: www.dbsalliance.org

Eating Disorder Referral and Information Center
Website: www.edreferral.com

Federation of Families for Children's Mental Health
9605 Medical Center Drive
Rockville, MD 20850
Phone: 240-403-1901
Fax: 240-403-1909
Website: www.ffcmh.org
E-mail: ffcmh@ffcmh.org

Geriatric Mental Health Foundation
7910 Woodmont Avenue
Suite 1050
Bethesda, MD 20814
Phone: 301-654-7850
Fax: 301-654-4137
Website: www.gmhfonline.org
E-mail: web@GMHFonline.org

Gift from Within
16 Cobb Hill Road
Camden, ME 04843
Phone: 207-236-8858
Fax: 207-236-2818
Website:
www.giftfromwithin.org
E-mail: JoyceB3955@aol.com

Human Services Research Institute
2336 Massachusetts Avenue
Cambridge, MA 02140
Phone: 617-876-0426
Fax: 617-492-7401
Website: www.hsri.org
E-mail: webmaster@hsri.org

International Society for the Study of Dissociation
8400 Westpark Drive
Second Floor
McLean, VA 22102
Phone: 703-610-9037
Fax: 703-610-0234
Website: www.issd.org
E-mail: info@isst-d.org

International Society for Traumatic Stress Studies
111 Deer Lake Road
Suite 100
Deerfield, IL 60015
Phone: 847-480-9028
Fax: 847-480-9282
Website: www.istss.org
E-mail: istss@istss.org

Mental Health America
2000 N. Beauregard Street,
Sixth Floor
Alexandria, VA 22311
Toll-Free: 800-969-6642
Phone: 703-684-7722
TTY: 800-433-5959
Fax: 703-684-5968
Website: www.nmha.org

National Alliance on Mental Illness
Toll-Free: 800-950-NAMI
(950-6264)
Website: www.nami.org

National Association of Anorexia Nervosa and Associated Disorders
P.O. Box 7
Highland Park, IL 60035
Phone: 847-831-3438
Fax: 847-831-3765
Website: www.anad.org
E-mail: anadhelp@anad.org

National Center for Children Exposed to Violence
Yale University
Child Study Center
230 South Frontage Road
New Haven, CT 06520-7900
Toll-Free: 877-49-NCCEV
(496-2238)
Phone: 203-785-7047
Fax: 203-785-4608
Website: www.nccev.org
E-mail: stacey.hobson@yale.edu

National Center for Juvenile Justice and Mental Health
345 Delaware Avenue
Delmar, NY 12054
Toll-Free: 866-9NCMHJJ
(962-6455)
Fax: 518-439-7612
Website: www.ncmhjj.com
E-mail: ncmhjj@prainc.com

National Eating Disorders Association
603 Stewart Street, Suite 803
Seattle, WA 98101
Toll-Free: 800-931-2237
(Helpline)
Phone: 206-382-3587
Fax: 206-829-8501
Website:
www.nationaleatingdisorders.org
E-mail:
info@NationalEatingDisorders.org

National Family Caregivers Association
10400 Connecticut Avenue
Suite 500
Kensington, MD 20895-3944
Toll-Free: 800-896-3650
Phone: 301-942-6430
Fax: 301-942-2302
Website:
www.thefamilycaregiver.org
E-mail:
info@thefamilycaregiver.org

National Resource Center on Psychiatric Advance Directives
Website: www.nrc-pad.org

National Sleep Foundation
1522 K Street, NW, Suite 500
Washington, DC 20005
Phone: 202-347-3471
Fax: 202-347-3472
Website:
www.sleepfoundation.org
E-mail: nsf@sleepfoundation.org

Nemours Foundation Center for Children's Health Media
1600 Rockland Road
Wilmington, DE 19803
Phone: 302-651-4000
Fax: 302-651-4055
Website: www.kidshealth.org
E-mail: info@kidshealth.org

Obsessive-Compulsive Foundation
P.O. Box 961029
Boston, MA 02196
Phone: 617-973-5801
Website: www.ocfoundation.org

Psychology Today
Website:
www.psychologytoday.com

Social Phobia/Social Anxiety Association
Website: www.socialphobia.org

Chapter 82

Directory of Patient Prescription Drug Assistance Programs for Free or Reduced-Cost Medications

Some pharmaceutical companies offer medication assistance programs to low-income individuals and families. These programs typically require a doctor's consent and proof of financial status. They may also require that you have either no health insurance, or no prescription drug benefit through your health insurance.

Please contact the pharmaceutical company directly for specific eligibility requirements and application information.

Note: Some of these companies may prefer to speak directly with your doctor.

For more information on Patient/Drug Assistance Programs access the following websites:

Partnership for Prescription Assistance
www.pparx.org

RxAssist: Accessing Pharmaceutical Patient Assistance Programs
www.rxassist.org

RxHope: The Heart of the Pharmaceutical Industry
www.rxhope.com

"Patient Prescription Drug Assistance Programs," © 2005 NAMI: The Nation's Voice on Mental Illness (www.nami.org). Reprinted with permission. Contact information was verified in January 2009.

Table 82.1. Programs for Prescription Drug Assistance

Brand Name	Pharmaceutical Company	Program Phone #
Abilify	Bristol-Myers Squibb Company	800-332-2056
BuSpar	Bristol-Myers Squibb Company	800-332-2056
Celexa	Forest Pharmaceuticals, Inc.	800-851-0758
clozapine (generic)	IVAX Pharmaceuticals, Inc.	800-327-4114 x4344
Clozaril	Novartis Pharmaceuticals	800-277-2254
Depakote	Abbott Laboratories	800-222-6885
Desyrel (150 & 300 mg pills only)	Bristol-Myers Squibb Company	800-332-2056
Effexor	Wyeth Pharmaceuticals	800-568-9938
Geodon	Pfizer Inc.	866-706-2400
Haldol, Haldol Decanoate	Ortho-McNeil Pharmaceutical, Inc.	800-652-6227
Isoptin	Abbott Laboratories	800-222-6885
Klonopin	Roche Pharmaceuticals	800-285-4484
Lexapro	Forest Pharmaceuticals, Inc.	800-851-0758
Neurontin	Pfizer Inc.	800-707-8990
Paxil	GlaxoSmithKline	866-728-4368
Prolixin, Prolixin Decanoate	Bristol-Myers Squibb Company	800-332-2056
Prozac	Eli Lilly and Company	800-545-6962
Risperdal	Janssen Pharmaceutica	800-652-6227
Serentil	Boehringer Ingelheim Pharmaceuticals	800-556-8317
Seroquel	AstraZeneca Pharmaceuticals	800-424-3727
Valium	Roche Pharmaceuticals	800-285-4484
Wellbutrin	GlaxoSmithKline	866-728-4368
Zoloft	Pfizer Inc.	800-707-8990
Zyprexa	Eli Lilly and Company	800-545-6962

Table 82.2. General Contact Information for Major Pharmaceutical Companies

Pharmaceutical Company Mailing Address	Phone # for Medical Information	Web Address
Abbott Laboratories 100 Abbott Park Rd. Abbott Park, IL 60064-3502	800-633-9110	www.abbott.com
AstraZeneca Pharmaceuticals 1800 Concord Pike P.O. Box 15437 Wilmington, DE 19850-5437	800-236-9933	www.astrazeneca-us.com
Aventis Pharmaceuticals, Inc. 300 Somerset Corporate Blvd. Bridgewater, NJ 08807-2854	800-633-1610	www.aventis.com
Boehringer Ingelheim Pharmaceuticals, Inc. 900 Ridgebury Rd. P.O. Box 368 Ridgefield, CT 06877-0368	800-542-6257	www.boehringer-ingelheim.com
Bristol-Myers Squibb Company 345 Park Avenue New York, NY 10154-0037	800-321-1335	www.bms.com
Eli Lilly and Company Lilly Corporate Center Indianapolis, IN 46285	800-545-5979	www.lilly.com
Forest Pharmaceuticals, Inc. 13600 Shoreline Drive St. Louis, MO 63045	800-678-1605	www.forestpharm.com
GlaxoSmithKline One Franklin Plaza P.O Box 7929 Philadelphia, PA 19101	888-825-5249	www.gsk.com
Janssen Pharmaceutica, Inc. 1125 Trenton-Harbourton Rd. Titusville, NJ 08560	800-526-7736 (800-JANSSEN)	www.janssen.com
Novartis Pharmaceuticals One Health Plaza East Hanover, NJ 07936-1080	888-669-6682	www.novartis.com

(continued on next page)

Table 82.2. General Contact Information for Major Pharmaceutical Companies (continued from previous page)

Pharmaceutical Company Mailing Address	Phone # for Medical Information	Web Address
Ortho-McNeil Pharmaceutical, Inc. 1125 Trenton-Harbourton Road P.O. Box 200 Titusville, NJ 08560-200	800-526-7736	www.ortho-mcneil.com
Pfizer Inc. 235 East 42nd St. New York, NY 10017-5755	800-438-1985	www.pfizer.com
Roche Pharmaceuticals 340 Kingsland St. Nutley, NJ 07110-1199	800-526-6367	www.roche.com
Schering-Plough Corporation 2000 Galloping Hill Rd. Kenilworth, NJ 07033	800-526-4099	www.sgp.com
Solvay Pharmaceuticals, Inc. 901 Sawyer Rd. Marietta, GA 30062	800-354-0026	www.solvay pharmaceuticals-us.com
Wyeth Laboratories 5 Giralda Farms Madison, NJ 07940	800-934-5556 option #1	www.wyeth.com

Index

Index

Page numbers followed by 'n' indicate a footnote. Page numbers in *italics* indicate a table or illustration.

A

B

E

F

G

H

I

J

K

L

M

O

P

Q

R

U

Health Reference Series

Complete Catalog

List price $93 per volume. School and library price $84 per volume.

Adolescent Health Sourcebook, 2nd Edition

Basic Consumer Health Information about the Physical, Mental, and Emotional Growth and Development of Adolescents, Including Medical Care, Nutritional and Physical Activity Requirements, Puberty, Sexual Activity, Acne, Tanning, Body Piercing, Common Physical Illnesses and Disorders, Eating Disorders, Attention Deficit Hyperactivity Disorder, Depression, Bullying, Hazing, and Adolescent Injuries Related to Sports, Driving, and Work

Along with Substance Abuse Information about Nicotine, Alcohol, and Drug Use, a Glossary, and Directory of Additional Resources

Edited by Joyce Brennfleck Shannon. 655 pages. 2007. 978-0-7808-0943-7.

"A particularly good resource for both parents and teens. The concise presentation of the material in brief and well-organized chapters creates an easy volume to browse."

—*School Library Journal, Jun '07*

"I don't believe there are any other books written in such easy to understand language that encompass such a breadth of topics. This is a complete revision of the book and is an excellent resource for parents and teens."

—*Doody's Review Service, 2007*

Adult Health Concerns Sourcebook

Basic Consumer Health Information about Medical and Mental Concerns of Adults, Including Facts about Choosing Healthcare Providers, Navigating Insurance Options, Maintaining Wellness, Preventing Cancer, Heart Disease, Stroke, Diabetes, and Osteoporosis, and Understanding Aging-Related Health Concerns, Including Menopause, Cognitive Changes, and Changes in the Coronary and Vascular Systems

Along with Tips on Caring for Aging Parents and Dealing with Health-Related Work and Travel Issues, a Glossary, and a Directory of Resources for Additional Help and Information

Edited by Sandra J. Judd. 648 pages. 2008. 978-0-7808-0999-4.

"Provides a thorough list of topics that are important to adult health and for caregivers."

—*CHOICE, Nov '08*

"Written in easy-to-understand language . . . the content is well-organized and is intended to aid adults in making health care-related decisions."

—*AORN Journal, Dec '08*

AIDS Sourcebook, 4th Edition

Basic Consumer Health Information about Human Immunodeficiency Virus (HIV) and Acquired Immunodeficiency Syndrome (AIDS), Featuring Updated Statistics and Facts about Risks, Prevention, Screening, Diagnosis, Treatments, Side Effects, and Complications, and Including a Section about the Impact of HIV/AIDS on the Health of Women, Children, and Adolescents

Along with Tips on Managing Life with AIDS, Reports on Current Research Initiatives and Clinical Trials, a Glossary of Related Terms, and Resource Directories for Further Help and Information

Edited by Ivy L. Alexander. 680 pages. 2008. 978-0-7808-0997-0.

SEE ALSO *Contagious Diseases Sourcebook, 2nd Edition*

Alcoholism Sourcebook, 2nd Edition

Basic Consumer Health Information about Alcohol Use, Abuse, and Dependence, Featuring Facts about the Physical, Mental, and Social Health Effects of Alcohol Addiction, Including Alcoholic Liver Disease, Pancreatic Disease, Cardiovascular Disease, Neurological Disorders, and the Effects of Drinking during Pregnancy

Along with Information about Alcohol Treatment, Medications, and Recovery Programs, in Addition to Tips for Reducing the Prevalence of Underage Drinking, Statistics about Alcohol Use, a Glossary of Related Terms, and Directories of Resources for More Help and Information

Edited by Amy L. Sutton. 625 pages. 2007. 978-0-7808-0942-0.

"A comprehensive look at the adverse effects of alcohol on people of all ages . . . It serves to whet the reader's appetite to continue learning using other resources. It is practical, easy to read, and enlightening, and is the first book a lay person should consult to learn about alcoholism."

—*Doody's Review Service, 2007*

"Should be a basic acquisition for any serious public or college-level library including health reference titles for general-interest readers."

—*California Bookwatch, Feb '07*

SEE ALSO *Drug Abuse Sourcebook, 2nd Edition*

Allergies Sourcebook, 3rd Edition

Basic Consumer Health Information about Allergic Disorders, Such as Anaphylaxis, Hives, Eczema, Rhinitis, Sinusitis, and Conjunctivitis, and Their Triggers, Including Pollen, Mold, Dust Mites, Animal Dander, Insects, Chemicals, Food, Food Additives, and Medications

Along with Advice about the Diagnosis and Treatment of Allergy Symptoms, a Glossary of Related Terms, a Directory of Resources for Help and Information, and Suggestions for Additional Reading

Edited by Amy L. Sutton. 588 pages. 2007. 978-0-7808-0950-5.

SEE ALSO *Asthma Sourcebook, 2nd Edition*

Alzheimer Disease Sourcebook, 4th Edition

Basic Consumer Health Information about Alzheimer Disease, Other Dementias, and Related Disorders, Including Multi-Infarct Dementia, Dementia with Lewy Bodies, Frontotemporal Dementia (Pick Disease), Wernicke-Korsakoff Syndrome (Alcohol-Related Dementia), AIDS Dementia Complex, Huntington Disease, Creutzfeldt-Jacob Disease, and Delirium

Along with Information about Coping with Memory Loss and Forgetfulness, Maintaining Skills, and Long-Term Planning for People with Dementia, and Suggestions Addressing Common Caregiver Concerns, Updated Information about Current Research Efforts, a Glossary of Related Terms, and Directories of Sources for Additional Help and Information

Edited by Karen Bellenir. 603 pages. 2008. 978-0-7808-1001-3.

"An invaluable resource for persons who have received a diagnosis, for caregivers, and for family members dealing with this insidious disease. It is recommended for public, community college, and ready-reference sections in academic libraries."

—*ARBAonline, Jul '08*

SEE ALSO *Brain Disorders Sourcebook, 2nd Edition*

Arthritis Sourcebook, 2nd Edition

Basic Consumer Health Information about Osteoarthritis, Rheumatoid Arthritis, Other Rheumatic Disorders, Infectious Forms of Arthritis, and Diseases with Symptoms Linked to Arthritis, Featuring Facts about Diagnosis, Pain Management, and Surgical Therapies

Along with Coping Strategies, Research Updates, a Glossary, and Resources for Additional Help and Information

Edited by Amy L. Sutton. 567 pages. 2004. 978-0-7808-0667-2.

"This easy-to-read volume is recommended for consumer health collections within public or academic libraries."

—*E-Streams, May '05*

"As expected, this updated edition continues the excellent reputation of this series in providing sound, usable health information. . . . Highly recommended."

—*American Reference Books Annual, 2005*

Asthma Sourcebook, 2nd Edition

Basic Consumer Health Information about the Causes, Symptoms, Diagnosis, and Treatment of Asthma in Infants, Children, Teenagers, and Adults, Including Facts about Different Types of Asthma, Common Co-Occurring Conditions, Asthma Management Plans, Triggers, Medications, and Medication Delivery Devices

Along with Asthma Statistics, Research Updates, a Glossary, a Directory of Asthma-Related Resources, and More

Edited by Karen Bellenir. 581 pages. 2006. 978-0-7808-0866-9.

Attention Deficit Disorder Sourcebook

Basic Consumer Health Information about Attention Deficit/Hyperactivity Disorder in Children and Adults, Including Facts about Causes, Symptoms, Diagnostic Criteria, and Treatment Options Such as Medications, Behavior Therapy, Coaching, and Homeopathy

Along with Reports on Current Research Initiatives, Legal Issues, and Government Regulations, and Featuring a Glossary of Related Terms, Internet Resources, and a List of Additional Reading Material

Edited by Dawn D. Matthews. 447 pages. 2002. 978-0-7808-0624-5.

"Recommended reference source."

—*Booklist, Jan '03*

SEE ALSO *Learning Disabilities Sourcebook, 3rd Edition*

Autism and Pervasive Developmental Disorders Sourcebook

Basic Consumer Health Information about Autism Spectrum and Pervasive Developmental Disorders, Such as Classical Autism, Asperger Syndrome, Rett Syndrome, and Childhood Disintegrative Disorder, Including Information about Related Genetic Disorders and Medical Problems and Facts about Causes, Screening Methods, Diagnostic Criteria, Treatments and Interventions, and Family and Education Issues

Along with a Glossary of Related Terms, Tips for Evaluating the Validity of Health Claims, and a Directory of Resources for Additional Help and Information

Edited by Sandra J. Judd. 603 pages. 2007. 978-0-7808-0953-6.

"Recommended for public libraries"

—*SciTech Book News, Mar '08*

SEE ALSO *Learning Disabilities Sourcebook, 3rd Edition*

Back and Neck Disorders Sourcebook, 2nd Edition

Basic Consumer Health Information about Spinal Pain, Spinal Cord Injuries, and Related Disorders, Such as Degenerative Disk Disease, Osteoarthritis, Scoliosis, Sciatica, Spina Bifida, and Spinal Stenosis, and Featuring Facts about Maintaining Spinal Health, Self-Care, Pain Management, Rehabilitative Care, Chiropractic Care, Spinal Surgeries, and Complementary Therapies

Along with Suggestions for Preventing Back and Neck Pain, a Glossary of Related Terms, and a Directory of Resources

Edited by Amy L. Sutton. 607 pages. 2004. 978-0-7808-0738-9.

"Recommended. ...An easy to use, comprehensive medical reference book."

—*E-Streams, Sep '05*

"For anyone who has back or neck problems, this book is ideal. Its easy-to-understand language and variety of topics makes this sourcebook a worthwhile read. The price...is reasonable for the amount of information contained in the book"

—*Occupational Therapy in Health Care, 2007*

Blood and Circulatory Disorders Sourcebook, 2nd Edition

Basic Consumer Health Information about the Blood and Circulatory System and Related Disorders, Such as Anemia and Other Hemoglobin Diseases, Cancer of the Blood and Associated Bone Marrow Disorders, Clotting and Bleeding Problems, and Conditions That Affect the Veins, Blood Vessels, and Arteries, Including Facts about the Donation and Transplantation of Bone Marrow, Stem Cells, and Blood and Tips for Keeping the Blood and Circulatory System Healthy

Along with a Glossary of Related Terms and Resources for Additional Help and Information

Edited by Amy L. Sutton. 634 pages. 2005. 978-0-7808-0746-4.

"Highly recommended pick for basic consumer health reference holdings at all levels."

—*The Bookwatch, Aug '05*

Brain Disorders Sourcebook, 2nd Edition

Basic Consumer Health Information about Acquired and Traumatic Brain Injuries, Infections of the Brain, Epilepsy and Seizure Disorders, Cerebral Palsy, and Degenerative Neurological Disorders, Including Amyotrophic Lateral Sclerosis (ALS), Dementias, Multiple Sclerosis, and More

Along with Information on the Brain's Structure and Function, Treatment and Rehabilitation Options, Reports on Current Research Initiatives, a Glossary of Terms Related to Brain Disorders and Injuries, and a Directory of Sources for Further Help and Information

Edited by Sandra J. Judd. 600 pages. 2005. 978-0-7808-0744-0.

"This easy-to-read volume provides up-to-date health information... Recommended for consumer health collections within public or academic libraries."

—*E-Streams, Feb '06*

SEE ALSO *Alzheimer Disease Sourcebook, 4th Edition*

Breast Cancer Sourcebook, 3rd Edition

Basic Consumer Health Information about Breast Health and Breast Cancer, Including Facts about Environmental, Genetic, and Other Risk Factors, Prevention Efforts, Screening and Diagnostic Methods, Surgical Treatment Options and Other Care Choices, Complementary and Alternative Therapies, and Post-Treatment Concerns

Along with Statistical Data, News about Research Advances, a Glossary of Related Terms, and Directories of Resources for Additional Information and Support

Edited by Karen Bellenir. 606 pages. 2009. 978-0-7808-1030-3.

SEE ALSO *Cancer Sourcebook for Women, 3rd Edition, Women's Health Concerns Sourcebook, 3rd Edition*

Breastfeeding Sourcebook

Basic Consumer Health Information about the Benefits of Breastmilk, Preparing to Breastfeed, Breastfeeding as a Baby Grows, Nutrition, and More, Including Information on Special Situations and Concerns Such as Mastitis, Illness, Medications, Allergies, Multiple Births, Prematurity, Special Needs, and Adoption

Along with a Glossary and Resources for Additional Help and Information

Edited by Jenni Lynn Colson. 367 pages. 2002. 978-0-7808-0332-9.

SEE ALSO *Pregnancy and Birth Sourcebook, 2nd Edition*

Burns Sourcebook

Basic Consumer Health Information about Various Types of Burns and Scalds, Including Flame, Heat, Cold, Electrical, Chemical, and Sun Burns

Along with Information on Short-Term and Long-Term Treatments, Tissue Reconstruction, Plastic Surgery, Prevention Suggestions, and First Aid

Edited by Allan R. Cook. 604 pages. 1999. 978-0-7808-0204-9.

"This is an exceptional addition to the series and is highly recommended for all consumer health collections, hospital libraries, and academic medical centers."

—*E-Streams, Mar '00*

"This key reference guide is an invaluable addition to all health care and public libraries in confronting this ongoing health issue."

—*American Reference Books Annual, 2000*

SEE ALSO *Dermatological Disorders Sourcebook, 2nd Edition*

Cancer Sourcebook, 5th Edition

Basic Consumer Health Information about Major Forms and Stages of Cancer, Featuring Facts about Head and Neck Cancers, Lung Cancers, Gastrointestinal Cancers, Genitourinary Cancers, Lymphomas, Blood Cell Cancers, Endocrine Cancers, Skin Cancers, Bone Cancers, Metastatic Cancers, and More

Along with Facts about Cancer Treatments, Cancer Risks and Prevention, a Glossary of Related Terms, Statistical Data, and a Directory of Resources for Additional Information

Edited by Karen Bellenir. 1105 pages. 2007. 978-0-7808-0947-5.

"The 5th, updated edition of *Cancer Sourcebook* should be in every public and health lending library collection... An unparalleled discussion essential for any health collections considering an all-in-one basic general reference."

—*California Bookwatch, Aug '07*

SEE ALSO *Breast Cancer Sourcebook, 3rd Edition, Cancer Sourcebook for Women, 3rd Edition, Cancer Survivorship Sourcebook, Leukemia Sourcebook*

Cancer Sourcebook for Women, 3rd Edition

Basic Consumer Health Information about Leading Causes of Cancer in Women, Featuring Facts about Gynecologic Cancers and Related Concerns, Such as Breast Cancer, Cervical Cancer, Endometrial Cancer, Uterine Sarcoma, Vaginal Cancer, Vulvar Cancer, and Common Non-Cancerous Gynecologic Conditions, in Addition to Facts about Lung Cancer, Colorectal Cancer, and Thyroid Cancer in Women

Along with Information about Cancer Risk Factors, Screening and Prevention, Treatment Options, and Tips on Coping with Life after Cancer Treatment, a Glossary of Cancer Terms, and a Directory of Resources for Additional Help and Information

Edited by Amy L. Sutton. 687 pages. 2006. 978-0-7808-0867-6.

"This excellent book provides the general public with information compiled in a way that will help them to gain the knowledge they need. 4 Stars!"

—*Doody's Review Service, Dec '06*

"An indispensable reference for health consumers and cancer patients. Recommended for public libraries and academic libraries with a medical department."

—*E-Streams, Sep '08*

Cancer Survivorship Sourcebook

Basic Consumer Health Information about the Physical, Educational, Emotional, Social, and Financial Needs of Cancer Patients from Diagnosis, through Cancer Treatment, and Beyond, Including Facts about Researching Specific Types of Cancer and Learning about Clinical Trials and Treatment Options, and Featuring Tips for Coping with the Side Effects of Cancer Treatments and Adjusting to Life after Cancer Treatment Concludes

Along with Suggestions for Caregivers, Friends, and Family Members of Cancer Patients, a Glossary of Cancer Care Terms, and Directories of Related Resources

Edited by Karen Bellenir. 633 pages. 2007. 978-0-7808-0985-7.

"Well organized and comprehensive in coverage, the book speaks to issues encountered both during and after cancer treatment. Recommended for consumer health and public libraries."

—*Library Journal, Aug 1 '07*

"*Cancer Survivorship Sourcebook* will be useful to anyone who has a friend or loved one with a cancer diagnosis."

—*American Reference Books Annual, 2008*

SEE ALSO *Cancer Sourcebook, 5th Edition*

Cardiovascular Diseases and Disorders Sourcebook, 3rd Edition

Basic Consumer Health Information about Heart and Vascular Diseases and Disorders, Such as Angina, Heart Attacks, Arrhythmias, Cardiomyopathy, Valve Disease, Atherosclerosis, and Aneurysms, with Information about Managing Cardiovascular Risk Factors and Maintaining Heart Health, Medications and Procedures Used to Treat Cardiovascular Disorders, and Concerns of Special Significance to Women

Along with Reports on Current Research Initiatives, a Glossary of Related Medical Terms, and a Directory of Sources for Further Help and Information

Edited by Sandra J. Judd. 687 pages. 2005. 978-0-7808-0739-6.

"This updated sourcebook is still the best first stop for comprehensive introductory information on cardiovascular diseases."

—*American Reference Books Annual, 2006*

"Recommended for public libraries and libraries supporting health care professionals."

—*E-Streams, Sep '05*

Caregiving Sourcebook

Basic Consumer Health Information for Caregivers, Including a Profile of Caregivers, Caregiving Responsibilities and Concerns, Tips for Specific Conditions, Care Environments, and the Effects of Caregiving

Along with Facts about Legal Issues, Financial Information, and Future Planning, a Glossary, and a Listing of Additional Resources

Edited by Joyce Brennfleck Shannon. 583 pages. 2001. 978-0-7808-0331-2.

"Essential for most collections."

—*Library Journal, Apr 1 '02*

"An ideal addition to the reference collection of any public library. Health sciences information professionals may also want to acquire the *Caregiving Sourcebook* for their hospital or academic library for use as a ready reference tool by health care workers interested in aging and caregiving."

—*E-Streams, Jan '02*

Child Abuse Sourcebook, 2nd Edition

Basic Consumer Health Information about the Physical, Sexual, and Emotional Abuse of Children, Neglect, Münchhausen Syndrome by Proxy (MSBP), and Shaken Baby Syndrome, and Featuring Facts about Withholding Medical Care, Corporal Punishment, Child Maltreatment in Youth Sports, and Parental Substance Abuse

Along with Information about Child Protective Services, Foster Care, Adoption, Parenting Challenges, Abuse Prevention Programs, and Intervention, Treatment, and Recovery Guidelines, a Glossary of Related Terms, and Resources for Additional Help and Information

Edited by Joyce Brennfleck Shannon. 600 pages. 2009. 978-0-7808-1037-2.

SEE ALSO *Domestic Violence Sourcebook, 3rd Edition*

Childhood Diseases and Disorders Sourcebook, 2nd Edition

Basic Consumer Health Information about the Physical, Mental, and Developmental Health of Pre-Adolescent Children, Including Facts about Infectious Diseases, Asthma, Allergies, Diabetes, and Other Acute and Chronic Conditions Affecting the Gastrointestinal Tract, Ears, Nose, Throat, Liver, Kidneys, Heart, Blood, Brain, Muscles, Bones, and Skin

Along with Reports on Recommended Childhood Vaccinations, Wellness Guidelines, a Glossary of Related Medical Terms, and a List of Resources for Parents

Edited by Sandra J. Judd. 694 pages. 2009. 978-0-7808-1031-0.

SEE ALSO *Healthy Children Sourcebook*

Colds, Flu and Other Common Ailments Sourcebook

Basic Consumer Health Information about Common Ailments and Injuries, Including Colds, Coughs, the Flu, Sinus Problems, Headaches, Fever, Nausea and Vomiting, Menstrual Cramps, Diarrhea, Constipation, Hemorrhoids, Back Pain, Dandruff, Dry and Itchy Skin, Cuts, Scrapes, Sprains, Bruises, and More

Along with Information about Prevention, Self-Care, Choosing a Doctor, Over-the-Counter Medications, Folk Remedies, and Alternative Therapies, and Including a Glossary of Important Terms and a Directory of Resources for Further Help and Information

Edited by Chad T. Kimball. 622 pages. 2001. 978-0-7808-0435-7.

"A good starting point for research on common illnesses. It will be a useful addition to public and consumer health library collections."

—*American Reference Books Annual, 2002*

"Will prove valuable to any library seeking to maintain a current, comprehensive reference collection of health resources. . . Excellent reference."

—*The Bookwatch, Aug '01*

Communication Disorders Sourcebook

Basic Information about Deafness and Hearing Loss, Speech and Language Disorders, Voice Disorders, Balance and Vestibular Disorders, and Disorders of Smell, Taste, and Touch

Edited by Linda M. Ross. 533 pages. 1996. 978-0-7808-0077-9.

"This is skillfully edited and is a welcome resource for the layperson. It should be found in every public and medical library."

—*Booklist Health Sciences Supplement, Oct '97*

Complementary and Alternative Medicine Sourcebook, 3rd Edition

Basic Consumer Health Information about Complementary and Alternative Medical Therapies, Including Acupuncture, Ayurveda, Traditional Chinese Medicine, Herbal Medicine, Homeopathy, Naturopathy, Biofeedback, Hypnotherapy, Yoga, Art Therapy, Aromatherapy, Clinical Nutrition, Vitamin and Mineral Supplements, Chiropractic, Massage, Reflexology, Crystal Therapy, Therapeutic Touch, and More

Along with Facts about Alternative and Complementary Treatments for Specific Conditions Such as Cancer, Diabetes, Osteoarthritis, Chronic Pain, Menopause, Gastrointestinal Disorders, Headaches, and Mental Illness, a Glossary, and a Resource List for Additional Help and Information

Edited by Sandra J. Judd. 630 pages. 2006. 978-0-7808-0864-5.

"A 'must' reference for any serious healthcare collection. Public library holdings, too, will welcome it as a popular reference."

—*California Bookwatch, Oct '06*

"Both basic and informative at the same time... a useful resource for health care professionals as well as consumers interested in learning more information about CAM therapies."

—*AORN Journal, Jan '08*

"A quality, indexed, referenced guideline for many alternative practices that are quite popular around the world...It is neatly organized to find facts quickly, is peer-reviewed, and stays current with the most recent advances."

—*Journal of Dental Hygiene, Jul '07*

Congenital Disorders Sourcebook, 2nd Edition

Basic Consumer Health Information about Nonhereditary Birth Defects and Disorders Related to Prematurity, Gestational Injuries, Congenital Infections, and Birth Complications, Including Heart Defects, Hydrocephalus, Spina Bifida, Cleft Lip and Palate, Cerebral Palsy, and More

Along with Facts about the Prevention of Birth Defects, Fetal Surgery and Other Treatment Options, Research Initiatives, a Glossary of Related Terms, and Resources for Additional Information and Support

Edited by Sandra J. Judd. 619 pages. 2007. 978-0-7808-0945-1.

"Congenital Disorders Sourcebook provides an excellent, non-technical overview of many aspects of pregnancy with the focus on congenital disorders."

—*American Reference Books Annual, 2008*

"An excellent readable reference aimed at the lay public for difficult to understand medical problems. An excellent starting point for the interested parent or family member who may then be motivated to seek more information."

—*Doody's Review Service, 2007*

SEE ALSO *Pregnancy and Birth Sourcebook, 2nd Edition*

Contagious Diseases Sourcebook, 2nd Edition

Basic Consumer Health Information about Diseases Spread from Person to Person through Direct Physical Contact, Airborne Transmissions, Sexual Contact, or Contact with Blood or Other Body Fluids, Including Pneumococcal, Staphylococcal, and Streptococcal Diseases, Colds, Influenza, Lice, Measles, Mumps, Tuberculosis, and Others

Along with Facts about Self-Care and Over-the-Counter Medications, Antibiotics and Drug Resistance, Disease Prevention, Vaccines, and Bioterrorism, a Glossary, and a Directory of Resources for More Information

Edited by Joyce Brennfleck Shannon. 600 pages. 2009. 978-0-7808-1075-4.

SEE ALSO *AIDS Sourcebook, 4th Edition, Hepatitis Sourcebook*

Cosmetic and Reconstructive Surgery Sourcebook, 2nd Edition

Basic Consumer Information about Plastic Surgery and Non-Surgical Appearance-Enhancing Procedures, Including Facts about Botulinum Toxin, Collagen Replacement, Dermabrasion,

Chemical Peels, Eyelid Surgery, Nose Reshaping, Lip Augmentation, Liposuction, Breast Enlargement and Reduction, Tummy Tucking, and Other Skin, Hair, Facial, and Body Shaping Procedures

Along with Information about Reconstructive Procedures for Congenital Disorders, Disfiguring Diseases, Burns, and Traumatic Injuries, a Glossary of Related Terms, and a Directory of Additional Resources

Edited by Karen Bellenir. 483 pages. 2007. 978-0-7808-0951-2.

"A practical guide for health care consumers and health care workers. . . . This easy-to-read reference guide would be useful for novice and veteran health care consumers, surgical technology students, nursing students, and perioperative nurses new to plastic and reconstructive surgery. It also may be helpful for medical-surgical nurses as a guide for patient teaching in their practices."

—*AORN Journal, Aug '08*

SEE ALSO *Surgery Sourcebook, 2nd Edition*

Death and Dying Sourcebook, 2nd Edition

Basic Consumer Health Information about End-of-Life Care and Related Perspectives and Ethical Issues, Including End-of-Life Symptoms and Treatments, Pain Management, Quality-of-Life Concerns, the Use of Life Support, Patients' Rights and Privacy Issues, Advance Directives, Physician-Assisted Suicide, Caregiving, Organ and Tissue Donation, Autopsies, Funeral Arrangements, and Grief

Along with Statistical Data, Information about the Leading Causes of Death, a Glossary, and Directories of Support Groups and Other Resources

Edited by Joyce Brennfleck Shannon. 626 pages. 2006. 978-0-7808-0871-3.

Dental Care and Oral Health Sourcebook, 3rd Edition

Basic Consumer Health Information about Dental Care and Oral Health Throughout the Lifespan, Including Facts about Cavities, Bad Breath, Cold and Canker Sores, Dry Mouth, Toothaches, Gum Disease, Malocclusion, Temporomandibular Joint and Muscle Disorders, Oral Cancers, and Dental Emergencies

Along with Information about Mouth Hygiene, Crowns, Bridges, Implants, and Fillings, Surgical, Orthodontic, and Cosmetic Dental Procedures, Pain Management, Health Conditions that Impact Oral Care, a Glossary of Related Terms, and a Directory of Additional Resources

Edited by Amy L. Sutton. 619 pages. 2008. 978-0-7808-1032-7.

Depression Sourcebook, 2nd Edition

Basic Consumer Health Information about Unipolar Depression, Bipolar Disorder, Dysthymia, Seasonal Affective Disorder, Postpartum Depression, and Other Depressive Disorders, Including Facts about Populations at Special Risk, Coexisting Medical Conditions, Symptoms, Treatment Options, and Suicide Prevention

Along with Statistical Data, a Glossary of Related Terms, and a Directory of Resources for Additional Help and Information

Edited by Sandra J. Judd. 646 pages. 2008. 978-0-7808-1003-7.

"Recommended for public libraries."

—*ARBAonline, Nov '08*

SEE ALSO *Mental Health Disorders Sourcebook, 4th Edition*

Dermatological Disorders Sourcebook, 2nd Edition

Basic Consumer Health Information about Conditions and Disorders Affecting the Skin, Hair, and Nails, Such as Acne, Rosacea, Rashes, Dermatitis, Pigmentation Disorders, Birthmarks, Skin Cancer, Skin Injuries, Psoriasis, Scleroderma, and Hair Loss, Including Facts about Medications and Treatments for Dermatological Disorders and Tips for Maintaining Healthy Skin, Hair, and Nails

Along with Information about How Aging Affects the Skin, a Glossary of Related Terms, and a Directory of Resources for Additional Help and Information

Edited by Amy L. Sutton. 617 pages. 2006. 978-0-7808-0795-2.

"Helpfully brings together. . . sources in one convenient place, saving the user hours of research time."

—*American Reference Books Annual, 2006*

SEE ALSO *Burns Sourcebook*

Diabetes Sourcebook, 4th Edition

Basic Consumer Health Information about Type 1 and Type 2 Diabetes Mellitus, Gestational Diabetes, Monogenic Forms of Diabetes, and Insulin Resistance, with Guidelines for Lifestyle Modifications and the Medical Management of Diabetes, Including Facts about Insulin, Insulin Delivery Devices, Oral Diabetes Medications, Self-Monitoring of Blood Glucose, Meal Planning, Physical Activity Recommendations, Foot Care, and Treatment Options for People with Kidney Failure

Along with a Section about Diabetes Complications and Co-Occurring Conditions, a Glossary of Related Terms, and Directories of Resources for Additional Help and Information

Edited by Karen Bellenir. 627 pages. 2008. 978-0-7808-1005-1.

"Completely and comprehensively covering almost everything a student or physician would need to know.... well worth the investment."

—*Internet Bookwatch, Dec '08*

SEE ALSO *Endocrine and Metabolic Disorders Sourcebook, 2nd Edition*

Diet and Nutrition Sourcebook, 3rd Edition

Basic Consumer Health Information about Dietary Guidelines and the Food Guidance System, Recommended Daily Nutrient Intakes, Serving Proportions, Weight Control, Vitamins and Supplements, Nutrition Issues for Different Life Stages and Lifestyles, and the Needs of People with Specific Medical Concerns, Including Cancer, Celiac Disease, Diabetes, Eating Disorders, Food Allergies, and Cardiovascular Disease

Along with Facts about Federal Nutrition Support Programs, a Glossary of Nutrition and Dietary Terms, and Directories of Additional Resources for More Information about Nutrition

Edited by Joyce Brennfleck Shannon. 605 pages. 2006. 978-0-7808-0800-3.

"A valuable resource tool for any individual."

—*Journal of Dental Hygiene, Apr '07*

"From different recommended eating habits to reduce disease and common ailments to nutrition advice for those with specific conditions, *Diet and Nutrition Sourcebook* is especially important because so much is changing in this area, and so rapidly."

—*California Bookwatch, Jun '06*

SEE ALSO *Digestive Diseases and Disorders Sourcebook, Eating Disorders Sourcebook, 2nd Edition, Gastrointestinal Diseases and Disorders Sourcebook, 2nd Edition, Vegetarian Sourcebook*

Digestive Diseases and Disorders Sourcebook

Basic Consumer Health Information about Diseases and Disorders that Impact the Upper and Lower Digestive System, Including Celiac Disease, Constipation, Crohn's Disease, Cyclic Vomiting Syndrome, Diarrhea, Diverticulosis and Diverticulitis, Gallstones, Heartburn, Hemorrhoids, Hernias, Indigestion (Dyspepsia), Irritable Bowel Syndrome, Lactose Intolerance, Ulcers, and More

Along with Information about Medications and Other Treatments, Tips for Maintaining a Healthy Digestive Tract, a Glossary, and Directory of Digestive Diseases Organizations

Edited by Karen Bellenir. 323 pages. 2000. 978-0-7808-0327-5.

"An excellent addition to all public or patient-research libraries."

—*American Reference Books Annual, 2001*

"Recommended reference source."

—*Booklist, May '00*

SEE ALSO *Diet and Nutrition Sourcebook, 3rd Edition, Gastrointestinal Diseases and Disorders Sourcebook, 2nd Edition*

Disabilities Sourcebook

Basic Consumer Health Information about Physical and Psychiatric Disabilities, Including Descriptions of Major Causes of Disability, Assistive and Adaptive Aids, Workplace Issues, and Accessibility Concerns

Along with Information about the Americans with Disabilities Act, a Glossary, and Resources for Additional Help and Information

Edited by Dawn D. Matthews. 602 pages. 2000. 978-0-7808-0389-3.

"A must for libraries with a consumer health section."

—*American Reference Books Annual, 2002*

"A much needed addition to the Omnigraphics *Health Reference Series*. A current reference work to provide people with disabilities, their families, caregivers or those who work with them, a broad range of information in one volume, has not been available until now. . . . It is recommended for all public and academic library reference collections."

—*E-Streams, May '01*

"An excellent source book in easy-to-read format covering many current topics; highly recommended for all libraries."

—*CHOICE, Jan '01*

Disease Management Sourcebook

Basic Consumer Health Information about Coping with Chronic and Serious Illnesses, Navigating the Health Care System, Communicating with Health Care Providers, Assessing Health Care Quality, and Making Informed Health Care Decisions, Including Facts about Second Opinions, Hospitalization, Surgery, and Medications

Along with a Section about Children with Chronic Conditions, Information about Legal, Financial, and Insurance Issues, a Glossary of Related Terms, and Directories of Additional Resources

Edited by Joyce Brennfleck Shannon. 621 pages. 2008. 978-0-7808-1002-0.

"Consumers need to know how to manage their health care the same way they manage anything else in their lives. The text is very readable and is written for the layperson and consumer. The cost is not prohibitive. This book should be in all collections of health care libraries and public libraries."

—*ARBAonline, Jul '08*

"The information is very current, and the selection of font and layout make the book easy to read. A hardback that will stand up to much usage, this is an excellent resource for consumers. . . . Recommended. General readers."

—*CHOICE, Nov '08*

"Intended for lay readers, this resource clarifies the many confusing and overwhelming details associated with chronic disease care. Meticulous and clearly explained, the book even includes diagrams intended to ease comprehension of over-the-counter medication labels. An essential guide to navigating the health-care rapids."

—*Library Journal, Aug '08*

Domestic Violence Sourcebook, 3rd Edition

Basic Consumer Health Information about Warning Signs, Risk Factors, and Health Consequences of Intimate Partner Violence, Sexual Violence and Rape, Stalking, Human Trafficking, Child Maltreatment, Teen Dating Violence, and Elder Abuse

Along with Facts about Victims and Perpetrators, Strategies for Violence Prevention, and Emergency Interventions, Safety Plans, and Financial and Legal Tips for Victims, a Glossary of Related Terms, and Directories of Resources for Additional Information and Support

Edited by Joyce Brennfleck Shannon. 600 pages. 2009. 978-0-7808-1038-9.

SEE ALSO *Child Abuse Sourcebook, 2nd Edition*

Drug Abuse Sourcebook, 2nd Edition

Basic Consumer Health Information about Illicit Substances of Abuse and the Misuse of Prescription and Over-the-Counter Medications, Including Depressants, Hallucinogens, Inhalants, Marijuana, Stimulants, and Anabolic Steroids

Along with Facts about Related Health Risks, Treatment Programs, Prevention Programs, a Glossary of Abuse and Addiction Terms, a Glossary of Drug-Related Street Terms, and a Directory of Resources for More Information

Edited by Catherine Ginther. 581 pages. 2004. 978-0-7808-0740-2.

"Commendable for organizing useful, normally scattered government and association-produced data into a logical sequence."

—*American Reference Books Annual, 2006*

"An excellent library reference."
—*The Bookwatch, May '05*

SEE ALSO *Alcoholism Sourcebook, 2nd Edition*

Ear, Nose, and Throat Disorders Sourcebook, 2nd Edition

Basic Consumer Health Information about Disorders of the Ears, Hearing Loss, Vestibular Disorders, Nasal and Sinus Problems, Throat and Vocal Cord Disorders, and Otolaryngologic Cancers, Including Facts about Ear Infections and Injuries, Genetic and Congenital Deafness, Sensorineural Hearing Disorders, Tinnitus, Vertigo, Ménière Disease, Rhinitis, Sinusitis, Snoring, Sore Throats, Hoarseness, and More

Along with Reports on Current Research Initiatives, a Glossary of Related Medical Terms, and a Directory of Sources for Further Help and Information

Edited by Sandra J. Judd. 631 pages. 2007. 978-0-7808-0872-0.

"A resource book for the general public that provides comprehensive coverage of basic up-to-date medical information about the causes, symptoms, diagnosis, and treatment of diseases and disorders that affect the ears, nose, sinuses, throat, and voice. . . . The majority of information is presented in question and answer format, much like questions a patient might ask of a health care provider. An extensive index facilitates the reader's ability to easily access information on any specific topic."
—*Journal of Dental Hygiene, Oct '07*

"A handy compilation of information on common and some not so common ailments of the ears, nose, and throat."
—*Doody's Review Service, 2007*

Eating Disorders Sourcebook, 2nd Edition

Basic Consumer Health Information about Anorexia Nervosa, Bulimia, Binge Eating, Compulsive Exercise, Female Athlete Triad, and Other Eating Disorders, Including Facts about Body Image and Other Cultural and Age-Related Risk Factors, Prevention Efforts, Adverse Health Effects, Treatment Options, and the Recovery Process

Along with Guidelines for Healthy Weight Control, a Glossary, and Directories of Additional Resources

Edited by Joyce Brennfleck Shannon. 557 pages. 2007. 978-0-7808-0948-2.

"Recommended for the reference collection of large public libraries."
—*American Reference Books Annual, 2008*

"A basic health reference any health or general library needs."
—*Internet Bookwatch, Jun '07*

SEE ALSO *Diet and Nutrition Sourcebook, 3rd Edition, Mental Health Disorders Sourcebook, 4th Edition*

Emergency Medical Services Sourcebook

Basic Consumer Health Information about Preventing, Preparing for, and Managing Emergency Situations, When and Who to Call for Help, What to Expect in the Emergency Room, the Emergency Medical Team, Patient Issues, and Current Topics in Emergency Medicine

Along with Statistical Data, a Glossary, and Sources of Additional Help and Information

Edited by Jenni Lynn Colson. 472 pages. 2002. 978-0-7808-0420-3.

"Handy and convenient for home, public, school, and college libraries. Recommended."
—*CHOICE, Apr '03*

"This reference can provide the consumer with answers to most questions about emergency care in the United States, or it will direct them to a resource where the answer can be found."
—*American Reference Books Annual, 2003*

SEE ALSO *Injury and Trauma Sourcebook*

Endocrine and Metabolic Disorders Sourcebook, 2nd Edition

Basic Consumer Health Information about Hormonal and Metabolic Disorders that Affect the Body's Growth, Development, and Functioning, Including Disorders of the Pancreas, Ovaries and Testes, and Pituitary, Thyroid, Parathyroid, and Adrenal Glands, with Facts about Growth Disorders, Addison Disease, Cushing Syndrome, Conn Syndrome, Diabetic Disorders, Multiple Endocrine Neoplasia, Inborn Errors of Metabolism, and More

Along with Information about Endocrine Functioning, Diagnostic and Screening Tests, a Glossary of Related Terms, and Directories of Additional Resources

Edited by Joyce Brennfleck Shannon. 597 pages. 2007. 978-0-7808-0952-9.

SEE ALSO *Diabetes Sourcebook, 4th Edition*

Environmental Health Sourcebook, 2nd Edition

Basic Consumer Health Information about the Environment and Its Effect on Human Health, Including the Effects of Air Pollution, Water Pollution, Hazardous Chemicals, Food Hazards, Radiation Hazards, Biological Agents, Household Hazards, Such as Radon, Asbestos, Carbon Monoxide, and Mold, and Information about Associated Diseases and Disorders, Including Cancer, Allergies, Respiratory Problems, and Skin Disorders

Along with Information about Environmental Concerns for Specific Populations, a Glossary of Related Terms, and Resources for Further Help and Information

Edited by Dawn D. Matthews. 650 pages. 2003. 978-0-7808-0632-0.

"Recommended for teenage and adult students and readers, and for public and academic libraries, as well as any library focusing on consumer health."

—*E-Streams, May '04*

"This recently updated edition continues the level of quality and the reputation of the numerous other volumes in Omnigraphics' *Health Reference Series*."

—*American Reference Books Annual, 2004*

Ethnic Diseases Sourcebook

Basic Consumer Health Information for Ethnic and Racial Minority Groups in the United States, Including General Health Indicators and Behaviors, Ethnic Diseases, Genetic Testing, the Impact of Chronic Diseases, Women's Health, Mental Health Issues, and Preventive Health Care Services

Along with a Glossary and a Listing of Additional Resources

Edited by Joyce Brennfleck Shannon. 648 pages. 2001. 978-0-7808-0336-7.

"Not many books have been written on this topic to date, and the *Ethnic Diseases Sourcebook* is a strong addition to the list. It will be an important introductory resource for health consumers, students, health care personnel, and social scientists. It is recommended for public, academic, and large hospital libraries."

—*American Reference Books Annual, 2002*

"Will prove valuable to any library seeking to maintain a current, comprehensive reference collection of health resources. . . . An excellent source of health information about genetic disorders which affect particular ethnic and racial minorities in the U.S."

—*The Bookwatch, Aug '01*

Eye Care Sourcebook, 3rd Edition

Basic Consumer Health Information about Eye Care and Eye Disorders, Including Facts about the Diagnosis, Prevention, and Treatment of Refractive Disorders, Cataracts, Glaucoma, Macular Degeneration, and Problems Affecting the Cornea, Retina, and Lacrimal Glands

Along with Advice about Preventing Eye Injuries and Tips for Living with Low Vision or Blindness, a Glossary of Related Terms, and Directories of Resources for More Help and Information

Edited by Amy L. Sutton. 646 pages. 2008. 978-0-7808-1000-6.

Family Planning Sourcebook

Basic Consumer Health Information about Planning for Pregnancy and Contraception, Including Traditional Methods, Barrier Methods, Hormonal Methods, Permanent Methods, Future Methods, Emergency Contraception, and Birth Control Choices for Women at Each Stage of Life

Along with Statistics, a Glossary, and Sources of Additional Information

Edited by Amy Marcaccio Keyzer. 503 pages. 2001. 978-0-7808-0379-4.

"Recommended for public, health, and undergraduate libraries as part of the circulating collection."

—*E-Streams, Mar '02*

"Will prove valuable to any library seeking to maintain a current, comprehensive reference collection of health resources. . . . Excellent reference."

—*The Bookwatch, Aug '01*

SEE ALSO *Pregnancy and Birth Sourcebook, 2nd Edition*

Fitness and Exercise Sourcebook, 3rd Edition

Basic Consumer Health Information about the Physical and Mental Benefits of Fitness, Including Cardiorespiratory Endurance, Muscular Strength, Muscular Endurance, and Flexibility, with Facts about Sports Nutrition and Exercise-Related Injuries and Tips about Physical Activity and Exercises for People of All Ages and for People with Health Concerns

Along with Advice on Selecting and Using Exercise Equipment, Maintaining Exercise Motivation, a Glossary of Related Terms, and a Directory of Resources for More Help and Information

Edited by Amy L. Sutton. 635 pages. 2007. 978-0-7808-0946-8.

"Updates the consumer information on the physical and mental benefits of physical activity throughout the lifespan offered in earlier editions. . . . Recommended. All readers; all levels."

—*CHOICE, Oct '07*

"An exceptionally well-rounded coverage perfect for any concerned about developing and understanding a fitness program."

—*California Bookwatch, Jun '07*

SEE ALSO *Sports Injuries Sourcebook, 3rd Edition*

Food Safety Sourcebook

Basic Consumer Health Information about the Safe Handling of Meat, Poultry, Seafood, Eggs, Fruit Juices, and Other Food Items, and Facts about Pesticides, Drinking Water, Food Safety Overseas, and the Onset, Duration, and Symptoms of Foodborne Illnesses, Including Types of Pathogenic Bacteria, Parasitic Protozoa, Worms, Viruses, and Natural Toxins

Along with the Role of the Consumer, the Food Handler, and the Government in Food Safety; a Glossary, and Resources for Additional Help and Information

Edited by Dawn D. Matthews. 327 pages. 1999. 978-0-7808-0326-8.

"Recommended reference source."

—*Booklist, May '00*

"This book takes the complex issues of food safety and foodborne pathogens and presents them in an easily understood manner. [It does] an excellent job of covering a large and often confusing topic."

— *American Reference Books Annual, 2000*

Forensic Medicine Sourcebook

Basic Consumer Information for the Layperson about Forensic Medicine, Including Crime Scene Investigation, Evidence Collection and Analysis, Expert Testimony, Computer-Aided Criminal Identification, Digital Imaging in the Courtroom, DNA Profiling, Accident Reconstruction, Autopsies, Ballistics, Drugs and Explosives Detection, Latent Fingerprints, Product Tampering, and Questioned Document Examination

Along with Statistical Data, a Glossary of Forensics Terminology, and Listings of Sources for Further Help and Information

Edited by Annemarie S. Muth. 574 pages. 1999. 978-0-7808-0232-2.

"Given the expected widespread interest in its content and its easy to read style, this book is recommended for most public and all college and university libraries."

—*E-Streams, Feb '01*

"A wealth of information, useful statistics, references are up-to-date and extremely complete. This wonderful collection of data will help students who are interested in a career in any type of forensic field. It is a great resource for attorneys who need information about types of expert witnesses needed in a particular case. It also offers useful information for fiction and nonfiction writers whose work involves a crime. A fascinating compilation. All levels."

—*CHOICE, Jan '00*

"There are several items that make this book attractive to consumers who are seeking certain forensic data. . . . This is a useful current

source for those seeking general forensic medical answers."
—American Reference Books Annual, 2000

Gastrointestinal Diseases and Disorders Sourcebook, 2nd Edition

Basic Consumer Health Information about the Upper and Lower Gastrointestinal (GI) Tract, Including the Esophagus, Stomach, Intestines, Rectum, Liver, and Pancreas, with Facts about Gastroesophageal Reflux Disease, Gastritis, Hernias, Ulcers, Celiac Disease, Diverticulitis, Irritable Bowel Syndrome, Hemorrhoids, Gastrointestinal Cancers, and Other Diseases and Disorders Related to the Digestive Process

Along with Information about Commonly Used Diagnostic and Surgical Procedures, Statistics, Reports on Current Research Initiatives and Clinical Trials, a Glossary, and Resources for Additional Help and Information

Edited by Sandra J. Judd. 654 pages. 2006. 978-0-7808-0798-3.

"The text is designed for the general reader seeking information on prevention, disease warning signs, diagnostic and therapeutic questions. . . . It is an excellent resource for the general reader to conveniently locate credible, coordinated and indexed information. . . . The sourcebook will prove very helpful for patients, caregivers and should be available in every physician waiting room."
—Doody's Review Service, 2006

SEE ALSO *Diet and Nutrition Sourcebook, 3rd Edition, Digestive Diseases and Disorders Sourcebook*

Genetic Disorders Sourcebook, 4th Edition

Basic Consumer Health Information about Hereditary Diseases and Disorders, Including Facts about the Human Genome, Genetic Inheritance Patterns, Disorders Associated with Specific Genes, Such as Sickle Cell Disease, Hemophilia, and Cystic Fibrosis, Chromosome Disorders, Such as Down Syndrome, Fragile X Syndrome, and Turner Syndrome, and Complex Diseases and Disorders Resulting from the Interaction of Environmental and Genetic Factors, Such as Allergies, Cancer, and Obesity

Along with Facts about Genetic Testing, Suggestions for Parents of Children with Special Needs, Reports on Current Research Initiatives, a Glossary of Genetic Terminology, and Resources for Additional Help and Information

Edited by Sandra J. Judd. 600 pages. 2009. 978-0-7808-1076-1.

Head Trauma Sourcebook

Basic Information for the Layperson about Open-Head and Closed-Head Injuries, Treatment Advances, Recovery, and Rehabilitation

Along with Reports on Current Research Initiatives

Edited by Karen Bellenir. 414 pages. 1997. 978-0-7808-0208-7.

Headache Sourcebook

Basic Consumer Health Information about Migraine, Tension, Cluster, Rebound and Other Types of Headaches, with Facts about the Cause and Prevention of Headaches, the Effects of Stress and the Environment, Headaches during Pregnancy and Menopause, and Childhood Headaches

Along with a Glossary and Other Resources for Additional Help and Information

Edited by Dawn D. Matthews. 342 pages. 2002. 978-0-7808-0337-4.

"Highly recommended for academic and medical reference collections."
—Library Bookwatch, Sep '02

SEE ALSO *Pain Sourcebook, 3rd Edition*

Healthy Aging Sourcebook

Basic Consumer Health Information about Maintaining Health through the Aging Process, Including Advice on Nutrition, Exercise, and Sleep, Help in Making Decisions about Midlife Issues and Retirement, and Guidance Concerning Practical and Informed Choices in Health Consumerism

Along with Data Concerning the Theories of Aging, Different Experiences in Aging by Minority Groups, and Facts about Aging Now and Aging in the Future; and Featuring a Glossary, a Guide to Consumer Help, Additional Suggested Reading, and Practical Resource Directory

Edited by Jenifer Swanson. 537 pages. 1999. 978-0-7808-0390-9.

"Recommended reference source."

—*Booklist, Feb '00*

SEE ALSO *Physical and Mental Issues in Aging Sourcebook*

Healthy Children Sourcebook

Basic Consumer Health Information about the Physical and Mental Development of Children between the Ages of 3 and 12, Including Routine Health Care, Preventative Health Services, Safety and First Aid, Healthy Sleep, Dental Care, Nutrition, and Fitness, and Featuring Parenting Tips on Such Topics as Bedwetting, Choosing Day Care, Monitoring TV and Other Media, and Establishing a Foundation for Substance Abuse Prevention

Along with a Glossary of Commonly Used Pediatric Terms and Resources for Additional Help and Information.

Edited by Chad T. Kimball. 624 pages. 2003. 978-0-7808-0247-6.

"Should be required reading for parents and teachers."

—*E-Streams, Jun '04*

"It is hard to imagine that any other single resource exists that would provide such a comprehensive guide of timely information on health promotion and disease prevention for children aged 3 to 12."

—*American Reference Books Annual, 2004*

"This easy-to-read volume is a tremendous resource."

—*AORN Journal, May '05*

SEE ALSO *Childhood Diseases and Disorders Sourcebook, 2nd Edition*

Healthy Heart Sourcebook for Women

Basic Consumer Health Information about Cardiac Issues Specific to Women, Including Facts about Major Risk Factors and Prevention, Treatment and Control Strategies, and Important Dietary Issues

Along with a Special Section Regarding the Pros and Cons of Hormone Replacement Therapy and Its Impact on Heart Health, and Additional Help, Including Recipes, a Glossary, and a Directory of Resources

Edited by Dawn D. Matthews. 321 pages. 2000. 978-0-7808-0329-9.

"A good reference source and recommended for all public, academic, medical, and hospital libraries."

—*Medical Reference Services Quarterly, Summer '01*

"Contains very important information about coronary artery disease that all women should know. The information is current and presented in an easy-to-read format. The book will make a good addition to any library."

—*American Medical Writers Association Journal, Summer '00*

SEE ALSO *Cardiovascular Diseases and Disorders Sourcebook, 3rd Edition, Women's Health Concerns Sourcebook, 3rd Edition*

Hepatitis Sourcebook

Basic Consumer Health Information about Hepatitis A, Hepatitis B, Hepatitis C, and Other Forms of Hepatitis, Including Autoimmune Hepatitis, Alcoholic Hepatitis, Nonalcoholic Steatohepatitis, and Toxic Hepatitis, with Facts about Risk Factors, Screening Methods, Diagnostic Tests, and Treatment Options

Along with Information on Liver Health, Tips for People Living with Chronic Hepatitis, Reports on Current Research Initiatives, a Glossary of Terms Related to Hepatitis, and a Directory of Sources for Further Help and Information

Edited by Sandra J. Judd. 570 pages. 2006. 978-0-7808-0749-5.

"The breadth of information found in this one book would not be readily found in another source. Highly recommended."

—*American Reference Books Annual, 2006*

SEE ALSO *Contagious Diseases Sourcebook*

Household Safety Sourcebook

Basic Consumer Health Information about Household Safety, Including Information about Poisons, Chemicals, Fire, and Water Hazards in the Home

Along with Advice about the Safe Use of Home Maintenance Equipment, Choosing Toys and Nursery Furniture, Holiday and Recreation Safety, a Glossary, and Resources for Further Help and Information

Edited by Dawn D. Matthews. 587 pages. 2002. 978-0-7808-0338-1.

"As a sourcebook on household safety this book meets its mark. It is encyclopedic in scope and covers a wide range of safety issues that are commonly seen in the home."

—*E-Streams, Jul '02*

Hypertension Sourcebook

Basic Consumer Health Information about the Causes, Diagnosis, and Treatment of High Blood Pressure, with Facts about Consequences, Complications, and Co-Occurring Disorders, Such as Coronary Heart Disease, Diabetes, Stroke, Kidney Disease, and Hypertensive Retinopathy, and Issues in Blood Pressure Control, Including Dietary Choices, Stress Management, and Medications

Along with Reports on Current Research Initiatives and Clinical Trials, a Glossary, and Resources for Additional Help and Information

Edited by Dawn D. Matthews and Karen Bellenir. 588 pages. 2004. 978-0-7808-0674-0.

"Academic, public, and medical libraries will want to add the *Hypertension Sourcebook* to their collections."

—*E-Streams, Aug '05*

"The strength of this source is the wide range of information given about hypertension."

—*American Reference Books Annual, 2005*

SEE ALSO *Stroke Sourcebook, 2nd Edition*

Immune System Disorders Sourcebook, 2nd Edition

Basic Consumer Health Information about Disorders of the Immune System, Including Immune System Function and Response, Diagnosis of Immune Disorders, Information about Inherited Immune Disease, Acquired Immune Disease, and Autoimmune Diseases, Including Primary Immune Deficiency, Acquired Immunodeficiency Syndrome (AIDS), Lupus, Multiple Sclerosis, Type 1 Diabetes, Rheumatoid Arthritis, and Graves' Disease

Along with Treatments, Tips for Coping with Immune Disorders, a Glossary, and a Directory of Additional Resources

Edited by Joyce Brennfleck Shannon. 643 pages. 2005. 978-0-7808-0748-8.

"Highly recommended for academic and public libraries."

—*American Reference Books Annual, 2006*

"The updated second edition is a 'must' for any consumer health library seeking a solid resource covering the treatments, symptoms, and options for immune disorder sufferers. . . . An excellent guide."

—*MBR Bookwatch, Jan '06*

SEE ALSO *AIDS Sourcebook, 4th Edition, Arthritis Sourcebook, 2nd Edition*

Infant and Toddler Health Sourcebook

Basic Consumer Health Information about the Physical and Mental Development of Newborns, Infants, and Toddlers, Including Neonatal Concerns, Nutrition Recommendations, Immunization Schedules, Common Pediatric Disorders, Assessments and Milestones, Safety Tips, and Advice for Parents and Other Caregivers

Along with a Glossary of Terms and Resource Listings for Additional Help

Edited by Jenifer Swanson. 570 pages. 2000. 978-0-7808-0246-9.

"As a reference for the general public, this would be useful in any library."

—*E-Streams, May '01*

"Recommended reference source."

—*Booklist, Feb '01*

Infectious Diseases Sourcebook

Basic Consumer Health Information about Non-Contagious Bacterial, Viral, Prion, Fungal, and Parasitic Diseases Spread by Food and Water, Insects and Animals, or Environmental Contact, Including Botulism, E. Coli, Encephalitis, Legionnaires' Disease, Lyme Disease, Malaria, Plague, Rabies, Salmonella, Tetanus, and Others, and Facts about Newly Emerging Diseases, Such as Hantavirus, Mad Cow Disease, Monkeypox, and West Nile Virus

Along with Information about Preventing Disease Transmission, the Threat of Bioterrorism, and Current Research Initiatives, with a Glossary and Directory of Resources for More Information

Edited by Karen Bellenir. 610 pages. 2004. 978-0-7808-0675-7.

"This reference continues the excellent tradition of the *Health Reference Series* in consolidating a wealth of information on a selected topic into a format that is easy to use and accessible to the general public."

—American Reference Books Annual, 2005

"Recommended for public and academic libraries."

—E-Streams, Jan '05

Injury and Trauma Sourcebook

Basic Consumer Health Information about the Impact of Injury, the Diagnosis and Treatment of Common and Traumatic Injuries, Emergency Care, and Specific Injuries Related to Home, Community, Workplace, Transportation, and Recreation

Along with Guidelines for Injury Prevention, a Glossary, and a Directory of Additional Resources

Edited by Joyce Brennfleck Shannon. 675 pages. 2002. 978-0-7808-0421-0.

"Practitioners should be aware of guides such as this in order to facilitate their use by patients and their families."

—Doody's Health Sciences Book Review Journal, Sep-Oct '02

"Recommended reference source."

—Booklist, Sep '02

"Highly recommended for academic and medical reference collections."

—Library Bookwatch, Sep '02

SEE ALSO *Emergency Medical Services Sourcebook, Sports Injuries Sourcebook, 3rd Edition*

Learning Disabilities Sourcebook, 3rd Edition

Basic Consumer Health Information about Dyslexia, Auditory and Visual Processing Disorders, Communication Disorders, Dyscalculia, Dysgraphia, and Other Conditions That Impede Learning, Including Attention Deficit/Hyperactivity Disorder, Autism Spectrum Disorders, Hearing and Visual Impairments, Chromosome-Based Disorders, and Brain Injury

Along with Facts about Brain Function, Assessment, Therapy and Remediation, Accommodations, Assistive Technology, Legal Protections, and Tips about Family Life, School Transitions, and Employment Strategies, a Glossary of Related Terms, and Directories of Additional Resources

Edited by Joyce Brennfleck Shannon. 613 pages. 2009. 978-0-7808-1039-6.

SEE ALSO *Attention Deficit Disorder Sourcebook, Autism and Pervasive Developmental Disorders Sourcebook*

Leukemia Sourcebook

Basic Consumer Health Information about Adult and Childhood Leukemias, Including Acute Lymphocytic Leukemia (ALL), Chronic Lymphocytic Leukemia (CLL), Acute Myelogenous Leukemia (AML), Chronic Myelogenous Leukemia (CML), and Hairy Cell Leukemia, and Treatments Such as Chemotherapy, Radiation Therapy, Peripheral Blood Stem Cell and Marrow Transplantation, and Immunotherapy

Along with Tips for Life During and After Treatment, a Glossary, and Directories of Additional Resources

Edited by Joyce Brennfleck Shannon. 564 pages. 2003. 978-0-7808-0627-6.

"Unlike other medical books for the layperson, . . . the language does not talk down to the reader. . . . This volume is highly recommended for all libraries."

—American Reference Books Annual, 2004

"A fine title which ranges from diagnosis to alternative treatments, staging, and tips for life during and after diagnosis."

—The Bookwatch, Dec '03

SEE ALSO *Cancer Sourcebook, 5th Edition*

Liver Disorders Sourcebook

Basic Consumer Health Information about the Liver and How It Works; Liver Diseases, Including Cancer, Cirrhosis, Hepatitis, and Toxic and Drug Related Diseases; Tips for Maintaining a Healthy Liver; Laboratory Tests, Radiology Tests, and Facts about Liver Transplantation

Along with a Section on Support Groups, a Glossary, and Resource Listings

Edited by Joyce Brennfleck Shannon. 580 pages. 2000. 978-0-7808-0383-1.

"This title is recommended for health sciences and public libraries with consumer health collections."

—E-Streams, Oct '00

"Recommended reference source."

—Booklist, Jun '00

SEE ALSO *Gastrointestinal Diseases and Disorders Sourcebook, 2nd Edition, Hepatitis Sourcebook*

Lung Disorders Sourcebook

Basic Consumer Health Information about Emphysema, Pneumonia, Tuberculosis, Asthma, Cystic Fibrosis, and Other Lung Disorders, Including Facts about Diagnostic Procedures, Treatment Strategies, Disease Prevention Efforts, and Such Risk Factors as Smoking, Air Pollution, and Exposure to Asbestos, Radon, and Other Agents

Along with a Glossary and Resources for Additional Help and Information

Edited by Dawn D. Matthews. 657 pages. 2002. 978-0-7808-0339-8.

"Highly recommended for academic and medical reference collections."

—Library Bookwatch, Sep '02

SEE ALSO *Respiratory Disorders Sourcebook, 2nd Edition*

Medical Tests Sourcebook, 3rd Edition

Basic Consumer Health Information about X-Rays, Blood Tests, Stool and Urine Tests, Biopsies, Mammography, Endoscopic Procedures, Ultrasound Exams, Computed Tomography, Magnetic Resonance Imaging (MRI), Nuclear Medicine, Genetic Testing, Home-Use Tests, and More

Along with Facts about Preventive Care and Screening Test Guidelines, Screening and Assessment Tests Associated with Such Specific Concerns as Cancer, Heart Disease, Allergies, Diabetes, Thyroid Disfunction, and Infertility, a Glossary of Related Terms, and a Directory of Resources for Additional Help and Information

Edited by Karen Bellenir. 627 pages. 2008. 978-0-7808-1040-2

"This volume has a wide scope that makes it useful . . . Can be a valuable reference guide."

—ARBAonline, Nov '08

Men's Health Concerns Sourcebook, 3rd Edition

Basic Consumer Health Information about Wellness in Men and Gender-Related Differences in Health, With Facts about Heart Disease, Cancer, Traumatic Injury, and Other Leading Causes of Death in Men, Reproductive Concerns, Sexual Dysfunction, Disorders of the Prostate, Penis, and Testes, Sex-Linked Genetic Disorders, and Other Medical and Mental Concerns of Men

Along with Statistical Data, a Glossary of Related Terms, and a Directory of Resources for Additional Information

Edited by Sandra J. Judd. 600 pages. 2009. 978-0-7808-1033-4.

SEE ALSO *Prostate and Urological Disorders Sourcebook*

Mental Health Disorders Sourcebook, 4th Edition

Basic Consumer Health Information about the Causes and Symptoms of Mental Health Problems, Including Depression, Bipolar Disorder, Anxiety Disorders, Posttraumatic Stress Disorder, Obsessive-Compulsive Disorder, Eating Disorders, Addictions, and Personality and Psychotic Disorders

Along with Information about Medications and Treatments, Mental Health Concerns in Children, Adolescents, and Adults, Tips on Living with Mental Health Disorders, a Glossary of Related Terms, and a Directory of Resources for Additional Help and Information

Edited by Amy L. Sutton. 600 pages. 2009. 978-0-7808-1041-9.

SEE ALSO *Depression Sourcebook, 2nd Edition, Stress-Related Disorders Sourcebook, 2nd Edition*

Mental Retardation Sourcebook

Basic Consumer Health Information about Mental Retardation and Its Causes, Including

Down Syndrome, Fetal Alcohol Syndrome, Fragile X Syndrome, Genetic Conditions, Injury, and Environmental Sources

Along with Preventive Strategies, Parenting Issues, Educational Implications, Health Care Needs, Employment and Economic Matters, Legal Issues, a Glossary, and a Resource Listing for Additional Help and Information

Edited by Joyce Brennfleck Shannon. 627 pages. 2000. 978-0-7808-0377-0.

"Public libraries will find the book useful for reference and as a beginning research point for students, parents, and caregivers."
—*American Reference Books Annual, 2001*

"The strength of this work is that it compiles many basic fact sheets and addresses for further information in one volume. It is intended and suitable for the general public."
—*E-Streams, Nov '00*

"An invaluable overview."
—*Reviewer's Bookwatch, Jul '00*

Movement Disorders Sourcebook, 2nd Edition

Basic Consumer Health Information about the Symptoms and Causes of Movement Disorders, Including Parkinson Disease, Amyotrophic Lateral Sclerosis, Cerebral Palsy, Muscular Dystrophy, Multiple Sclerosis, Myasthenia, Myoclonus, Spina Bifida, Dystonia, Essential Tremor, Choreatic Disorders, Huntington Disease, Tourette Syndrome, and Other Disorders That Cause Slowed, Absent, or Excessive Movements

Along with Information about Surgical and Nonsurgical Interventions, Physical Therapies, Strategies for Independent Living, a Glossary of Related Terms, and a Directory of Resources for Additional Help and Information

Edited by Amy L. Sutton. 600 pages. 2009. 978-0-7808-1034-1.

SEE ALSO *Multiple Sclerosis Sourcebook, Muscular Dystrophy Sourcebook*

Multiple Sclerosis Sourcebook

Basic Consumer Health Information about Multiple Sclerosis (MS) and Its Effects on Mobility, Vision, Bladder Function, Speech, Swallowing, and Cognition, Including Facts about Risk Factors, Causes, Diagnostic Procedures, Pain Management, Drug Treatments, and Physical and Occupational Therapies

Along with Guidelines for Nutrition and Exercise, Tips on Choosing Assistive Equipment, Information about Disability, Work, Financial, and Legal Issues, a Glossary of Related Terms, and a Directory of Additional Resources

Edited by Joyce Brennfleck Shannon. 553 pages. 2007. 978-0-7808-0998-7.

SEE ALSO *Movement Disorders Sourcebook, 2nd Edition*

Muscular Dystrophy Sourcebook

Basic Consumer Health Information about Congenital, Childhood-Onset, and Adult-Onset Forms of Muscular Dystrophy, Such as Duchenne, Becker, Emery-Dreifuss, Distal, Limb-Girdle, Facioscapulohumeral (FSHD), Myotonic, and Ophthalmoplegic Muscular Dystrophies, Including Facts about Diagnostic Tests, Medical and Physical Therapies, Management of Co-Occurring Conditions, and Parenting Guidelines

Along with Practical Tips for Home Care, a Glossary, and Directories of Additional Resources

Edited by Joyce Brennfleck Shannon. 552 pages. 2004. 978-0-7808-0676-4.

"This book is highly recommended for public and academic libraries as well as health care offices that support the information needs of patients and their families."
—*E-Streams, Apr '05*

"Excellent reference."
—*The Bookwatch, Jan '05*

SEE ALSO *Movement Disorders Sourcebook, 2nd Edition*

Obesity Sourcebook

Basic Consumer Health Information about Diseases and Other Problems Associated with Obesity, and Including Facts about Risk Factors, Prevention Issues, and Management Approaches

Along with Statistical and Demographic Data, Information about Special Populations,

Research Updates, a Glossary, and Source Listings for Further Help and Information

Edited by Wilma Caldwell and Chad T. Kimball. 360 pages. 2001. 978-0-7808-0333-6.

"The book synthesizes the reliable medical literature on obesity into one easy-to-read and useful resource for the general public."
—*American Reference Books Annual, 2002*

"Well suited for the health reference collection of a public library or an academic health science library that serves the general population."
—*E-Streams, Sep '01*

Osteoporosis Sourcebook

Basic Consumer Health Information about Primary and Secondary Osteoporosis and Juvenile Osteoporosis and Related Conditions, Including Fibrous Dysplasia, Gaucher Disease, Hyperthyroidism, Hypophosphatasia, Myeloma, Osteopetrosis, Osteogenesis Imperfecta, and Paget's Disease

Along with Information about Risk Factors, Treatments, Traditional and Non-Traditional Pain Management, a Glossary of Related Terms, and a Directory of Resources

Edited by Allan R. Cook. 568 pages. 2001. 978-0-7808-0239-1.

"This resource is recommended as a great reference source for public, health, and academic libraries, and is another triumph for the editors of Omnigraphics."
—*American Reference Books Annual, 2002*

"Will prove valuable to any library seeking to maintain a current, comprehensive reference collection of health resources. . . . From prevention to treatment and associated conditions, this provides an excellent survey."
—*The Bookwatch, Aug '01*

SEE ALSO *Healthy Aging Sourcebook, Women's Health Concerns Sourcebook, 3rd Edition*

Pain Sourcebook, 3rd Edition

Basic Consumer Health Information about Acute and Chronic Pain, Including Nerve Pain, Bone Pain, Muscle Pain, Cancer Pain, and Disorders Characterized by Pain, Such as Arthritis, Temporomandibular Muscle and Joint (TMJ) Disorder, Carpal Tunnel Syndrome, Headaches, Heartburn, Sciatica, and Shingles, and Facts about Diagnostic Tests and Treatment Options for Pain, Including Over-the-Counter and Prescription Drugs, Physical Rehabilitation, Injection and Infusion Therapies, Implantable Technologies, and Complementary Medicine

Along with Tips for Living with Pain, a Glossary of Related Terms, and a Directory of Additional Resources

Edited by Joyce Brennfleck Shannon. 644 pages. 2008. 978-0-7808-1006-8.

"Excellent for ready-reference users and can be used for beginning students in health fields . . . appropriate for the consumer health collection in both public and academic libraries."
—*ARBAonline, Nov '08*

Pediatric Cancer Sourcebook

Basic Consumer Health Information about Leukemias, Brain Tumors, Sarcomas, Lymphomas, and Other Cancers in Infants, Children, and Adolescents, Including Descriptions of Cancers, Treatments, and Coping Strategies

Along with Suggestions for Parents, Caregivers, and Concerned Relatives, a Glossary of Cancer Terms, and Resource Listings

Edited by Edward J. Prucha. 575 pages. 1999. 978-0-7808-0245-2.

"An excellent source of information. Recommended for public, hospital, and health science libraries with consumer health collections."
—*E-Streams, Jun '00*

"A valuable addition to all libraries specializing in health services and many public libraries."
—*American Reference Books Annual, 2000*

SEE ALSO *Childhood Diseases and Disorders Sourcebook, 2nd Edition, Healthy Children Sourcebook*

Physical and Mental Issues in Aging Sourcebook

Basic Consumer Health Information on Physical and Mental Disorders Associated with the Aging Process, Including Concerns about Cardiovascular Disease, Pulmonary Disease, Oral Health, Digestive Disorders, Musculoskeletal and Skin Disorders, Metabolic

Changes, Sexual and Reproductive Issues, and Changes in Vision, Hearing, and Other Senses

Along with Data about Longevity and Causes of Death, Information on Acute and Chronic Pain, Descriptions of Mental Concerns, a Glossary of Terms, and Resource Listings for Additional Help

Edited by Jenifer Swanson. 660 pages. 1999. 978-0-7808-0233-9.

"This is a treasure of health information for the layperson."
—*CHOICE Health Sciences Supplement, May '00*

"Recommended for public libraries."
—*American Reference Books Annual, 2000*

SEE ALSO *Healthy Aging Sourcebook*

Podiatry Sourcebook, 2nd Edition

Basic Consumer Health Information about Disorders, Diseases, and Deformities that Affect the Foot and Ankle, Including Sprains, Corns, Calluses, Bunions, Plantar Warts, Plantar Fasciitis, Neuromas, Clubfoot, Flat Feet, Achilles Tendonitis, and Much More

Along with Information about Selecting a Foot Care Specialist, Foot Fitness, Shoes and Socks, Diagnostic Tests and Corrective Procedures, Financial Assistance for Corrective Devices, a Glossary of Related Terms, and a Directory of Resources for Additional Help and Information

Edited by Ivy L. Alexander. 516 pages. 2007. 978-0-7808-0944-4.

"An excellent resource. . . . Although there have been various types of 'foot books' published in the past, none are as comprehensive as this one. 5 Stars (out of 5)!"
—*Doody's Review Service, 2007*

"Perfect for both health libraries and general-interest lending collections."
—*Internet Bookwatch, Jul '07*

Pregnancy and Birth Sourcebook, 3rd Edition

Basic Consumer Health Information about Pregnancy and Fetal Development, Including Facts about Fertility and Conception, Physical and Emotional Changes during Pregnancy, Prenatal Care and Diagnostic Tests, High-Risk Pregnancies and Complications, Labor, Delivery, and the Postpartum Period

Along with Tips on Maintaining Health and Wellness during Pregnancy and Caring for Newborn Infants, a Glossary of Related Terms, and Directories of Resources for Additional Help and Information

Edited by Amy L. Sutton. 600 pages. 2009. 978-0-7808-1074-7.

SEE ALSO *Breastfeeding Sourcebook, Congenital Disorders Sourcebook, 2nd Edition, Family Planning Sourcebook, Women's Health Concerns Sourcebook, 3rd Edition*

Prostate and Urological Disorders Sourcebook

Basic Consumer Health Information about Urogenital and Sexual Disorders in Men, Including Prostate and Other Andrological Cancers, Prostatitis, Benign Prostatic Hyperplasia, Testicular and Penile Trauma, Cryptorchidism, Peyronie Disease, Erectile Dysfunction, and Male Factor Infertility, and Facts about Commonly Used Tests and Procedures, Such as Prostatectomy, Vasectomy, Vasectomy Reversal, Penile Implants, and Semen Analysis

Along with a Glossary of Andrological Terms and a Directory of Resources for Additional Information

Edited by Karen Bellenir. 604 pages. 2006. 978-0-7808-0797-6.

"Certain to be a popular pick among library reference holdings. . . . No prior knowledge is assumed for any of the conditions or terms herein, making it a most accessible general-interest reference."
—*California Bookwatch, Apr '06*

SEE ALSO *Men's Health Concerns Sourcebook, 3rd Edition, Urinary Tract and Kidney Diseases and Disorders Sourcebook, 2nd Edition*

Prostate Cancer Sourcebook

Basic Consumer Health Information about Prostate Cancer, Including Information about the Associated Risk Factors, Detection, Diagnosis, and Treatment of Prostate Cancer

Along with Information on Non-Malignant Prostate Conditions, and Featuring a Section

Listing Support and Treatment Centers and a Glossary of Related Terms

Edited by Dawn D. Matthews. 340 pages. 2001. 978-0-7808-0324-4.

"Recommended reference source."

—*Booklist, Jan '02*

"A valuable resource for health care consumers seeking information on the subject. . . . All text is written in a clear, easy-to-understand language that avoids technical jargon. Any library that collects consumer health resources would strengthen their collection with the addition of the *Prostate Cancer Sourcebook.*"

—*American Reference Books Annual, 2002*

SEE ALSO *Cancer Sourcebook, 5th Edition, Men's Health Concerns Sourcebook, 3rd Edition*

Rehabilitation Sourcebook

Basic Consumer Health Information about Rehabilitation for People Recovering from Heart Surgery, Spinal Cord Injury, Stroke, Orthopedic Impairments, Amputation, Pulmonary Impairments, Traumatic Injury, and More, Including Physical Therapy, Occupational Therapy, Speech/Language Therapy, Massage Therapy, Dance Therapy, Art Therapy, and Recreational Therapy

Along with Information on Assistive and Adaptive Devices, a Glossary, and Resources for Additional Help and Information

Edited by Dawn D. Matthews. 519 pages. 2000. 978-0-7808-0236-0.

"This is an excellent resource for public library reference and health collections."

—*American Reference Books Annual, 2001*

"Recommended reference source."

—*Booklist, May '00*

Respiratory Disorders Sourcebook, 2nd Edition

Basic Consumer Health Information about Infectious, Inflammatory, and Chronic Conditions Affecting the Lungs and Respiratory System, Including Pneumonia, Bronchitis, Influenza, Tuberculosis, Sarcoidosis, Asthma, Cystic Fibrosis, Chronic Obstructive Pulmonary Disease, Lung Abscesses, Pulmonary Embolism, Occupational Lung Diseases, and Other Bacterial, Viral, and Fungal Infections

Along with Facts about the Structure and Function of the Lungs and Airways, Methods of Diagnosing Respiratory Disorders, and Treatment and Rehabilitation Options, a Glossary of Related Terms, and a Directory of Resources for Additional Help and Information

Edited by Sandra L. Judd. 638 pages. 2008. 978-0-7808-1007-5.

"A great addition for public and school libraries because it provides concise health information . . . readers can start with this reference source and get satisfactory answers before proceeding to other medical reference tools for more in depth information . . . A good guide for health education on lung disorders."

—*ARBAonline, Nov '08*

SEE ALSO *Lung Disorders Sourcebook*

Sexually Transmitted Diseases Sourcebook, 4th Edition

Basic Consumer Health Information about Chlamydial Infections, Gonorrhea, Hepatitis, Herpes, HIV/AIDS, Human Papillomavirus, Pubic Lice, Scabies, Syphilis, Trichomoniasis, Vaginal Infections, and Other Sexually Transmitted Diseases, Including Facts about Risk Factors, Symptoms, Diagnosis, Treatment, and the Prevention of Sexually Transmitted Infections

Along with Updates on Current Research Initiatives, a Glossary of Related Terms, and Resources for Additional Help and Information

Edited by Laura Larsen. 600 pages. 2009. 978-0-7808-1073-0.

SEE ALSO *AIDS Sourcebook, 4th Edition, Contagious Diseases Sourcebook, 2nd Edition, Men's Health Concerns Sourcebook, 3rd Edition, Women's Health Concerns Sourcebook, 3rd Edition*

Sleep Disorders Sourcebook, 2nd Edition

Basic Consumer Health Information about Sleep and Sleep Disorders, Including Insomnia, Sleep Apnea, Restless Legs Syndrome, Narcolepsy, Parasomnias, and Other Health Problems That Affect Sleep, Plus Facts about Diagnostic Procedures, Treatment Strategies,

Sleep Medications, and Tips for Improving Sleep Quality

Along with a Glossary of Related Terms and Resources for Additional Help and Information

Edited by Amy L. Sutton. 567 pages. 2005. 978-0-7808-0743-3.

"This book will be useful for just about everybody, especially the 40 million Americans with sleep disorders."

—*American Reference Books Annual, 2006*

"A welcome addition to public libraries and consumer health libraries."

—*Medical Reference Services Quarterly, Summer '06*

Smoking Concerns Sourcebook

Basic Consumer Health Information about Nicotine Addiction and Smoking Cessation, Featuring Facts about the Health Effects of Tobacco Use, Including Lung and Other Cancers, Heart Disease, Stroke, and Respiratory Disorders, Such as Emphysema and Chronic Bronchitis

Along with Information about Smoking Prevention Programs, Suggestions for Achieving and Maintaining a Smoke-Free Lifestyle, Statistics about Tobacco Use, Reports on Current Research Initiatives, a Glossary of Related Terms, and Directories of Resources for Additional Help and Information

Edited by Karen Bellenir. 595 pages. 2004. 978-0-7808-0323-7.

"Provides everything needed for the student or general reader seeking practical details on the effects of tobacco use."

—*The Bookwatch, Mar '05*

"Public libraries and consumer health care libraries will find this work useful."

—*American Reference Books Annual, 2005*

SEE ALSO *Respiratory Disorders Sourcebook, 2nd Edition*

Sports Injuries Sourcebook, 3rd Edition

Basic Consumer Health Information about Sprains and Strains, Fractures, Growth Plate Injuries, Overtraining Injuries, and Injuries to the Head, Face, Shoulders, Elbows, Hands, Spinal Column, Knees, Ankles, and Feet, and with Facts about Heat-Related Illness, Steroids and Sport Supplements, Protective Equipment, Diagnostic Procedures, Treatment Options, and Rehabilitation

Along with a Glossary of Related Terms and a Directory of Resources for Additional Help and Information

Edited by Sandra J. Judd. 623 pages. 2007. 978-0-7808-0949-9.

SEE ALSO *Fitness and Exercise Sourcebook, 3rd Edition*

Stress-Related Disorders Sourcebook, 2nd Edition

Basic Consumer Health Information about Stress and Stress-Related Disorders, Including Types of Stress, Sources of Acute and Chronic Stress, the Impact of Stress on the Body's Systems, and Mental and Emotional Health Problems Associated with Stress, Such as Depression, Anxiety Disorders, Substance Abuse, Posttraumatic Stress Disorder, and Suicide

Along with Advice about Getting Help for Stress-Related Disorders, Information about Stress Management Techniques, a Glossary of Stress-Related Terms, and a Directory of Resources for Additional Help and Information

Edited by Amy L. Sutton. 608 pages. 2007. 978-0-7808-0996-3.

"Accessible to the lay reader. Highly recommended for medical and psychiatric collections."

—*Library Journal, Mar '08*

"Well-written for a general readership, the 2nd Edition of *Stress-Related Disorders Sourcebook* is a useful addition to the health reference literature."

—*American Reference Books Annual, 2008*

SEE ALSO *Mental Health Disorders Sourcebook, 4th Edition*

Stroke Sourcebook, 2nd Edition

Basic Consumer Health Information about Stroke, Including Ischemic, Hemorrhagic, and Mini Strokes, as Well as Risk Factors, Prevention Guidelines, Diagnostic Tests, Medications and

Surgical Treatments, and Complications of Stroke

Along with Rehabilitation Techniques and Innovations, Tips on Staying Healthy and Maintaining Independence after Stroke, a Glossary of Related Terms, and a Directory of Resources for Stroke Survivors and Their Families

Edited by Amy L. Sutton. 626 pages. 2008. 978-0-7808-1035-8.

"An encyclopedic handbook on stroke that is written in a language the layperson can understand. . . . This is one of the most helpful, readable books on stroke. This volume is highly recommended and should be in every medical, hospital and public library; in addition, every family practitioner should have a copy in his or her office."

—*ARBAonline Dec '08*

SEE ALSO *Hypertension Sourcebook*

Surgery Sourcebook, 2nd Edition

Basic Consumer Health Information about Common Inpatient and Outpatient Surgeries, Including Critical Care and Trauma, Gastrointestinal, Gynecologic and Obstetric, Cardiac and Vascular, Neurologic, Ophthalmologic, Orthopedic, Reconstructive and Cosmetic, and Other Major and Minor Surgeries

Along with Information about Anesthesia and Pain Relief Options, Risks and Complications, Postoperative Recovery Concerns, and Innovative Surgical Techniques and Tools, a Glossary of Related Terms, and a Directory of Additional Resources

Edited by Amy L. Sutton. 645 pages. 2008. 978-0-7808-1004-4.

"Large public libraries and medical libraries would benefit from this material in their reference collections."

—*ARBAonline Aug '08*

SEE ALSO *Cosmetic and Reconstructive Surgery Sourcebook, 2nd Edition*

Thyroid Disorders Sourcebook

Basic Consumer Health Information about Disorders of the Thyroid and Parathyroid Glands, Including Hypothyroidism, Hyperthyroidism, Graves Disease, Hashimoto Thyroiditis, Thyroid Cancer, and Parathyroid Disorders, Featuring Facts about Symptoms, Risk Factors, Tests, and Treatments

Along with Information about the Effects of Thyroid Imbalance on Other Body Systems, Environmental Factors That Affect the Thyroid Gland, a Glossary, and a Directory of Additional Resources

Edited by Joyce Brennfleck Shannon. 573 pages. 2005. 978-0-7808-0745-7.

"Recommended for consumer health collections."

—*American Reference Books Annual, 2006*

"Highly recommended pick for basic consumer health reference holdings at all levels."

—*The Bookwatch, Aug '05*

SEE ALSO *Endocrine and Metabolic Disorders Sourcebook, 2nd Edition*

Transplantation Sourcebook

Basic Consumer Health Information about Organ and Tissue Transplantation, Including Physical and Financial Preparations, Procedures and Issues Relating to Specific Solid Organ and Tissue Transplants, Rehabilitation, Pediatric Transplant Information, the Future of Transplantation, and Organ and Tissue Donation

Along with a Glossary and Listings of Additional Resources

Edited by Joyce Brennfleck Shannon. 610 pages. 2002. 978-0-7808-0322-0.

"Recommended for libraries with an interest in offering consumer health information."

—*E-Streams, Jul '02*

"This is a unique and valuable resource for patients facing transplantation and their families."

—*Doody's Review Service, Jun '02*

Traveler's Health Sourcebook

Basic Consumer Health Information for Travelers, Including Physical and Medical Preparations, Transportation Health and Safety, Essential Information about Food and Water, Sun Exposure, Insect and Snake Bites, Camping and Wilderness Medicine, and Travel with Physical or Medical Disabilities

Along with International Travel Tips, Vaccination Recommendations, Geographical Health Issues, Disease Risks, a Glossary, and a Listing of Additional Resources

Edited by Joyce Brennfleck Shannon. 619 pages. 2000. 978-0-7808-0384-8.

"Recommended reference source."
—*Booklist, Feb '01*

"This book is recommended for any public library, any travel collection, and especially any collection for the physically disabled."
—*American Reference Books Annual, 2001*

SEE ALSO *Worldwide Health Sourcebook*

Urinary Tract and Kidney Diseases and Disorders Sourcebook, 2nd Edition

Basic Consumer Health Information about the Urinary System, Including the Bladder, Urethra, Ureters, and Kidneys, with Facts about Urinary Tract Infections, Incontinence, Congenital Disorders, Kidney Stones, Cancers of the Urinary Tract and Kidneys, Kidney Failure, Dialysis, and Kidney Transplantation

Along with Statistical and Demographic Information, Reports on Current Research in Kidney and Urologic Health, a Summary of Commonly Used Diagnostic Tests, a Glossary of Related Terms, and a Directory of Resources for Additional Help and Information

Edited by Ivy L. Alexander. 621 pages. 2005. 978-0-7808-0750-1.

"A good choice for a consumer health information library or for a medical library needing information to refer to their patients."
—*American Reference Books Annual, 2006*

SEE ALSO *Prostate and Urological Disorders Sourcebook*

Vegetarian Sourcebook

Basic Consumer Health Information about Vegetarian Diets, Lifestyle, and Philosophy, Including Definitions of Vegetarianism and Veganism, Tips about Adopting Vegetarianism, Creating a Vegetarian Pantry, and Meeting Nutritional Needs of Vegetarians, with Facts Regarding Vegetarianism's Effect on Pregnant and Lactating Women, Children, Athletes, and Senior Citizens

Along with a Glossary of Commonly Used Vegetarian Terms and Resources for Additional Help and Information

Edited by Chad T. Kimball. 337 pages. 2002. 978-0-7808-0439-5.

"Organizes into one concise volume the answers to the most common questions concerning vegetarian diets and lifestyles. This title is recommended for public and secondary school libraries."
—*E-Streams, Apr '03*

"Invaluable reference for public and school library collections alike."
—*Library Bookwatch, Apr '03*

"The articles in this volume are easy to read and come from authoritative sources. The book does not necessarily support the vegetarian diet but instead provides the pros and cons of this important decision. . . . Recommended for public libraries and consumer health libraries."
—*American Reference Books Annual, 2003*

SEE ALSO *Diet and Nutrition Sourcebook, 3rd Edition*

Women's Health Concerns Sourcebook, 3rd Edition

Basic Consumer Health Information about Issues and Trends in Women's Health and Health Conditions of Special Concern to Women, Including Endometriosis, Uterine Fibroids, Menstrual Irregularities, Menopause, Sexual Dysfunction, Infertility, Cancer in Women, and Other Such Chronic Disorders as Lupus, Fibromyalgia, and Thyroid Disease

Along with Statistical Data, Tips for Maintaining Wellness, a Glossary, and a Directory of Resources for Further Help and Information

Edited by Sandra J. Judd. 600 pages. 2009. 978-0-7808-1036-5.

SEE ALSO *Breast Cancer Sourcebook, 3rd Edition, Cancer Sourcebook for Women, 3rd Edition, Healthy Heart Sourcebook for Women, Osteoporosis Sourcebook*

Workplace Health and Safety Sourcebook

Basic Consumer Health Information about Workplace Health and Safety, Including the Effect of Workplace Hazards on the Lungs,

Skin, Heart, Ears, Eyes, Brain, Reproductive Organs, Musculoskeletal System, and Other Organs and Body Parts

Along with Information about Occupational Cancer, Personal Protective Equipment, Toxic and Hazardous Chemicals, Child Labor, Stress, and Workplace Violence

Edited by Chad T. Kimball. 610 pages. 2000. 978-0-7808-0231-5.

"As a reference for the general public, this would be useful in any library."

—*E-Streams, Jun '01*

"Provides helpful information for primary care physicians and other caregivers interested in occupational medicine. . . . General readers; professionals."

—*CHOICE, May '01*

Worldwide Health Sourcebook

Basic Information about Global Health Issues, Including Malnutrition, Reproductive Health, Disease Dispersion and Prevention, Emerging Diseases, Risky Health Behaviors, and the Leading Causes of Death

Along with Global Health Concerns for Children, Women, and the Elderly, Mental Health Issues, Research and Technology Advancements, and Economic, Environmental, and Political Health Implications, a Glossary, and a Resource Listing for Additional Help and Information

Edited by Joyce Brennfleck Shannon. 597 pages. 2001. 978-0-7808-0330-5.

"Named an Outstanding Academic Title."

—*CHOICE, Jan '02*

"Yet another handy but also unique compilation in the extensive *Health Reference Series*, this is a useful work because many of the international publications reprinted or excerpted are not readily available. Highly recommended."

—*CHOICE, Nov '01*

SEE ALSO *Traveler's Health Sourcebook*

Teen Health Series

Complete Catalog

List price $69 per volume. School and library price $62 per volume.

Abuse and Violence Information for Teens

Health Tips about the Causes and Consequences of Abusive and Violent Behavior

Including Facts about the Types of Abuse and Violence, the Warning Signs of Abusive and Violent Behavior, Health Concerns of Victims, and Getting Help and Staying Safe

Edited by Sandra Augustyn Lawton. 411 pages. 2008. 978-0-7808-1008-2.

"A useful resource for schools and organizations providing services to teens and may also be a starting point in research projects."

—*Reference and Research Book News, Aug '08*

"Violence is a serious problem for teens. . . . This resource gives teens the information they need to face potential threats and get help—either for themselves or for their friends."

—*ARBAonline, Aug '08*

Accident and Safety Information for Teens

Health Tips about Medical Emergencies, Traumatic Injuries, and Disaster Preparedness

Including Facts about Motor Vehicle Accidents, Burns, Poisoning, Firearms, Natural Disasters, National Security Threats, and More

Edited by Karen Bellenir. 420 pages. 2008. 978-0-7808-1046-4.

SEE ALSO *Sports Injuries Information for Teens, 2nd Edition*

Alcohol Information for Teens, 2nd Edition

Health Tips about Alcohol and Alcoholism

Including Facts about Alcohol's Effects on the Body, Brain, and Behavior, the Consequences of Underage Drinking, Alcohol Abuse Prevention and Treatment, and Coping with Alcoholic Parents

Edited by Lisa Bakewell. 400 pages. 2009. 978-0-7808-1043-3.

SEE ALSO *Drug Information for Teens, 2nd Edition*

Allergy Information for Teens

Health Tips about Allergic Reactions Such as Anaphylaxis, Respiratory Problems, and Rashes

Including Facts about Identifying and Managing Allergies to Food, Pollen, Mold, Animals, Chemicals, Drugs, and Other Substances

Edited by Karen Bellenir. 410 pages. 2006. 978-0-7808-0799-0.

"This is a comprehensive, readable text on the subject of allergic diseases in teenagers. 5 Stars (out of 5)!"

—*Doody's Review Service, Jun '06*

"This authoritative and useful self-help title is a solid addition to YA collections, whether for personal interest or reports."

—*School Library Journal, Jul '06*

Asthma Information for Teens

Health Tips about Managing Asthma and Related Concerns

Including Facts about Asthma Causes, Triggers, Symptoms, Diagnosis, and Treatment

Edited by Karen Bellenir. 386 pages. 2005. 978-0-7808-0770-9.

"Highly recommended for medical libraries, public school libraries, and public libraries."

—*American Reference Books Annual, 2006*

"Although this volume is nearly 400 pages long, it is so clearly written and well organized that even hesitant readers will be able to find the facts they need, whether for reports or personal information. . . . A succinct but complete resource."

—*School Library Journal, Sep '05*

Body Information for Teens

Health Tips about Maintaining Well-Being for a Lifetime

Including Facts about the Development and Functioning of the Body's Systems, Organs, and Structures and the Health Impact of Lifestyle Choices

Edited by Sandra Augustyn Lawton. 458 pages. 2007. 978-0-7808-0443-2.

■

Cancer Information for Teens, 2nd Edition

Health Tips about Cancer Awareness, Symptoms, Prevention, Diagnosis, and Treatment

Including Facts about Common Cancers Affecting Teens, Causes, Detection, Coping Strategies, Clinical Trials, Nutrition and Exercise, Cancer in Friends or Family, and More

Edited by Karen Bellenir and Lisa Bakewell. 400 pages. 2009. 978-0-7808-1085-3.

■

Complementary and Alternative Medicine Information for Teens

Health Tips about Non-Traditional and Non-Western Medical Practices

Including Information about Acupuncture, Chiropractic Medicine, Dietary and Herbal Supplements, Hypnosis, Massage Therapy, Prayer and Spirituality, Reflexology, Yoga, and More

Edited by Sandra Augustyn Lawton. 407 pages. 2007. 978-0-7808-0966-6.

"This volume covers CAM specifically for teenagers but of general use also. It should be a welcome addition to both public and academic libraries."

—*American Reference Books Annual, 2008*

"This volume provides a solid foundation for further investigation of the subject, making it useful for both public and high school libraries."

—*VOYA: Voice of Youth Advocates, Jun '07*

■

Diabetes Information for Teens

Health Tips about Managing Diabetes and Preventing Related Complications

Including Information about Insulin, Glucose Control, Healthy Eating, Physical Activity, and Learning to Live with Diabetes

Edited by Sandra Augustyn Lawton. 410 pages. 2006. 978-0-7808-0811-9.

"A comprehensive instructional guide for teens. . . . some of the material may also be directed towards parents or teachers. 5 stars (out of 5)!"

—*Doody's Review Service, 2006*

"Students dealing with their own diabetes or that of a friend or family member or those writing reports on the topic will find this a valuable resource."

—*School Library Journal, Aug '06*

"This text is directed to the teen population and would be an excellent library resource for a health class or for the teacher as a reference for class preparation. It can, however, serve a much wider audience. The clinical educator on diabetes may find it valuable to educate the newly diagnosed client regardless of age. It also would be an excellent reference and education tool for a preventive medicine seminar on diabetes."

—*Physical Therapy, Mar '07*

■

Diet Information for Teens, 2nd Edition

Health Tips about Diet and Nutrition

Including Facts about Dietary Guidelines, Food Groups, Nutrients, Healthy Meals, Snacks, Weight Control, Medical Concerns Related to Diet, and More

Edited by Karen Bellenir. 432 pages. 2006. 978-0-7808-0820-1.

"A very quick and pleasant read in spite of the fact that it is very detailed in the information it gives. . . . A book for anyone concerned about diet and nutrition."

—*American Reference Books Annual, 2007*

SEE ALSO *Eating Disorders Information for Teens, 2nd Edition*

■

Drug Information for Teens, 2nd Edition

Health Tips about the Physical and Mental Effects of Substance Abuse

Including Information about Marijuana, Inhalants, Club Drugs, Stimulants, Hallucinogens,

Opiates, Prescription and Over-the-Counter Drugs, Herbal Products, Tobacco, Alcohol, and More

Edited by Sandra Augustyn Lawton. 468 pages. 2006. 978-0-7808-0862-1.

"As with earlier installments in Omnigraphics' *Teen Health Series, Drug Information for Teens* is designed specifically to meet the needs and interests of middle and high school students. . . . Strongly recommended for both academic and public libraries."

—*American Reference Books Annual, 2007*

"Solid thoughtful advice is given about how to handle peer pressure, drug-related health concerns, and treatment strategies."

—*School Library Journal, Dec '06*

SEE ALSO *Alcohol Information for Teens, 2nd Edition, Tobacco Information for Teens*

Eating Disorders Information for Teens, 2nd Edition

Health Tips about Anorexia, Bulimia, Binge Eating, And Other Eating Disorders

Including Information about Risk Factors, Diagnosis and Treatment, Prevention, Related Health Concerns, and Other Issues

Edited by Sandra Augustyn Lawton. 377 pages. 2009. 978-0-7808-1044-0.

SEE ALSO *Diet Information for Teens, 2nd Edition*

Fitness Information for Teens, 2nd Edition

Health Tips about Exercise, Physical Well-Being, and Health Maintenance

Including Facts about Conditioning, Stretching, Strength Training, Body Shape and Body Image, Sports Nutrition, and Specific Activities for Athletes and Non-Athletes

Edited by Lisa Bakewell. 432 pages. 2009. 978-0-7808-1045-7.

SEE ALSO *Diet Information for Teens, 2nd Edition, Sports Injuries Information for Teens, 2nd Edition*

Learning Disabilities Information for Teens

Health Tips about Academic Skills Disorders and Other Disabilities That Affect Learning

Including Information about Common Signs of Learning Disabilities, School Issues, Learning to Live with a Learning Disability, and Other Related Issues

Edited by Sandra Augustyn Lawton. 400 pages. 2006. 978-0-7808-0796-9.

"This book provides a wealth of information for any reader interested in the signs, causes, and consequences of learning disabilities, as well as related legal rights and educational interventions. . . . Public and academic libraries should want this title for both students and general readers."

—*American Reference Books Annual, 2006*

Mental Health Information for Teens, 2nd Edition

Health Tips about Mental Wellness and Mental Illness

Including Facts about Mental and Emotional Health, Depression and Other Mood Disorders, Anxiety Disorders, Conduct Disorder, Self-Injury, Psychosis, Schizophrenia, and More

Edited by Karen Bellenir. 424 pages. 2006. 978-0-7808-0863-8.

"This excellent overview of the psychological disorders that affect teens provides clear definitions and descriptions, and discusses resources, therapies, coping mechanisms, and medications."

—*School Library Journal Curriculum Connections, Fall '07*

"A well done reference for a specific, often under-represented group."

—*Doody's Review Service, 2006*

SEE ALSO *Stress Information for Teens*

Pregnancy Information for Teens

Health Tips about Teen Pregnancy and Teen Parenting

Including Facts about Prenatal Care, Pregnancy Complications, Labor and Delivery,

Postpartum Care, Pregnancy-Related Lifestyle Concerns, and More

Edited by Sandra Augustyn Lawton. 434 pages. 2007. 978-0-7808-0984-0.

SEE ALSO *Sexual Health Information for Teens, 2nd Edition*

Sexual Health Information for Teens, 2nd Edition

Health Tips about Sexual Development, Reproduction, Contraception, and Sexually Transmitted Infections

Including Facts about Puberty, Sexuality, Birth Control, Chlamydia, Gonorrhea, Herpes, Human Papillomavirus, Syphilis, and More

Edited by Sandra Augustyn Lawton. 430 pages. 2008. 978-0-7808-1010-5.

"This offering represents the most up-to-date information available on an array of topics including abstinence-only sexual education and pregnancy-prevention methods. . . . The range of coverage—from puberty and anatomy to sexually transmitted diseases—is thorough and extensive. Each chapter includes a bibliographic citation, and the three back sections containing additional resources, further reading, and the index are all first-rate. . . . This volume will be well used by students in need of the facts, whether for educational or personal reasons."

—*School Library Journal, Nov '08*

SEE ALSO *Pregnancy Information for Teens*

Skin Health Information for Teens, 2nd Edition

Health Tips about Dermatological Concerns and Skin Cancer Risks

Including Facts about Acne, Warts, Allergies, and Other Conditions and Lifestyle Choices, Such as Tanning, Tattooing, and Piercing, That Affect the Skin, Nails, Scalp, and Hair

Edited by Edited by Kim Wohlenhaus. 400 pages. 2009. 978-0-7808-1042-6.

Sleep Information for Teens

Health Tips about Adolescent Sleep Requirements, Sleep Disorders, and the Effects of Sleep Deprivation

Including Facts about Why People Need Sleep, Sleep Patterns, Circadian Rhythms, Dreaming, Insomnia, Sleep Apnea, Narcolepsy, and More

Edited by Karen Bellenir. 355 pages. 2008. 978-0-7808-1009-9.

SEE ALSO *Body Information for Teens*

Sports Injuries Information for Teens, 2nd Edition

Health Tips about Acute, Traumatic, and Chronic Injuries in Adolescent Athletes

Including Facts about Sprains, Fractures, and Overuse Injuries, Treatment, Rehabilitation, Sport-Specific Safety Guidelines, Fitness Suggestions, and More

Edited by Karen Bellenir. 429 pages. 2008. 978-0-7808-1011-2.

"An engaging selection of informative articles about the prevention and treatment of sports injuries. . . The value of this book is that the articles have been vetted and are often augmented with inserts of useful facts, definitions of technical terms, and quick tips. Sensitive topics like injuries to genitalia are discussed openly and responsibly. This revised edition contains updated articles and defines sport more broadly than the first edition."

—*School Library Journal, Nov '08*

"This work will be useful in the young adult collections of public libraries as well as high school libraries. . . . A useful resource for student research."

—*ARBAonline, Aug '08*

SEE ALSO *Accident and Safety Information for Teens*

Stress Information for Teens

Health Tips about the Mental and Physical Consequences of Stress

Including Information about the Different Kinds of Stress, Symptoms of Stress, Frequent Causes of Stress, Stress Management Techniques, and More

Edited by Sandra Augustyn Lawton. 392 pages. 2008. 978-0-7808-1012-9.

"Understanding what stress is, what causes it, how the body and the mind are impacted by it,

and what teens can do are the general categories addressed here. . . . The chapters are brief but informative, and the list of community-help organizations is exhaustive. Report writers will find information quickly and easily, as will those who have personal concerns. The print is clear and the format is readable, making this an accessible resource for struggling readers and researchers."

—*School Library Journal, Dec '08*

"The articles selected will specifically appeal to young adults and are designed to answer their most common questions."

—*ARBAonline, Aug '08*

SEE ALSO *Mental Health Information for Teens, 2nd Edition*

Suicide Information for Teens

Health Tips about Suicide Causes and Prevention

Including Facts about Depression, Risk Factors, Getting Help, Survivor Support, and More

Edited by Joyce Brennfleck Shannon. 368 pages. 2005. 978-0-7808-0737-2.

"Highly Recommended for libraries serving teenagers as well as those who work with them."

—*E-Streams, Apr '06*

SEE ALSO *Mental Health Information for Teens, 2nd Edition*

Tobacco Information for Teens

Health Tips about the Hazards of Using Cigarettes, Smokeless Tobacco, and Other Nicotine Products

Including Facts about Nicotine Addiction, Immediate and Long-Term Health Effects of Tobacco Use, Related Cancers, Smoking Cessation, Tobacco Use Prevention, and Tobacco Use Statistics

Edited by Karen Bellenir. 440 pages. 2007. 978-0-7808-0976-5.

"A comprehensive resource. Each chapter is written to stand alone, so students can dip in and use the information in each section for reports or to answer personal questions without having to read the entire book. . . . The book is packed full of statistics, with sources to help students look up more."

—*School Library Journal, Sep '07*

"Pulls together a wide variety of authoritative sources to provide a comprehensive overview of tobacco use for this age group. . . . This reasonably priced reference title should be considered a necessary purchase for all public libraries and school media centers, along with academic libraries supporting teacher education."

—*American Reference Books Annual, 2008*

SEE ALSO *Drug Information for Teens, 2nd Edition*

Health Reference Series

Adolescent Health Sourcebook, 2nd Edition
Adult Health Concerns Sourcebook
AIDS Sourcebook, 4th Edition
Alcoholism Sourcebook, 2nd Edition
Allergies Sourcebook, 3rd Edition
Alzheimer Disease Sourcebook, 4th Edition
Arthritis Sourcebook, 2nd Edition
Asthma Sourcebook, 2nd Edition
Attention Deficit Disorder Sourcebook
Autism & Pervasive Developmental Disorders Sourcebook
Back & Neck Sourcebook, 2nd Edition
Blood & Circulatory Disorders Sourcebook, 2nd Edition
Brain Disorders Sourcebook, 2nd Edition
Breast Cancer Sourcebook, 3rd Edition
Breastfeeding Sourcebook
Burns Sourcebook
Cancer Sourcebook, 5th Edition
Cancer Sourcebook for Women, 3rd Edition
Cancer Survivorship Sourcebook
Cardiovascular Diseases & Disorders Sourcebook, 3rd Edition
Caregiving Sourcebook
Child Abuse Sourcebook
Childhood Diseases & Disorders Sourcebook, 2nd Edition
Colds, Flu & Other Common Ailments Sourcebook
Communication Disorders Sourcebook
Complementary & Alternative Medicine Sourcebook, 3rd Edition
Congenital Disorders Sourcebook, 2nd Edition
Contagious Diseases Sourcebook
Cosmetic & Reconstructive Surgery Sourcebook, 2nd Edition
Death & Dying Sourcebook, 2nd Edition
Dental Care & Oral Health Sourcebook, 3rd Edition
Depression Sourcebook, 2nd Edition
Dermatological Disorders Sourcebook, 2nd Edition
Diabetes Sourcebook, 4th Edition
Diet & Nutrition Sourcebook, 3rd Edition
Digestive Diseases & Disorder Sourcebook
Disabilities Sourcebook
Disease Management Sourcebook
Domestic Violence Sourcebook, 3rd Edition
Drug Abuse Sourcebook, 2nd Edition
Ear, Nose & Throat Disorders Sourcebook, 2nd Edition
Eating Disorders Sourcebook, 2nd Edition
Emergency Medical Services Sourcebook
Endocrine & Metabolic Disorders Sourcebook, 2nd Edition
Environmental Health Sourcebook, 2nd Edition
Ethnic Diseases Sourcebook
Eye Care Sourcebook, 3rd Edition
Family Planning Sourcebook
Fitness & Exercise Sourcebook, 3rd Edition
Food Safety Sourcebook
Forensic Medicine Sourcebook
Gastrointestinal Diseases & Disorders Sourcebook, 2nd Edition
Genetic Disorders Sourcebook, 3rd Edition
Head Trauma Sourcebook
Headache Sourcebook
Health Insurance Sourcebook
Healthy Aging Sourcebook
Healthy Children Sourcebook
Healthy Heart Sourcebook for Women
Hepatitis Sourcebook
Household Safety Sourcebook
Hypertension Sourcebook
Immune System Disorders Sourcebook, 2nd Edition
Infant & Toddler Health Sourcebook
Infectious Diseases Sourcebook
Injury & Trauma Sourcebook